OCCIPITAL SEIZURES AND EPILEPSIES IN CHILDREN

OCCIPITAL SEIZURES AND EPILEPSIES IN CHILDREN

Colloquium of the Pierfranco e Luisa Mariani Foundation

Edited by
F. Andermann, A. Beaumanoir, L. Mira, J. Roger and
C.A. Tassinari

Mariani Foundation Paediatric Neurology series: 1

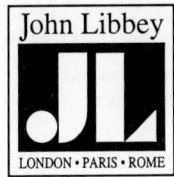

British Library Cataloguing in Publication Data

Occipital Seizures and Epilepsies in Children
– Mariani Foundation Paediatric Neurology series: 1

    I. Andermann, Frederick   II. Series
    618.92
ISSN: 0969-0301
ISBN: 0 86196 385 7

Published by

John Libbey & Company Ltd, 13 Smiths Yard, Summerley Street, London SW18 4HR, England.
Telephone: 081-947 2777: Fax 081-947 2664
John Libbey Eurotext Ltd, 6 rue Blanche, 92120 Montrouge, France.
John Libbey - C.I.C. s.r.l., via Lazzaro Spallanzani 11, 00161 Rome, Italy

© 1993 John Libbey & Company Ltd. All rights reserved.
Unauthorised duplication contravenes applicable laws.

Printed in Great Britain by Whitstable Litho Ltd, Whitstable, Kent, UK

Contents

	Preface	vii
	Introduction	1
Chapter 1	Ontogenesis of the occipital lobe *Michel Imbert*	3
Chapter 2	Ontogenesis of the GABAergic system *Roberto Spreafico and Maria Cristina Regondi*	9
Chapter 3	Age-dependent changes in susceptibility to seizures and to seizure-induced brain damage *Raman Sankar, Roi Ann Wallis, Kerry Thompson, Cheng Xin Yang, Toshiaki Akira and Claude Wasterlain*	15
Chapter 4	Structures and functions of the occipital lobe *Giuliano Avanzini*	31
Chapter 5	Visual testing in the first 2 years of life *Lieven Lagae and Paul Casaer*	43
Chapter 6	Neurophysiological examinations of visual function in the development of the infant *Samuel Sokol*	49
Chapter 7	VEP in children with damage of vision *Piernanda Vigliano, Giorgio Capizzi and Lorella Tornetta*	59
Chapter 8	EEG in children with visual pathway damage *Laura Mira and Andrée Van Lierde*	65
Chapter 9	Semiology of occipital seizures in infants and children *Anne Beaumanoir*	71
Chapter 10	The semiology of migraine attacks in childhood *Giovani Lanzi and Umberto Balottin*	87
Chapter 11	Migraine–epilepsy syndrome: intercalated seizures in benign occipital epilepsy *Mario Giovanni Terzano, Liborio Parrino, Vladimiro Pietrini and Laura Galli*	93

Chapter 12	An EEG contribution to the study of migraine *Anne Beaumanoir*	101
Chapter 13	Occipital epileptic abnormalities in mitochondrial disorders *Frederick Andermann*	111
Chapter 14	Occipital epilepsy in neonates and infants *Anne Lortie, Perrine Plouin, Jean Marc Pinard and Olivier Dulac*	121
Chapter 15	Benign occipital epilepsy of childhood with prolonged seizures and autonomic symptoms *Federico Vigevano and Stefano Ricci*	133
Chapter 16	Television-induced occipital seizures *Roberto Michelucci and Carlo Alberto Tassinari*	141
Chapter 17	Neurophysiological investigations in photosensitive epilepsies *Guido Rubboli and Fabrizio Salvi*	145
Chapter 18	Benign childhood epilepsy with occipital paroxysms *Chrysostomos P. Panayiotopoulos*	151
Chapter 19	Outcome of idiopathic childhood epilepsy with occipital paroxysms *Renzo Guerrini, Agatino Battaglia, Charlotte Dravet, Michelle Bureau and Pierre Genton*	165
Chapter 20	The partial occipital epilepsies in childhood *Bernardo Dalla Bernardina, Elena Fontana, Ornella Cappellaro, Emanuele Zullini, Francesca Darra, Vito Colamaria and Roberto Caraballo*	173
Chapter 21	Occipital symptomatic epilepsy: epidemiological aspects *Giorgio Capizzi, Piernanda Vigliano, Anna Maria Pengo and Maria Baiona*	183
Chapter 22	Coeliac disease, epilepsy and cerebral calcifications: a multicentric study Coordinators: *Furio Bouquet, Giuseppe Gobbi, Luigi Greco, Andrea Lambertini, Carlo Alberto Tassinari, Alessandro Ventura and Maria Gilda Zaniboni*	189
Chapter 23	Medical management of occipital epilepsies *Margherita Santucci, Giuseppe Gobbi, Lorella Minotti, Emanuela Donati, Daniele Giovanni Poggioli, Elisabetta Tarsi and Paola Giovanardi Rossi*	197
Chapter 24	Occipital seizures with childhood onset in severe partial epilepsy: a surgical perspective *Claudio Munari, Laura Tassi, Stefano Francione, Philippe Kahane, Chariklia Malapani, Giorgio Lo Russo and Dominique Hoffmann*	203
Chapter 25	Occipital lobe epilepsy in children *Frederick Andermann, Vicenta Salanova, André Olivier and Theodore Rasmussen*	213
Chapter 26	Evolution of the semiology of childhood occipital seizures *Joseph Roger*	221
	Discussion	225
	Synopsis by *Anne Beaumanoir*	237
	Author Index	239
	Subject Index	241

Preface

The Mariani Foundation is dedicated to paediatric neurology: Luisa Mariani was, for over thirty years, especially close to the problems and needs of the Children's Division in the 'Carlo Besta' National Neurological Institute of Milan. Shortly after the death of her husband, Pierfranco, she sought to create a more permanent legacy of his very productive life by devoting the fruits of its prosperity to the benefit of suffering children.

So, in 1984, this Foundation was established with the purpose of assisting children with afflictions of the nervous system. The goal was not, and is not, only to provide material assistance here and now, but, rather, to be instrumental in complementing the overall educational and research programs in paediatric neurology.

The Foundation's activities in the educational field range from an intensive series of didactic conferences, among which are the annual Post-graduate Courses organized in cooperation with the 'Carlo Besta' National Neurological Institute, to seminars and workshops targeted to the acquisition and application of advanced skills.

The experience of such a practice-orientated electrophysiology workshop, the seminar on methodology for the clinical use of electroencephalography (now in its sixth consecutive year), inaugurated our very successful association with Dr. Anne Beaumanoir, whose recognized didactic gifts, combined with her exceptional drive and initiative, prompted the project of this first Mariani Foundation Colloquium on paediatric epilepsy.

The scientific success of the meeting is the source and the substance of this publication; our conviction of its value is expressed in the commitment to continue this new Paediatric Neurology series with other volumes, representing the Mariani Foundation's focal points of interest, such as infantile epilepsy, motor development, or research on rare diseases which might otherwise be overlooked by publicly funded projects.

We hope that the exchange of knowledge and ideas that constituted the basis of this Colloquium, combining the advantages of a highly competent body of specialists with an opportunity to compare informally experiences and perspectives, will inspire similar projects in related or different fields: thus, the Foundation also wishes the emphasize the importance of private intervention in health and social issues.

Antonio Magnocavallo
Chairman, Mariani Foundation

Introduction

The Pierfranco and Luisa Mariani Foundation, upon suggestion of its Scientific Committee, chose the subject of Occipital Seizures and Epilepsies in Children for the first colloquium on infantile epilepsy, which took place in Milan on 26 and 27 March 1992 at the 'Vittore Buzzi' Children's Hospital.

The purpose of this meeting was to identify and clarify any characteristics peculiar to the seizures of the occipital cortex and to the epileptic syndromes of the occipital lobes, in relation to the stages of development of the visual systems, both sensory and sensory-motor.

Although more work has to be done to achieve this goal, as Imbert observed, nonetheless a further cooperation has been achieved between basic scientists and clinical specialists, who are in agreement in designating the child's occipital epilepsy as a stimulating model to investigate the ontogenesis of epileptic seizures and epilepsies.

This publication presents the individual lectures of the Colloquium, as well as the final discussion; and the Scientific Committee of the Colloquium should be considered its collective Editor. However, the most comprehensive curator's work has been accomplished by Maria Majno, coordinator of the Mariani Foundation, without whose competence and cheerful energy the Colloquium would not have been the scientific success it indeed was. Dr. Laura Mira, head of the Neurology and Neurophysiology Service at the 'Vittore Buzzi' Children's Hospital, has played a major contribution in this undertaking, first as Scientific Secretary of the Colloquium, then as Editor of its proceedings.

Anne Beaumanoir
Colloquium President and Scientific Committee Member

Chapter 1

Ontogenesis of the occipital lobe

Michel Imbert

Université Pierre et Marie Curie, Laboratoire des Neurosciences de la Vision, CNRS, Université Paris VI, 9 quai Saint Bernard, 75005 Paris, France

Summary

In a series of experiments, summarized in this short review, extraocular muscle proprioception was shown to play a crucial role in the postnatal development of some specific properties of the primary visual cortical neurons. In particular, bilateral or unilateral sectioning of the ophthalmic branch of the trigeminal nerve, which carries extraocular proprioceptive afferents, when performed at 6–8 weeks of age in the cat, prevented the development of normal binocular depth perception thresholds. It has also been shown that after extraocular muscle proprioceptive deafferentation, most cortical area 17 neurons lose their ability to discriminate changes in binocular spatial disparity.

The general conclusion which can be drawn from these experiments is that the normal maturation of the brain, during a critical period of postnatal development, depends on the existence of visual and proprioceptive interactions. These interactions, which occur at a relatively low level of visual information processing, indicate that early sensorimotor experience may unite the input system and the control system of the sensory initiated motor responses.

Introduction

Numerous neurophysiological studies, instigated by Hubel and Wiesel as of the early 1960s (summarized in Hubel & Wiesel, 1977), have demonstrated that neurons in the mammalian occipital cortex responded specifically to precise visual patterns. These neurons are activated when small spots of light are shone on to a restricted region of the animal's visual field. The more precise spatial configuration the stimulus has, the more important the response will be. These forms are generally linear edges whose orientation within the receptive field is relatively precise and specific. Different cortical cells prefer different orientations, but considering the whole population of cortical neurons, no particular orientation – neither vertical nor horizontal for example – is favoured. Besides orientation selectivity, the visual cortical cells are for the most part binocularly activated. Yet, if the parameters of the effective stimulus, especially its orientation, are analogous for both retinae, the visual cortical neurons are generally influenced differently, on a quantitative level, by the two eyes. Moreover, for there to be binocular activation, the stimulus must be presented in such a way that the two retinal images are situated in relation to each other in a precise relationship of disparity (Barlow *et al.*, 1967). This relationship varies from one neuron to the next and could account for the stereoscopic vision of the third dimension.

The complex interneuronal connections that, from the retina to the occipital cortex, endow the cortical neurons with such properties, are susceptible to modifications. If the visual world of an immature animal is altered by eliminating certain characteristics in the visible environment, the corresponding feature characteristics of the cortical visual neurons will be modified in such a way as to be limited to the parameters present in the first months of postnatal life (review in Imbert, 1979; Frégnac & Imbert, 1984). Therefore, manipulating the visual input of an animal during a critical period of postnatal development can induce profound modifications in the response properties of neurons in the striate occipital cortex. However, such drastic alterations in response properties are only seen when the animal is allowed to actively explore its impoverished visual environment, suggesting a specific relation between motor processes and vision during development (Imbert & Frégnac, 1983; Imbert, 1985a, b).

Such an idea of a connection between motor processes and spatial perception has a long history that can be traced to the eighteenth century, and which has been fully established, on experimental grounds, by the description of perceptual deficits in congenitally blind humans who acquired vision after late cataract surgery (reviewed by von Senden in 1960) and by the study of the behaviour of visually deprived chimpanzees (Riesen, 1947).

The relation between motor processes and vision gained a scientific status with Donald Hebb who declared in his influential book *The Organization of Behavior* 'activation of the oculomotor system, overt or implicit, contributes essentially to the development of visual integration without being sufficient to it ...' (Hebb, 1949). This proposition has been taken up by many experimenters studying the influence of voluntary motility in the elaboration of visuomotor programmes (see Held & Hein, 1963). As of the 1960s, it was clear and well accepted that depriving a neonate animal, either a monkey or a kitten, of free movement induced detrimental effects on visuomotor coordination.

However, the demonstration that some of the very specific visual properties of individual striate neurons themselves, and not only the global visuomotor behaviour, were also dependent on oculomotricity was established only in the late 1970s.

The first indication came from an experiment by Lamberto Maffei and Sylvia Bisti, published in 1976. These authors showed that a unilateral strabismus produced by severing the extraocular rectus medialis muscle caused a disruption of ocular dominance distribution in area 17 in kittens, who were kept in complete darkness for several weeks after the surgery until the electrophysiological exploration of their visual cortex took place. In surgical strabismus, Hubel & Wiesel concluded, in their study of 1965, 'that a lack of synergy in the input from the two eyes is sufficient to cause a profound disruption in the connections that subserve binocular interactions'.

Originally applied by Hubel & Wiesel to purely visual signals, this conclusion was extended by Maffei & Bisti, suggesting that an imbalance of proprioceptive information from extraocular muscles of each eye could suffice to account for the disruption of binocularity in strabismic cats. Although this effect could not be replicated by others, the hypothesis put forward by Maffei & Bisti has nevertheless been largely corroborated by experiments carried out in our laboratory in collaboration with P. Buisseret, Yves Frégnac, Elyane Gary-Bobo and Yves Trotter.

These experiments show the role played by extraocular muscle proprioception in the postnatal development of visual cortical properties, then their implication in depth perception, and finally their crucial role in the ability showed by the primary visual cortical neurons to discriminate changes in disparity.

Postnatal development of orientation selectivity

When carefully studying the evolution of response properties of visual cortical neurons during the first weeks in kittens either normally reared or reared in complete darkness, it is possible to bring forth a number of significant points.

As soon as a definite visual response can be recorded, that is around the end of the second postnatal week, a rather significant proportion of these neurons (about 50 per cent) exhibit a true orientation selectivity. For about half of these, this selectivity is as precise as the one shown by cortical neurons recorded in adult animals.

The relative proportion of orientation selective cells and non-specific cells is not different until the end of the third week in animals reared in whatever conditions, in normally lit environment or in complete darkness. As of the turn of the third week, the properties of the neurons develop differently: in normally reared kittens, the number of oriented cells increases rapidly; on the other hand, in dark-reared kittens, the number of oriented cells decreases in favour of non-oriented cells, which will be the only ones to remain after 6 weeks spent in total darkness.

However, a spectacular recovery of orientation selectivity is observed when the 6-week-old dark-reared animal is allowed to have a few hours of active visual experience. Vision *per se* is not the only factor involved in the recovery of visual properties by the population of area 17 neurons. Indeed, if oculomotor activity is prevented during visual experience, by using for example a muscular relaxant, no recovery of orientation selectivity occurs. In contrast, provided that ocular motility is preserved, a striking restoration can be observed (Buisseret *et al.*, 1978).

At this point two possibilities can be invoked for explaining the recovery of orientation selectivity; the factor controlling the recovery is either the motor command itself, or the reafferent signals which accompany eye movements, that is to say the proprioceptive afferents from the extraocular muscles.

It was possible to test this last possibility directly. Indeed it is known that in the cat, and also in the monkey, the majority of the proprioceptive afferences from the extraocular muscle follow the ophthalmic branch of the trigeminal nerve in its intracranial trajectory (Batini & Buisseret, 1974). Therefore, by sectioning this nerve before it enters Gasser's ganglia, it is possible to dissociate the proprioceptive afferences of the motor efferences, without interfering with oculomotricity.

These experiments confirm the hypothesis that the factor related to ocular motility, indispensable for the recovery of orientation selectivity, is of extraocular proprioceptive origin (Trotter *et al.*, 1979).

Postnatal development of binocular interaction

The other principal property of area 17 neurons, namely binocular interaction, as measured by the standard ocular dominance distribution histograms, is also subject to modifications following proprioceptive deafferentation.

In order to describe more precisely the role of afferents running through the VI nerve during development of the so-called 'cortical binocularity', unilateral sectioning of the VI in normally and in dark-reared kittens of different ages was performed.

The issue at stake in these experiments was to determine whether the physiological effects one could observe depended on visual experience or not, and to determine the precise time course of this cortical modification.

The main results obtained in this series of experiments can be summarized as follows:

- a disruption of ocular dominance was produced by the unilateral sectioning of the VI nerve performed at the peak of the period of sensitivity to monocular lid suture, i.e. between 4 and 8 weeks of age;
- this effect was observed several weeks after surgery and once established remained present even after a delay of several years;
- this effect seems largely independent of visual experience, since it was observed in both normally reared and dark-reared kittens, operated on at 6 weeks and maintained in the dark for several weeks after the surgery. The absence of modification in ocular dominance

following bilateral sectioning of the VI nerve suggests that the asymmetry of extraocular muscle proprioception inflow was responsible for the disruption of cortical binocularity.

Therefore it seems clear that the asymmetry on the proprioceptive feedback from the extraocular muscles of each eye interferes with the maintenance of cortical binocularity (Trotter et al., 1987)

The development of depth perception: behavioural studies

One might wonder whether reduction in the proprioceptive inflow could impair the initial development of binocularly mediated behaviour. Since relative perception of depth is closely linked with binocular vision and *a fortiori* with the integrity of its underlying neuronal mechanisms, it seems natural to envision implication of proprioceptive afferences of the extraocular muscles in the development of this perceptive capacity.

This hypothesis has been verified in our laboratory with a behavioural method, inspired by Lashley and developed by Mitchell, the so-called forced choice jump method (Mitchell et al., 1979). The development of depth perception has been assessed in normally reared kittens and can be summarized as follows (Graves et al. 1987):

- at 5 weeks, binocular depth perception threshold was about 45 minutes of arc;
- then the threshold decreases steadily until 10–11 weeks, at this age it reaches an adult level of about 5 minutes of arc. The monocular threshold also decreases with age to reach adult values of 20 minutes of arc at about 15–18 weeks.

Now for kittens that underwent unilateral sectioning of the VI nerve, binocular depth perception failed to reach normal adult levels: the depth discrimination capacity is greatly reduced in kittens unilaterally deprived of proprioceptive afferents. Indeed, their binocular perception threshold is approximately 15 to 20 minutes of arc, i.e. three to four times higher than that of control animals (5 minutes of arc).

This deficit is not a consequence of possible strabismus, since the sectioning of the ophthalmic branch of the trigeminal nerve does not modify the interocular alignment, and the deficit is specific to the sectioning of the VI. Moreover, once established, the deficit remains permanent, but there is no effect when the sectioning is performed in the adult.

Therefore we thought it would be of interest to assess the exact temporal limits within which the sectioning of the VI was able to induce this spectacular effect on depth perception. In order to study the temporal limits of the susceptibility of depth perception to proprioceptive deafferentation of the extraocular muscles, unilateral and bilateral sectioning of the VI were systematically performed in kittens of different ages: 3, 10–11, 14 weeks. We thereby showed that the severing of the VI nerve only produced significant impairment of the binocular depth perception thresholds when performed after 8 weeks and before 10–13 weeks of age (Trotter et al., 1991).

The fact that in kittens completely deprived of vision, the unilateral sectioning of the VI produces a disruption of the ocular dominance distribution, seems to indicate that extraocular proprioception *per se* participates in the development or in the maintenance of neural binocular interactions.

This interpretation gains support from recent physiological experiments which concern the neuronal stereoscopic processing after extraocular muscle deafferentation. These experiments show a low level of binocularity and disparity sensitivity in the primary visual cortex after sectioning of extraocular muscle proprioceptive afferents during a critical period. After unilateral sectioning most cortical area 17 cells lose their ability to discriminate changes in binocular spatial disparity. This loss is permanent and is due to a reduction of binocular suppression and to a selective increase in the variability of the binocular response (Trotter et al., 1990).

During this sensitive period, extraocular muscle proprioceptive inputs should provide feedback signals necessary for spatial ocular disparity calibration and for the visuomotor integration so that a permanent adjustment of visuomotor coordinates may take place. If proprioceptive inputs are missing, retinal maps and motor maps would lack this eye position reference, and consequently some functional disorders would occur. These experiments demonstrate that, during a critical period of postnatal development, the extraocular muscle proprioception contributes critically to the normal development of highly specific visual properties of primary visual neurons.

Conclusions

The general conclusion which can be drawn from the experiments summarized in the present chapter is that the normal maturation of the brain during the postnatal period depends in large part on early sensorimotor experience. In the case of the occipital cortex, the fact that the processes of development of the very specific visual properties of the cortical neurons are critically dependent on the proprioceptive afferents ensuing from ocular movements indicates that multisensory interactions, in this case visual and proprioceptive, exist at a relatively low level of visual information processing and reveals that early experience may unite the input system and the control system of the sensory initiated motor responses (Imbert, 1985b).

The demonstration that the perceptivo-motor relationship that an immature organism has with its surroundings influences its brain development is particularly relevant to a meeting devoted to the study of occipital seizures and epilepsies in children.

References

Barlow, H.B., Blakemore, C. & Pettigrew, J.D. (1967): The neural mechanism of binocular depth perception. *J. Physiol.* **193**, 327–432.

Batini, C. & Buisseret, P. (1974): Sensory peripheral pathway from extrinsic eye muscles. *Arch. Ital. Biol.* **112**, 18–32.

Buisseret, P., Gary-Bobo, E. & Imbert, M. (1978): Ocular motility may be involved in recovery of orientational properties of visual cortical neurons in dark-reared kittens. *Nature* **272**, 816–817.

Frégnac, Y. & Imbert, M. (1984): Development of neuronal selectivity in primary visual cortex of cat. *Physiol. Rev.* **64**, 325–434.

Graves, A.L., Trotter, Y. & Frégnac, Y. (1987): Role of extraocular muscle proprioception in the development of depth perception in cats. *J. Neurophysiol.* **58**, 816–831.

Hebb, D.O. (1949): *The organization of behavior.* New York: John Wiley & Sons.

Held, R. & Hein, A. (1963): Movement-produced stimulation in the development of visually guided behavior. *J. Comp. Physiol. Psychol.*, **56**, 872–876.

Hubel, D.H. & Wiesel, T.N. (1965): Binocular interaction in striate cortex of kittens reared with artificial squint. *J. Neurophysiol.* **28**, 1041–1059.

Hubel, D.H. & Wiesel, T.N. (1977): Ferrier lecture: Functional architecture of macaque visual cortex. *Proc. Roy. Soc. Lond. B* **198**, 1–59.

Imbert, M. (1979): Maturation of visual cortex with and without visual experience. In: *Developmental neurobiology of vision*, ed. R.D. Freeman, pp. 43–49. New York, London: Plenum Pub. Corp.

Imbert, M. (1985a): Extraretinal factors controlling the development of neuronal selectivity. In: *Brain plasticity, learning and memory*, vol. 28, eds. B.E. Will, P. Schmitt & J.C. Dalrymple-Alford, pp. 61–69. New York, London: Plenum Press.

Imbert, M. (1985b): Physiological underpinnings of perceptual development. In: *Guggenheim Foundation symposium on neonate and infant cognition*, pp. 69–88. Hillsdale, New Jersey: Lawrence Erlbaum Ass.

Imbert, M. & Frégnac, Y. (1983): Specification of cortical neurons by visuomotor experience. *Prog. Brain Res.* **58**, 427–436.

Maffei, L. & Bisti, S. (1976): Binocular interaction in strabismic kittens deprived of vision. *Science* **191**, 579–580.

Mitchell, D.E., Kaye, M. & Timney, B. (1979): Assessment of depth perception in cats. *Perception* **8**, 389–396.

Riesen, A.H. (1947): The development of perception in man and chimpanzee. *Science* **106**, 107–108.

Trotter, Y., Beaux, J.C., Pouget, A. & Imbert, M. (1991): Temporal limits of the susceptibility of depth perception to proprioceptive deafferentations of extraocular muscles. *Dev. Brain Res.* **59**, 23–29.

Trotter, Y., Celebrini, S., Beaux, J. & Grandjean, B. (1990): Neuronal stereoscopic processing following extraocular proprioception deafferentation. *NeuroReport* **1**, 187–190.

Trotter, Y., Frégnac, Y. & Buisseret, P. (1987): The period of susceptibility of visual cortical binocularity to unilateral proprioceptive deafferentation of extraocular muscles. *J. Neurophysiol.* **58**, 795–815.

Trotter, Y., Gary-Bobo, E. & Buisseret, P. (1979): Restoration of orientation specificity of the visual cells in kittens after section of the ophthalmic branches of the Vth nerve. *Neurosci. Lett.* **53**, 296.

von Senden, M. (1960): *Space and sight*. London: Methuen.

Chapter 2

Ontogenesis of the GABAergic system

Roberto Spreafico and Maria Cristina Regondi

Department of Neurophysiology, Istituto Nazionale Neurologico 'Carlo Besta', via Celoria 11, 20133 Milan, Italy

Summary

During development, different processes such as proliferation, migration, differentiation and maturation contribute to the formation of the final structure of the neocortex through the formation of transient cortical structures. These general mechanisms are similar for the two main neuronal populations residing in the cortex: the projecting neurons and the interneurons. Since this latter group of cells has a peculiar morphology and uses GABA as neurotransmitter, the availability of different neuroanatomical methods, including immunocytochemistry, allows the detailed study of the morphological and functional development of this class of neurons. Despite the similarity of proliferative and migratory events between projecting and local circuit neurons, differentiation and maturation of the latter differ from the former. Projecting neurons, known as excitatory elements in the neocortex, develop before the local circuit neurons and their synapses are recognized before the inhibitory ones. Moreover, the distribution of GABA positive neurons in the neocortex reaches the adult configuration in the rat only between the second and third postnatal week. The GABA receptor seems to undergo maturational rearrangements during the postnatal weeks before reaching the final adult pattern. Since during the embryonic stages both GABA and its receptor are visible particularly in transient cortical structures, it has been postulated that GABA during developmental stages could also subserve morphogenetic mechanisms. In addition, the different timing in maturation between excitatory and inhibitory elements could at least in part explain the particular vulnerability and hyperexcitability of the immature neocortex.

Introduction

During the ontogenesis of the cerebral cortex, the formation of transient structures occurs before the establishment of the final layered configuration observed in mature mammals. In humans, the formation of telencephalic vesicles is recognized around the 40th postovulatory day at the rostral end of the prosencephalon and a progressive enlargement of this brain component is observed following a ventro-dorsolateral and antero-posterior gradient. Through mechanisms of development, differentiation and maturation, the neocortex will grow from 3 per cent to 80 per cent of the whole telencephalon by the time of birth (Jenkins, 1921). At the beginning, the cerebral vesicles are formed by densely packed undifferentiated cells, a pseudostratified neuroepithelium, lying between the pial surface and the lateral ventricles. This aggregation of cells, the matrix, will give rise to the whole cellular component of the future neocortex. Thus the final neocortical configuration will be established from matrix cells through processes of proliferation, migration, differentiation, maturation and programmed cell death. This implies that matrix cells will be transformed into different cellular elements of the neocortex.

Recent experimental studies, performed in different animal species, have suggested that two mechanisms are involved in defining the cortical cell fate: intrinsic information and environmental determinants (McConnell, 1992); in particular the environmental influences seem to play an essential role in the definition of neuronal phenotypes. Moreover, a single cell, during its development, makes sequential decisions, each one of which progressively restricts its successive developmental potential until its ultimate fate (McConnell, 1988, 1992).

After the appearance of the cerebral vesicles, the first afferent fibres, presumably originating from the brainstem, reach the neocortical wall (approximately around the 45th–50th postovulatory day in the human embryo), marking the beginning of the neocortical development (Marin-Padilla, 1988). From this point a series of events can be observed and transient structures are recognized within the developing cortex. A group of early generated neurons leaves the ventricular zone and is positioned just below the pial surface, forming a thin layer named marginal zone (MZ). Following the hypothesis of Marin-Padilla (1988), this primitive cortical organization should be renamed primordial plexiform layer (PPL) since this first transformation occurs after the arrival of the corticopetal fibres, forming a fibrillo-neural organization.

The subsequent arrival of migrating postmitotic neuroblasts, generating the cortical plate (CP), will split the PPL into two components. The first one, close to the pial surface, is the embryonic formation of the future layer I and thus is named prospective layer I (PLI). The second, below the newly formed and expanding CP, is a transient structure named subplate (SP). Below the SP a narrow layer of embryonic white matter, the intermediate zone (IZ), is recognized dividing the SP from the ventricular zone (VZ). The only functioning cortical areas during the early embryonic stages are the PLI and the SP, where the first synapses are recognized (Marin-Padilla, 1988). In the further embryonic stages, the PLI and the SP are progressively separated from each other by the continuous expansion of the CP which, during the early cortical ontogenesis, remains undifferentiated. As the maturation of the cortex proceeds, the transient structures (i.e. the IZ, the VZ and later on the SP) will disappear and the layered cortex with the underlying white matter will remain.

With the exception of layer I and of the lower tier of layer VI, which are derivative of the PPL, all the other layers of neocortex, from II to the upper tier of VI, will derive from the CP.

The CP is formed and enlarged by successive waves of migrating neuroblasts which begin their travel after the last mitotic division. The first group of migrated neuroblasts, located just below the PLI, will be displaced downward by a second migratory wave. The subsequent migrating neuroblasts must therefore cross the layers of previously migrated neurons which will be in turn further displaced downward. Thus, as has been experimentally demonstrated, the neurons of the adult deep cortical layers are generated and migrate before those in the superficial layers. The mechanism of migration, therefore, follows an inside-out sequence (Rakic, 1972).

The migrating neuroblasts are radially oriented and it has been demonstrated that they migrate climbing the processes of the radially oriented glial cells and maintaining a close contact with those fibres until they reach their final target within the CP (Rakic, 1971). This migratory principle is followed by both projecting and local circuit neurons (lcn) and also proliferation and differentiation events occur concomitantly. Projecting neurons and interneurons (lcn), found in the adult layers II–VI of the neocortex, develop in tandem (Miller, 1988).

The possibility of investigating the ontogenetic pattern of different neuronal phenotypes derives from the availability of technical methods allowing the simultaneous study of the morphological maturation and the presence of specific neurochemical contents of the cellular element.

The morphological differentiation of lcn begins after the completion of their migration and continues through the early postnatal period. The peculiarity of these neurons, beside their morphological characteristics, is that they use the γ-aminobutyric acid (GABA) as neurotransmitter which can be revealed using a specific antibody against GABA or against its synthetic enzyme, glutamic acid decarboxylase (GAD). This immunocytochemical procedure, combined with autoradiographic methods using tritiated thymidine, addressed to identify the date of birth of neurons during the embryonic stages, have provided evidence for the generation timing of lcn in some animal species (Miller, 1986; Peduzzi, 1986). In particular, in the rat Miller (1986) demonstrated that lcn, migrating within the CP following an inside-out sequence, are generated starting from the end of the second gestational week, until birth. (It must be remembered that, in the rat, gestation is 21 days.)

Although some studies referring to the morphogenesis of cortical neurons in humans are present in the literature, the most complete data so far available have been obtained using Golgi impregnation methods in rats and cats. Thus, the maturation events of lcn will be explained here by reference to these animals. These neurons, despite their different morphological characteristics, have two common features: their dendrites are aspinous or sparsely spinous and their axon is confined to the gray matter arborizing at a relatively short distance from the cell body. These aspects, as well as the dendritic arborization clearly detectable in the adult cortex, are difficult to distinguish during the embryonic (E) period since the perykaria, the axonal and the dendritic patterns are evolving toward their final configuration in the postnatal (P) period.

In the rat, stellate neurons are the first lcn identifiable in the immature cortex (Parnavelas et al., 1978) with the exception of the Cajal–Retius cell detectable much earlier in the PPL (Marin-Padilla, 1984). Recent reports confirm this later finding, demonstrating that the first GABAergic neurons are present, in the rat, in the subpial region, corresponding to the PPL, by E14 and after the appearance of the CP which is identifiable as a band of non-GABA-positive neurons.

Cells containing GABA are also visible in the SP and in the IZ (Cobas et al., 1991). The SP region is considered of particular importance during the embryonic period since it has been defined as the waiting compartment of cortical afferent fibres during maturation of the cortex (see Shatz, 1992 for ref.). When the maturation is achieved, most of the GABAergic neurons of the subplate die, through a mechanism of programmed cell death, leaving the afferent fibres free to reach their ultimate target. Only few SP GABAergic neurons survive and will be incorporated in the subcortical white matter as 'interstitial neurons' (Valverde & Facal Valverde, 1988).

Within layers II–VI the morphogenesis of the lcn in the deeper layers precedes that of lcn in the superficial layers.

In the rat the lcn achieve their mature size and the mature complexity of dendrites at the end of the third postnatal week (P21), but the intracellular maturation of cytoplasmic organells is not completed before the fourth postnatal week.

Soon after birth the axons are growing very slowly but it is only between P10 and P20 that the complexity of axonal branches markedly increases. With the expansion of the axonal arborization, a parallel increment of synapses is observed. The first axoplasmatic synapses are recognized on the soma of pyramidal neurons in layers II–III and V by P3 and a progressive increment is detected until P30. It must be pointed out that the presence of morphologically defined synapses, as observed during the early stages of cortical maturation, does not imply that they are functioning at least with the same role as we observed in the adult neocortex.

In addition to the appearance, migration and morphological differentiation of lcn, as revealed by their morphology and by their GABA content, other aspects of the development must be considered, such as neurochemical differentiation. This includes the maturation of systems responsible for the uptake, synthesis, release, reception and degradation of the GABA.

Despite the appearance of the GABA positive neurons during the early stages of development in the PPL and in the SP, it is only around the day of birth that the first GABA-positive neurons are detected and located in layer VI. The neurons progressively increase during the first postnatal days also in the most superficial layers and it is only by P12 that GABA-positive neurons reach the adult distribution. Thus, with the exception of some neurons originating from the PPL, GABA starts to be expressed around the day of birth. When the GAD antibody is used, the results obtained in developmental studies differ from those based on GABA immunohistochemistry. In fact neurons, positive for the GABA synthesizing enzyme (GAD), appear later and are much fewer than GABA immunoreactive cells. This implies either the presence of an embryonic form of GAD not recognized by the adult form used for the ICC, or the presence of an alternative route of synthesis not present in the adult (Spreafico *et al.*, 1988).

The immunocytochemical data are in line with pharmacological and biochemical experiments, showing a discrepancy between GABA and GAD content in neonatal cortex as compared to the adult. Moreover, GAD activity reaches the adult level by the end of third postnatal week, while GABA has already reached the mature level by the second week.

The development of GABA release is particularly difficult to assess because of the presence of glial cells, but it has been suggested that Ca^{2+} dependent GABA release, virtually absent during the first postnatal week, increases progressively during the second and third postnatal weeks.

Another important issue is the maturation of receptors. The $GABA_A$ receptor is the major variety of GABA receptor in the cerebral cortex and its development in the neocortex has been studied by autoradiographic binding methods and more recently by immunological procedures (Vitorica *et al.*, 1990). Data obtained from GABA binding showed that at postnatal week 1 only 10 per cent of the adult binding activity is present; the adult level being reached by week 6 (Coyle, 1982). Recent data, comparing the distribution of GABA-positive neurons and $GABA_A$ receptors, showed a precocious appearance (around E14) of the receptor in the PPL (Cobas *et al.*, 1991). A concomitant appearance of $GABA_A$ receptor and GABA neurons in the CP is observed by E20. However, the authors showed that during the development of the CP the receptor immunoreactivity precedes the axogenesis of cortical interneurons and the formation of symmetrical synapses. Recent reports agree in suggesting that the morphogenetic role of GABA during development is mediated by its specific receptors (Cobas *et al.*, 1991; Lipton & Kater, 1989). In this respect it must be noticed that GABA is one of the most precocious neurotransmitters appearing during development (Lauder *et al.*, 1986).

In conclusion, the GABAergic system must not be regarded, at least in the neocortex, as functionally homogenous during development. The inhibitory effects of GABA that we are used to consider in the adult cortex are not evident during the early stages of development where the GABA system is subserving other mechanisms such as morphogenetic roles. Thus the function of GABA evolves and differentiates in tandem with the evolution and differentiation of the cortical mantle.

Acknowledgements

The authors are grateful to Ms. Marina Denegri for typing the manuscript. This work was partially supported by Associazione P. Zorzi per le Neuroscienze.

References

Cobas, A., Fairen, A., Alvarez-Bolado, G. & Sanchez, M.P. (1991): Prenatal development of the intrinsic neurons of the rat neocortex: a comparative study of the distribution of GABA-immunoreactive cells and the $GABA_A$ receptor. *Neuroscience* **40**, 205–212.

Coyle, J.T. (1982): Development of neurotransmitters in the neocortex. *Neurosci. Res. Progr. Bull.* **20**, 479–507.

Jenkins, G.B. (1921): Relative weight and volume of the component parts of the brain of the human embryo at different stages of development. *Contrib. Embryol. Carnegie Inst.* **13**, 41–60.

Lauder, J.M., Han, V.K.M., Henderson, P., Verdoorn, T. & Towle, A.C. (1986): Prenatal ontogeny of the GABAergic system in the rat brain: an immunocytochemical study. *Neuroscience* **19**, 465–493.

Lipton, S.A. & Kater, S.B. (1989): Neurotransmitter regulation of neuronal outgrowth, plasticity and survival. *Trends Neurosci.* **12**, 265–270.

Marin-Padilla, M. (1984): Neurons of layer I: a developmental analysis. In: *Cerebral cortex*, vol. 1, eds. A. Peters & E.G. Jones, pp. 447–478. New York, London: Plenum Press.

Marin-Padilla, M. (1988): Early ontogenesis of the human cerebral cortex. In: *Cerebral cortex*, vol. 7, eds. A. Peters & E.G. Jones, pp. 1–34. New York, London: Plenum Press.

McConnell, S. (1988): Development and decision-making in the mammalian cerebral cortex. *Brain Res. Rev.* **13**, 1–23.

McConnell, S. (1992): The control of neuronal identity in the developing cerebral cortex. *Curr. Opin. Neurobiol.* **2**, 23–27.

Miller, M.V. (1986): The migration and neurochemical differentiation of γ-aminobutyric acid (GABA)-immunoreactive neurons in the rat visual cortex as demonstrated by immunocytochemical-autoradiographic technique. *Dev. Brain Res.* **25**, 271–285.

Miller, M.V. (1988): Development of projection and local circuit neurons in neocortex. In: *Cerebral cortex*, Vol. 7, eds. A. Peters & E.G. Jones, pp. 133–175. New York, London: Plenum Press.

Parnavelas, J.G., Bradford, R., Mounty, E.J. & Lieberman, A.R. (1978): The development of non pyramidal neurons in the visual cortex of the rat. *Anat. Embryol.* **155**, 1–14.

Peduzzi, J.D. (1986): Genesis of GABA immunoreactive neurons in the ferret visual cortex. *Soc. Neurosci. Abstr.* **12**, 1372.

Rakic, P. (1971): Guidance of neurons migrating to the fetal monkey neocortex. *Brain Res.* **33**, 471–476.

Rakic, P. (1972): Mode of cell migration to the superficial layers of fetal monkey neocortex. *J. Comp. Neurol.* **145**, 61–84.

Shatz, C.J. (1992): How are specific connections formed between thalamus and cortex? *Curr. Opin. Neurobiol.* **2**, 78–82.

Spreafico, R., Di Biasi, S., Frassoni, C. & Battaglia, G. (1988): A comparison of GAD and GABA immunoreactive neurons in the first somatosensory area (SI) of the cortex. *Brain Res.* **474**, 192–196.

Valverde, F. & Facal Valverde, M.V. (1988): Postnatal development of interstitial (subplate) cells in the white matter of the temporal cortex of kittens: a correlated Golgi and electron microscopic study. *J. Comp. Neurol.* **269**, 168–192.

Vitorica, J., Park, D., Chiu, G. & de Blas, A.L. (1990): Characterization with antibodies of the γ-aminobutyric acid$_A$/benzodiazepine receptor complex during development of the rat brain. *J. Neurochem.* **54**, 187–194.

Chapter 3

Age-dependent changes in susceptibility to seizures and to seizure-induced brain damage

Raman Sankar, Roi Ann Wallis, Kerry Thompson, Cheng Xin Yang, Toshiaki Akira and Claude Wasterlain

Epilepsy Research Laboratory, VA Medical Center, Sepulveda, CA 91343, USA; Departments of Neurology and Pediatrics and the Brain Research Institute, UCLA School of Medicine; USA

Summary

Seizures induce the release of large amounts of excitatory amino acids (EAA) and the energy failure sometimes associated with status epilepticus can interfere with reuptake of those neurotransmitters and with other aspects of neuronal homeostasis. The resulting opening of ionic channels can flood the cell with calcium or other ions which can injure neurons. Recent evidence suggests that several mechanisms enhance and prolong this essentially toxic sequence of events. The activation of protein kinases, such as calmodulin kinase II, which is activated by calcium but becomes calcium-independent, and the liberation of nitric oxide can prolong excitotoxic actions and enhance cell injury.

Several factors make the immature brain particularly susceptible to seizure spread and to the transition from single seizures to status epilepticus: the potassium released by seizures into the extracellular space reaches much higher concentrations in the immature brain than in the adult and these concentrations are highly epileptogenic. Electrotonic coupling via GAP junctions can be quite prominent in the immature brain. In the very young, the presence of large numbers of excitatory $GABA_A$ synapses could also play an important role. The transient overexpression of EAA receptors during stages in development and the ontogeny of the expression of calcium buffering proteins can result in distinctive and age-dependent patterns of injury in the developing brain. Seizures cause the release of EAAs which may modify the expression of axonal growth cone markers, such as GAP-43, during periods of enhanced plasticity and affect development. The response to seizures of the immature brain varies greatly with age and differs markedly from the response of the mature organ. Results from various laboratories are discussed and an attempt is made to correlate these with clinical experience.

Introduction

Several types of catastrophic epilepsies of childhood are associated with occipital or posterior cortical foci and carry a very poor prognosis for developmental outcome (Adler *et al.*, 1991; Reynolds, 1981; Engel & Shewmon, 1991). By contrast, many occipital epilepsies of childhood have an excellent prognosis and poor developmental outcomes, if they occur at all, are quite unusual.

The relationship between seizure activity and brain development has not received a great deal of attention but it is already evident that age-dependent effects can be quite specific, for a particular seizure type, a particular brain region, or a specific stage of development.

This review will only outline a few of the basic principles suggested by experimental work on the effect of seizures on brain development.

Excitotoxic mechanisms of brain damage

The excitotoxic theory, first proposed by John Olney (1978), postulates that release of excitatory amino acid neurotransmitters plays a key role in several types of cell injury. A considerable amount of evidence has accumulated in favour of the view that neurotransmitter release can mediate neuronal injury (Rothman, 1984) and that in tissue culture this is expressed through the NMDA subtype of glutamate receptors (Choi, 1985) and is blocked by NMDA antagonists (Choi et al., 1988) – and by dissociative anaesthetics (Goldberg et al., 1987). When seizures are induced in hippocampal slices with high concentrations of glutamate and glycine in the perfusion fluid, severe injury of the CA1 neurons can be measured by the progressive loss of evoked population spike in CA1 following stimulation of the Schaffer collaterals. Similarly, exposure for just a few minutes to high concentrations of the glutamate agonist NMDA produces a loss of CA1 spikes which is time- and concentration-dependent, showing that CA1 injury can be produced by specific stimulation of NMDA receptors (Table 1). This injury is unaffected by blockers of non-NMDA receptors, is independent of the liberation of intracellular calcium stores and fulfils most criteria for an excitotoxic type of insult. In the absence of extracellular calcium, injury is considerably slower, demonstrating that calcium influx through the ionic channels associated with NMDA receptors plays a major role in CA1 injury. However, it is important to remember that injury still occurs in the absence of extracellular calcium and that NMDA-mediated injury, while it is probably the single most important mechanism of damage from status epilepticus and the most rapid mechanism of injury in most brain regions, is not the only mechanism of neuronal death (Table 1).

Table 1. Acute NMDA injury in CA1

Treatment	n	% recovery
NMDA	5	10 ± 6
NMDA + 0 Ca^{2+}	3	88 ± 5*
NMDA + TTX	4	13 ± 13
NMDA + glucose	3	7 ± 4
NMDA + dantrolene	3	15 ± 6
NMDA + CNQX	3	0
NMDA + MK-801	6	109 ± 27*

Hippocampal slices were exposed for 8 min to NMDA (20 µM), tetrodotoxin (0.1 mM), glucose (20 mM), dantrolene (20 µM), CNQX (100 µM) or MK-801 (32 µM). The CA1 population spike upon stimulation of Schaffer collaterals was measured before and 60 min after exposure. * $P < 0.05$ compared to NMDA alone.

Table 2. Acute AMPA injury in CA1

Treatment	n	% recovery
AMPA	15	2 ± 2
AMPA + 0 Ca^{2+}	4	12 ± 6
AMPA + MK-801	4	11 ± 1
AMPA + DNQX	6	102 ± 11*
AMPA + dantrolene	4	0 ± 3
AMPA + nifedipine	4	14 ± 5

Hippocampal slices were exposed for 8 min to AMPA (50 µM), DNQX (100 µM), nifedipine (10 µM). Other conditions as in Table 1. *$P < 0.05$ compared to AMPA alone.

Exposure to AMPA causes injury which is blocked by non-NMDA antagonists, unaffected by the removal of extracellular calcium and is also independent of the liberation of intracellular calcium stores (Table 2). This injury reflects a high specificity for non-NMDA receptors. By contrast, kainic acid produces a cell injury in CA1 which is not reduced by trimming the CA3 sector from the slice (Table 3), is blocked by non-NMDA antagonists but also reduced by decreasing extracellular calcium and by blocking NMDA synapses. It is partially reduced by dantrolene, which blocks the release of intracellular calcium stores. This complex picture may in part reflect the fact that kainic acid is not totally selective to the kainic receptors but can also stimulate other excitatory amino acid receptors. Table 4 summarizes the sequence of events that leads to the dominant mechanism of neuronal injury in most brain regions during status epilepticus; the release of large amounts of excitatory amino acids neurotransmitters glutamate and aspartate is coupled with inhibition of the reuptake of these neurotransmitters due to depletion of energy reserves in both glial cells and neurons. This results in persistent occupancy of receptor sites, which open ionic channels. The resulting influx of calcium through NMDA-associated channels appears to represent the dominant mechanism of injury, with a small contribution of calcium flux through L-type voltage gated ionic channels. In specific brain regions, however, different mechanisms come into play where for example calcium influx through non-NMDA channels is the most important process.

Table 3. Acute kainate injury in CA1

Treatment	n	% recovery
Kainic acid	15	17 ± 6
KA + DNQX	3	$69 \pm 18*$
KA + 0 Ca^{2+}	4	$60 \pm 22*$
KA + MK-801	6	33 ± 9
KA + dantrolene	4	$80 \pm 12*$
KA + cut CA_3	3	8 ± 5
KA + azelastine	4	0

Hippocampal slices were exposed for 8 min to kainic acid (65 μM). Conditions as in Table 2.

Table 4. A mechanism of cell injury in SE

Cell firing releases glutamate
Energy failure inhibits reuptake
Glutamate binds to NMDA receptors
Depolarization removes Mg^{2+} block
Ca^{2+} enters through NMDAR ion channels
Some Ca^{2+} enters through voltage-gated channels
High free $[Ca^{2+}]_i$ cause cell injury to neurons

These excitotoxic mechanisms have been demonstrated not only in experimental epilepsy but in excitotoxic damage from domoic acid poisoning in man and a similar role is also implied by the studies of the temporal lobes removed at surgery for intractable epilepsy in humans.

Activation of protein kinases

Recent evidence indicates that status epilepticus induces autophosphorylation of calmodulin kinase II, with a major increase of calcium-independent enzyme together with a decrease of calcium-stimulated enzyme activity (Fig. 1). This calcium-independent enzyme continues to display enhanced activity even if intracellular calcium returns to normal. This enhancement of activity persists for several hours after the end of status epilepticus. It is associated with the translocation of the enzyme from the soluble portion to the membrane (Table 5). One of the likely consequences of this change is a continuation of the phosphorylation by calmodulin kinase II of synapsin I, a vesicle wall protein (Fig. 2). Synapsin I falls off the wall of the vesicle which then tends to fuse with the synaptic

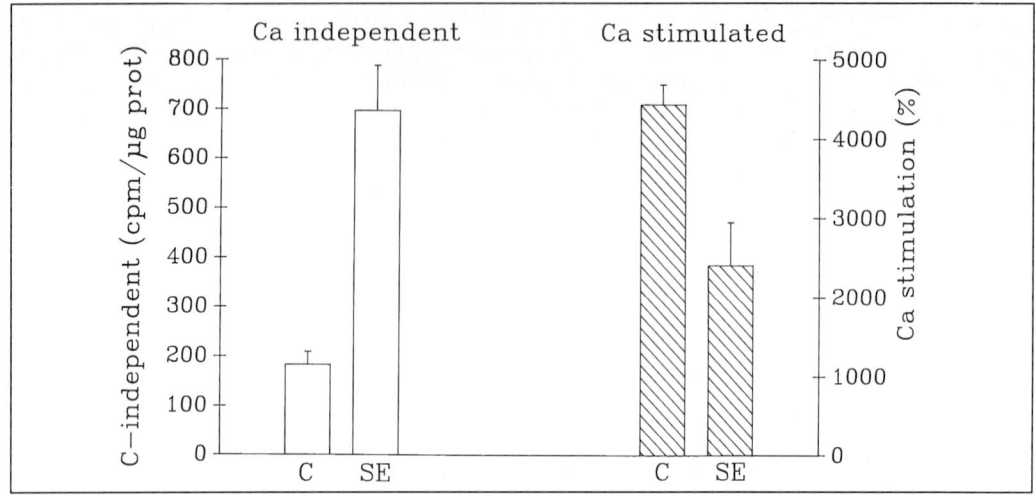

Fig. 1. Effect of autophosphorylation on the activity of calmodulin kinase II. 1.5 µCi of purified enzyme was preincubated under phosphorylation conditions with 5 µCi unlabelled ATP and 100 µM free calcium at 4 °C for times ranging from 0 through 30 min. Calmodulin kinase was active at this temperature, while phosphatases showed little activity. Calcium-calmodulin-dependent and independent kinase activities were assayed by adding myelin basic protein (5 µM), γ-^{32}P-ATP (final ATP concentration 80 µM with specific activity of 0.3–1.0 µCi-nmole) and either water or EGTA (free-calcium concentration 10^{-4} and 10^{-8} respectively). Reactions were run in duplicate and express the radioactivity incorporated into myelin basic protein.

Reproduced with permission from the J. Neurochem.

cleft and to release its neurotransmitter. This could both increase the likelihood of status epilepticus becoming selfsustaining and participate in the maturation phase of cell injury following severe seizures.

Table 5. Translocation of calmodulin kinase II during SE

	CKII-LI	^{125}I-CM binding	
		50 kD	60 kD
Soluble	78 ± 14	58 ± 12	62 ± 17
Membrane	193 ± 31	190 ± 24	169 ± 37

SE values are expressed as % of controls (mean ± SEM). Calmodulin kinase II-like immunoreactivity (CKII-LI) was measured with ^{125}I-protein A using a Western blot technique. Calmodulin binding used an overlay technique.

Activation of nitric oxide synthase

Recent evidence (Dawson et al., 1991) indicates that in dissociated cortical cultures, neuronal injury induced by activation of NMDA receptors involves the generation of nitric oxide, a novel, highly diffusible neurotransmitter (Bredt et al., 1991). Nitric oxide is generated by oxidation of L-arginine through the enzyme nitric oxide synthase, a process which requires molecular oxygen and can be inhibited by the competitive blockers nitroarginine or monomethylarginine. Recent evidence in our laboratory suggests that both in hypoxia (Wallis et al., 1992) and in seizures induced by exposure to high concentrations of glutamate and glycine in hippocampal slices (Akira et al., 1992), the opening of NMDA receptor-gated ionic channels and the CA1 neuronal injury which is associated with sustained opening of those channels are greatly reduced by inhibitors of nitric oxide synthesis

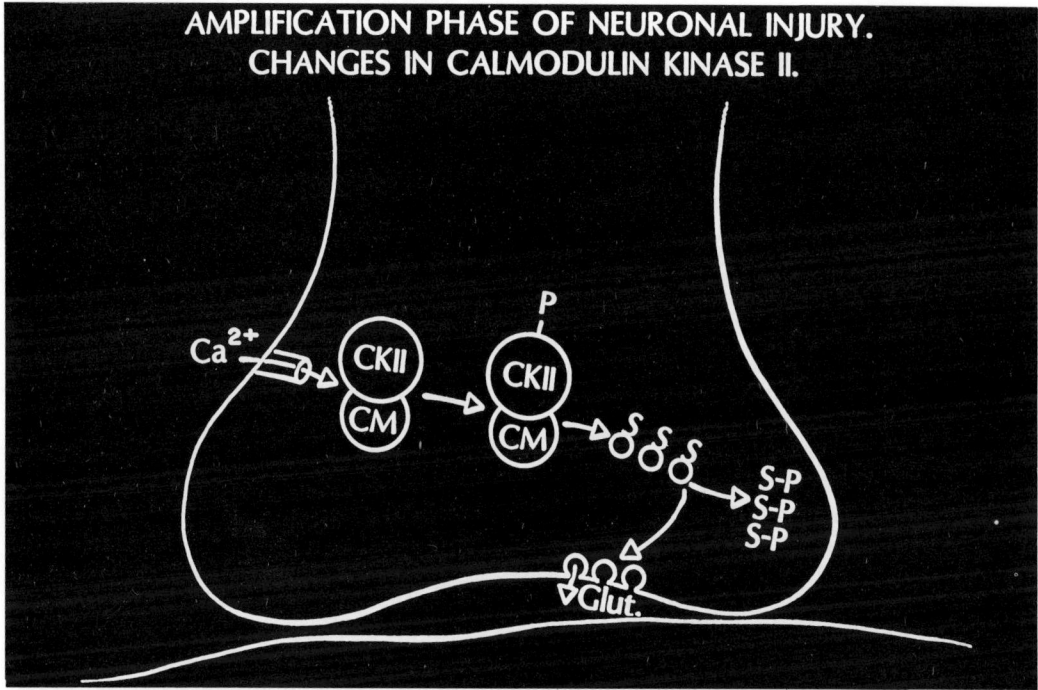

Fig. 2. Autophosphorylation of calmodulin kinase II may enhance transmitter release even after intraneural calcium returns to normal, and this may contribute to making SE self-sustaining.

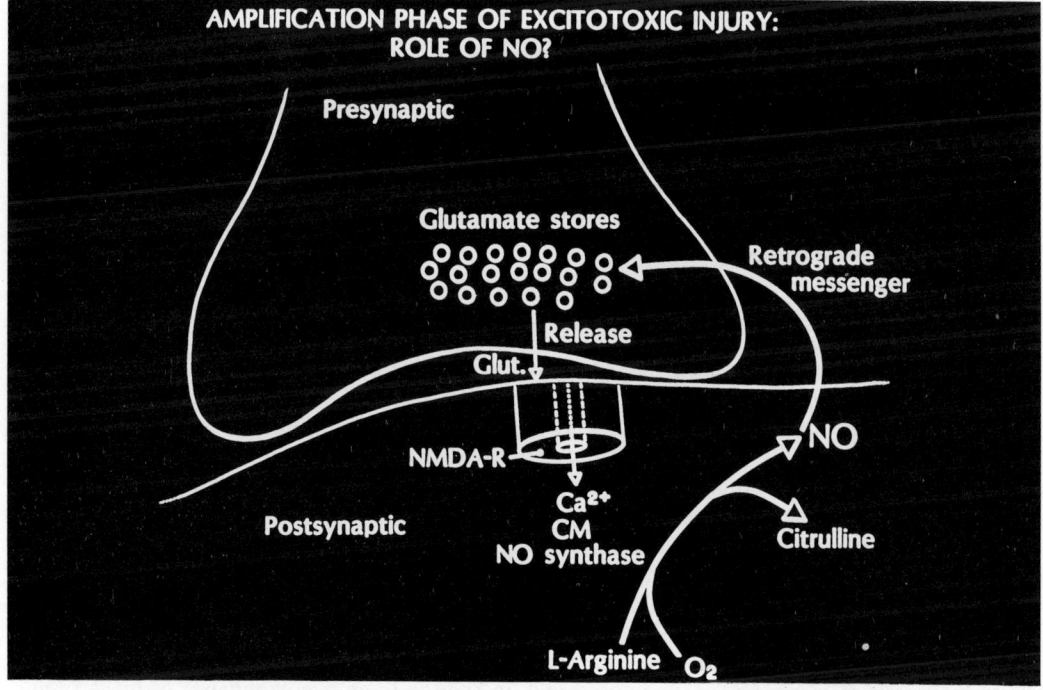

Fig. 3. Postulated mechanism of participation of NO in neuronal injury during SE.

and that this inhibition is competitively reversed by an excess of the substrate L-arginine (Akira et al., 1992). This process seems to involve increased release of excitatory amino acid neurotransmitters and is blocked by extracellular haemoglobin, suggesting that it requires nitric oxide diffusion through the extracellular spaces. These results are compatible with the following model: calcium influx through NMDA receptors activates nitric oxide synthase, generating nitric oxide in the post-synaptic cell. Nitric oxide would diffuse back to the pre-synaptic terminal and would function there as a retrograde messenger to increase the release of excitatory amino acid neurotransmitters (Fig. 3). The only known action of nitric oxide is to directly stimulate guanylate cyclase, the enzyme that generates cyclic GMP. Whether and how this might result in an enhanced transmitter release is unknown at present. Nevertheless, these mechanisms appear to play an important role in excitotoxic neuronal injury in many areas of the brain.

The immature brain is highly susceptible to status epilepticus

A number of factors combine to make the immature brain particularly susceptible to seizure spread (Table 6). Among the synaptic mechanisms that contribute to this susceptibility are the overexpression of NMDA and AMPA receptors, which is transient and coincides with the phase of rapid brain growth and differentiation. At the same time, many of the GABA synapses in the immature brain are excitatory and this may play a major role in tilting the balance between excitation and inhibition in favour of the former (Cherubini et al., 1990). The immaturity of the substantia nigra of immature animals also eliminates a powerful break to seizure mechanisms, both in single seizures and in status epilepticus (Gale, 1985; Baxter et al., 1991; Wasterlain et al., 1991).

Table 6. Factors contributing to neuronal injury in the immature brain

In SE, the immature brain is:
    More resistant:
        Lower metabolic rate
        Less lactate build-up
        Fewer kainate receptors
        Less EAA release
    More vulnerable:
        Cerebral glucopenia
        Less calcium-binding proteins
        More NMDA + AMPA receptors
        Age-specific growth factors

Extra synaptic mechanisms also play an important role in facilitating seizure spread in the immature brain. The limited capacity for glucose transport across the immature blood–brain barrier makes neonates very susceptible to glucose depletion and leads to cerebral glucopoenia which can compound cell injury from seizures (Dwyer & Wasterlain, 1985; Morin et al., 1988). Increased electrotonic coupling in the immature brain could play an important role in seizure spread (Connors et al., 1983; Dudek et al., 1990). The role of potassium, due in part to reduced potassium intake by immature glia and in part to other factors, is partially illustrated in Fig. 4, from the work of Swann and collaborators. Similar stimulation results in much higher elevation of extracellular potassium in the immature brain, compared to mature tissue (Hablitz & Heinemann, 1987; Swann et al., 1988). Rises of extracellular potassium up to 18 mM have been reported in seizing immature brain and such concentrations, when perfused into hippocampal slices, cause sustained seizure activity in the absence of any further stimulation. Thus it appears that spread of seizures through neurotransmitter-induced depolarization and the resulting increase in extracellular potassium may play a major role in local seizure spread in the immature brain, in additon to an overabundance of local-circuit recurrent excitatory synapses (Swann et al., 1991).

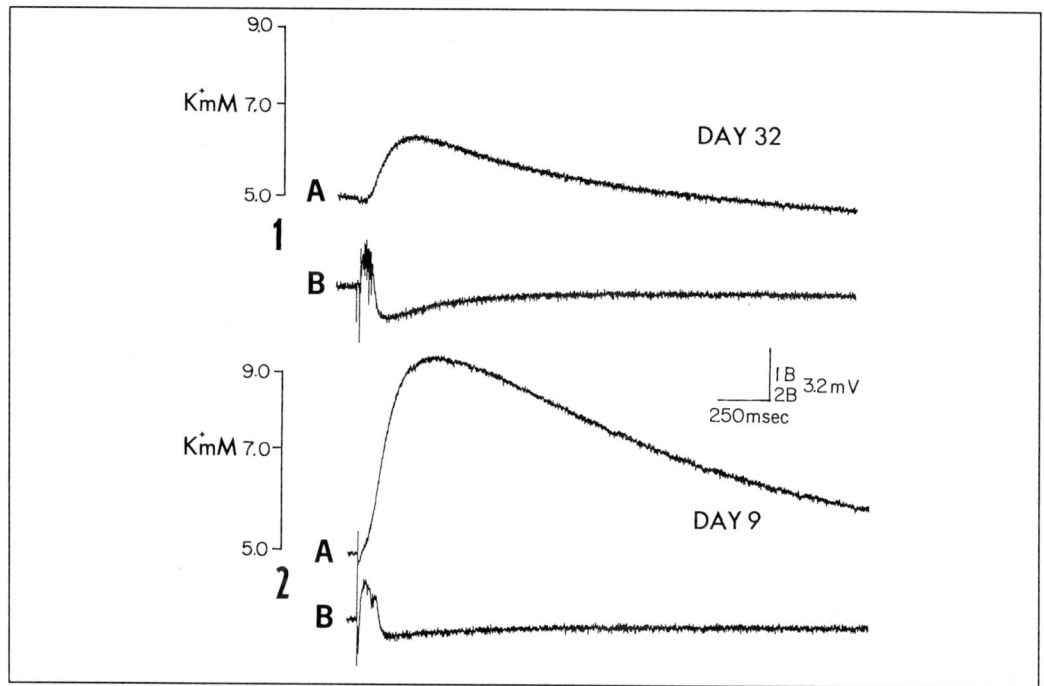

Fig. 4. Comparison of K^+ sensitive microelectrode signals recorded on postnatal day 9 and 32 during epileptiform burst generation (A). Recordings were made in the proximal portion of the basilar dendritic layer using hippocampal slices. Extracellular field potentials (B) recorded simultaneously are also shown (from Swann et al., 1988 with permission).

The immature brain is quite resistant to some types of seizures

In adult animals, status epilepticus induced by systemic kainic acid severely damages the population of CA3-CA4 cells which have kainic acid receptors (Fig. 5). However, status epilepticus induced by kainic acid in immature rats (Moshe, 1987, Sperber et al., 1991) completely spares CA3-CA4 cells. This may be associated with the fact that kainic acid receptors develop quite late during ontogeny (Campochiaro & Coyle, 1978) so that few receptors for kainic acid are present in 15-day-old rat hippocampus. In other words, the immature brain is quite resistant to kainic acid seizures and this may be associated with the normal ontogenic programme characterized by the late maturation of this type of receptor. An alternative explanation might be that the smaller dosages of kainic acid needed to induce sustained seizures in immature animals actually result in seizures less severe than those observed in the adult. Nevertheless, it seems that in some ways the immature brain is less susceptible to seizure-induced injury than the fully mature brain. Whether this resistance to damage is in any way related to the benign outcome of some type of childhood epilepsies is entirely speculative.

Transient overexpression of NMDA receptors and NMDA-mediated excitotoxicity in the immature brain

During postnatal brain development in the rat, there is transient overexpression of the NMDA subtype of glutamate receptors (Tremblay et al., 1988). This is associated with a transient over-expression of damage induced by NMDA or by other excitotoxic agents in rat neocortex or hippocampus (Yang et al., 1989). Seven- to 15-day-old rats developed lesions of larger volume than

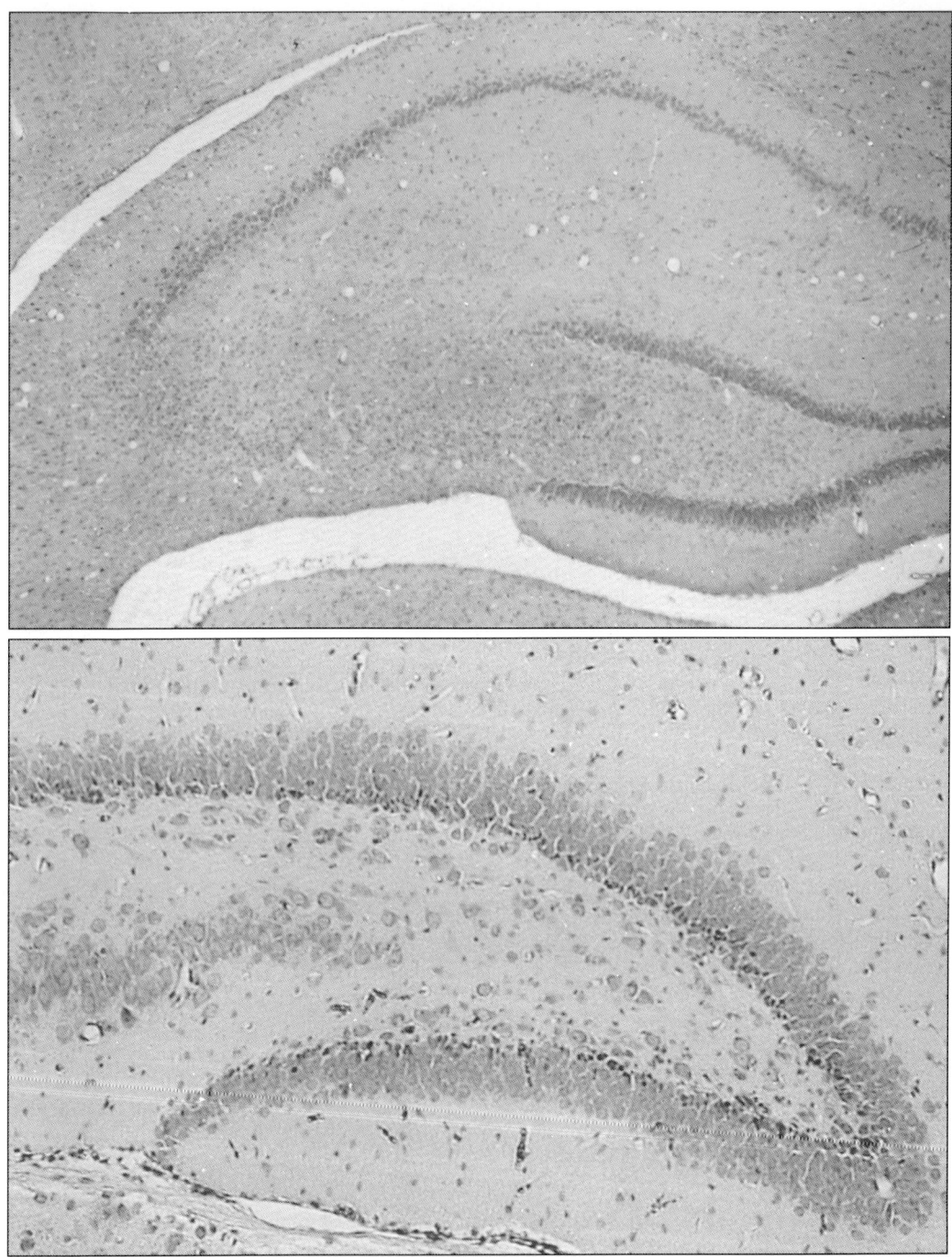

Fig. 5. (a) An adult male Wistar rat received i.p. kainic acid (10 mg/kg), resulting in several hours of limbic seizures and was perfused-fixed 3 days later. Haematoxylin and eosin. The CA3–4 sector of the hippocampus shows severe damage. (b) A 14-day-old male Wistar rat received i.p. kainic acid (3 mg/kg), resulting in several hours of limbic seizures, and was perfused-fixed 3 days later. However, the hippocampus shows no damage.

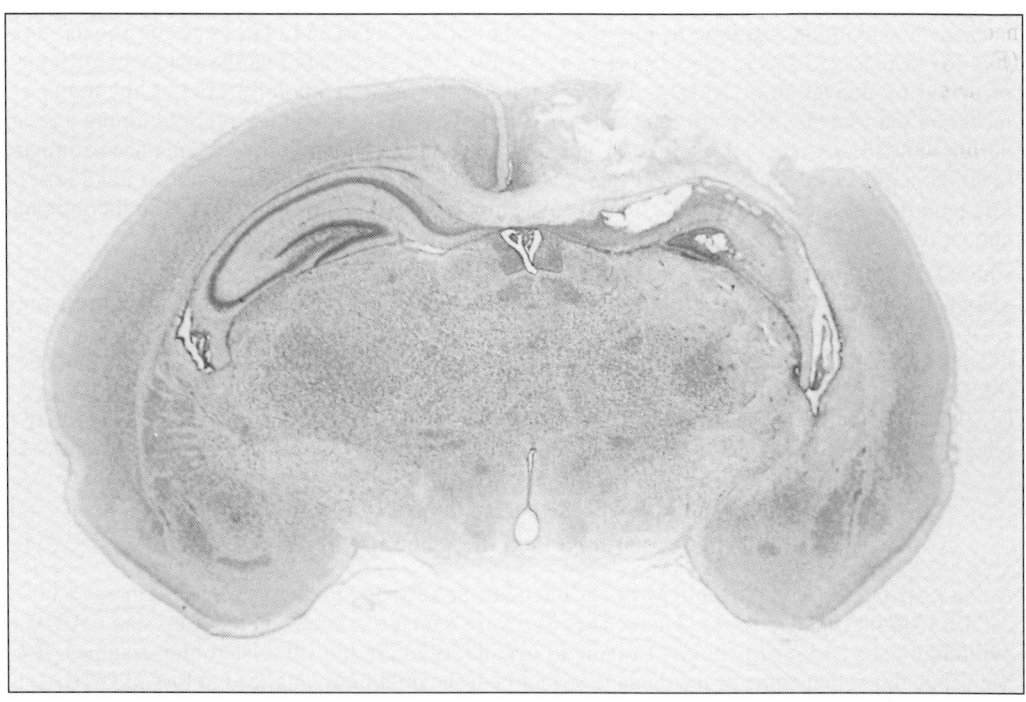

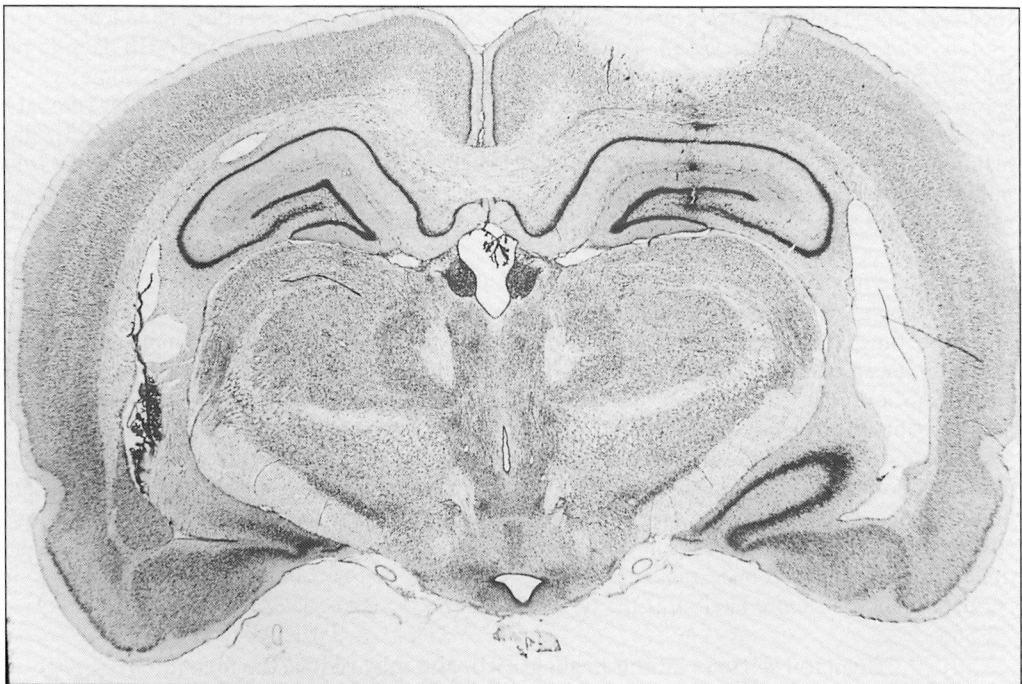

Fig. 6. 50 nmoles of NMDA (volume: 0.5 μl) were injected into the cortex and hippocampus of a 7-day-old rat (a) and of an adult rat (b) 3 days before sacrifice. Lesion volume and severity were significantly greater in the immature brain.

neonates or adults in response to injections of the same volume and concentration of excitotoxin (Fig. 6) (McDonald et al., 1988; Yang et al., 1989). Thus it appears that the ontogeny of injuries mediated by activation of NMDA receptors follows the same temporal profile as the number of receptors themselves. They are transiently overexpressed in the immature brain, defining a period during which EAA receptor expression and EAA excitotoxic vulnerability are enhanced compared to either neonates or adults. Whether this enhanced vulnerability occurs in humans is unknown, but it is tempting to speculate that the highly adverse outcome of some seizure types in the immature human brain could be related to similar developmental factors.

Animal data in various species also suggest that there is a developmental lag between post-synaptic glutamate binding and high-affinity uptake of glutamate during this period of overexpression of EAA receptors (McDonald et al., 1988). The transient overproduction of EAA synaptic terminals relates temporally to heightened synaptic plasticity and consolidation of synaptic connections (McDonald & Johnston, 1990). Taken together, this could imply that during certain stages of development, the brain is less equipped to rapidly take up the large quantities of EAA that may be released during seizures and that this could happen at a time of heightened synaptic plasticity.

Sustained stimulation of the perforant path has different results in the mature and in the immature brain

A classical model of status epilepticus in the adult involves stimulation of the perforant path for 2–24 h (Sloviter, 1987, 1991). This results in severe damage to hilar interneurons and CA3–CA4 pyramidal cells and results in loss of paired pulse inhibition in the stimulated hippocampus. It has been speculated that some of the damage to interneurons might not only lead to loss of GABAergic inhibition (Sloviter, 1991) but also to aberrrant regeneration which might set up an excitatory reverberating circuit in which granule cells would excite granule cells, resulting in epileptogenesis (Sutula et al., 1989; Sutula, 1990). Our studies of perforant path stimulation in 14–16-day-old rats (an age at which those animals are quite resistant to hippocampal damage from some type of seizures; Sperber et al., 1991) shows that perforant path stimulation leads to long-lasting, probably permanent, loss of paired pulse inhibition in the stimulated hippocampus. This is associated with a histological pattern quite different from the adult. There is no damage to CA3-CA4 pyramidal cells, but instead there is oedema and apparent selective necrosis of some granule cells in the inner layers of the dentate gyrus and of a few hilar interneurons. While it is too early to speculate on the significance of those results, they clearly show that the resistance of the brain, and particularly of the immature hippocampus, to certain types of seizures is not complete nor absolute. Clearly, some type of seizures can produce some damage with both physiological and anatomical expression. At the same time, they confirm the great resistance of pyramidal cells in the immature brain to seizure-induced damage. Similarly, flurothyl seizures in 2-week-old marmoset monkeys produce some CA3 lesions but completely spare CA1. In fact, we know of no seizure model in immature animals which shows any CA1 damage. The inescapable conclusion is that Ammon's horn sclerosis, the most common substrate of epilepsy in the human brain, is unlikely to result from seizures occurring during the perinatal period. In fact, perinatal ischaemia also spares CA1 and is an equally unlikely source of Ammon's horn sclerosis. Since this histological change is so common in human epilepsy, it must be either the result of unknown damage to the foetal hippocampus occurring at a time when its cells are even more resistant to ischaemia and seizures than they are during the perinatal period, or more likely it is the result of seizures occurring later in life.

Neonatal seizures inhibit brain growth and may reduce the formation of neuron to neuron connections

The effect of seizures on brain growth may be more important than their effects on neuronal survival. Eighty per cent of the cells in the human brain are generated postnatally (pn) and mitotic

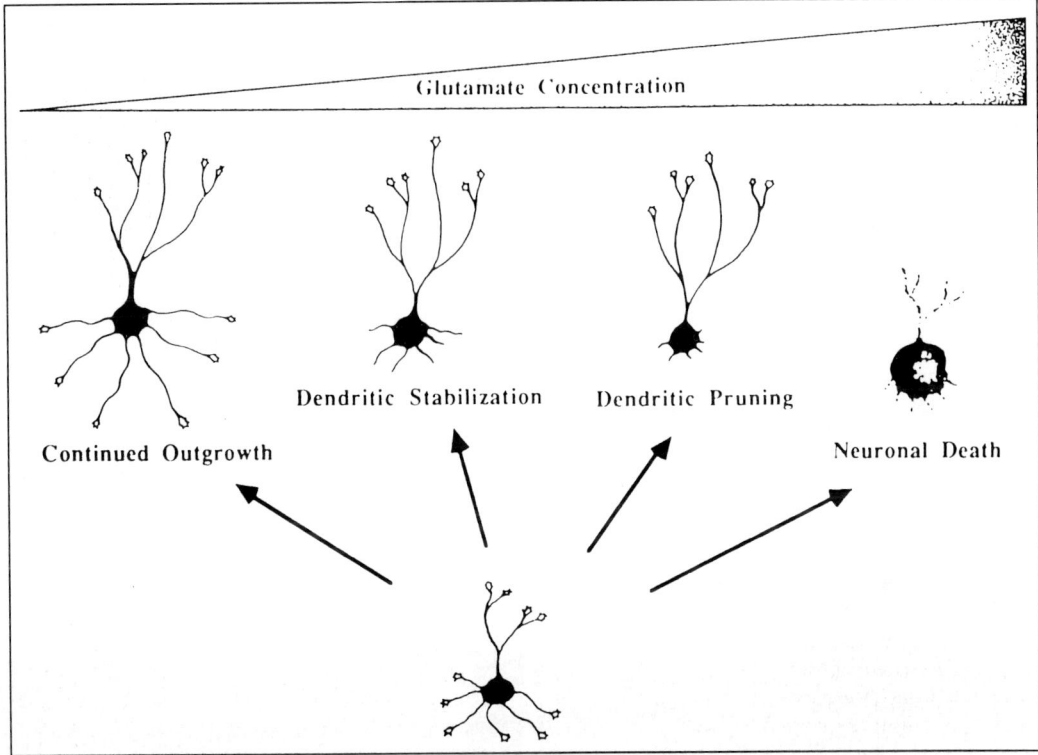

Fig. 7. Neurotransmitter control of growth cone behaviour (Lipton & Kater, 1989).

activity continues in the rat forebrain until day 20 pn, in rat cerebellum until day 18 pn and in human cerebellum until at least 1 year of age. Postnatal mitotic activity occurs in granule neurons of both the human and rat hippocampus and glial proliferation is largely a postnatal phenomenon in both species. Many cell populations have a limited time span during which they can undergo mitotic activity and if that opportunity is bypassed the resulting deficit in cell numbers cannot be made up. For example, the basket cells of the cerebellum are generated almost exclusively during the first postnatal week in the rat. If mitosis or migration of those cells is prevented by a disease such as hypothyroidism, correction of the metabolic defect after the first week of life occurs too late and the result is a cerebellum devoid of basket cells. Seizures are known to inhibit protein synthesis and to arrest mitosis (Suga & Wasterlain, 1980). Their presence at the tail end of the period of cell division in a brain region can result in permanent reduction of brain size and cellularity (Wasterlain, 1976).

The establishment of synaptic connections and the programmed elimination of excess synaptic terminals are also normal growth processes that can be affected by metabolic brain disease and potentially by seizure activity. When seizures occur during a period of active brain myelination in the rat, they result in a selective deficit in myelin-specific lipids, which is greater than the concomitant reduction of cell numbers (Dwyer & Wasterlain, 1982). A reduction of protein markers of synaptic terminals by seizures in those immature brains is also observed (Jorgensen *et al.*, 1980) suggesting a curtailment of the growth of synaptic connections (Wasterlain *et al.*, 1990).

The behaviour of growth cones is in large part determined by their synaptic input; for example, dissociated cortical neurons in culture have rapidly expanding growth cones when extracellular glutamate concentration is low (as it would be in the extracellular space of a healthy brain). Modest increases in extracellular glutamate concentration lead to arrest of that growth with synaptic stabilization. Greater increases result in retraction and pruning of growth cones (Fig. 7) (Lipton & Kater, 1989).

Preliminary studies of the expression of the axonal growth cone marker protein GAP-43 show a significant reduction of the concentration of the protein in the hippocampus 2 days after a 2 h episode of flurothyl-induced status epilepticus, possibly suggesting that seizures inhibit the expression of growth cone proteins and the establishment of new synaptic connections (Fig. 8).

The nature and extent of seizure-associated damage varies with age

In summary, experimental studies show great age-dependent variations in the nature and severity of brain damage associated with seizure activity. The immature brain is far more resistant than the adult to damage induced by lactic acid build up, or kainate-induced status epilepticus and its lower metabolic rate and lesser tendency to release large amounts of excitatory amino acid during seizures (because of the immaturity of its presynaptic terminals) protect the brain from damage. At the same time, its limited ability to transport glucose across the blood–brain barrier, the absence in some neurons of the calcium buffering capacity conferred by the presence of the calcium buffering protein calbindin D28k, the overexpression of NMDA and AMPA receptors and the adverse effect of inhibiting brain growth make it far more vulnerable than the adult to some types of insults.

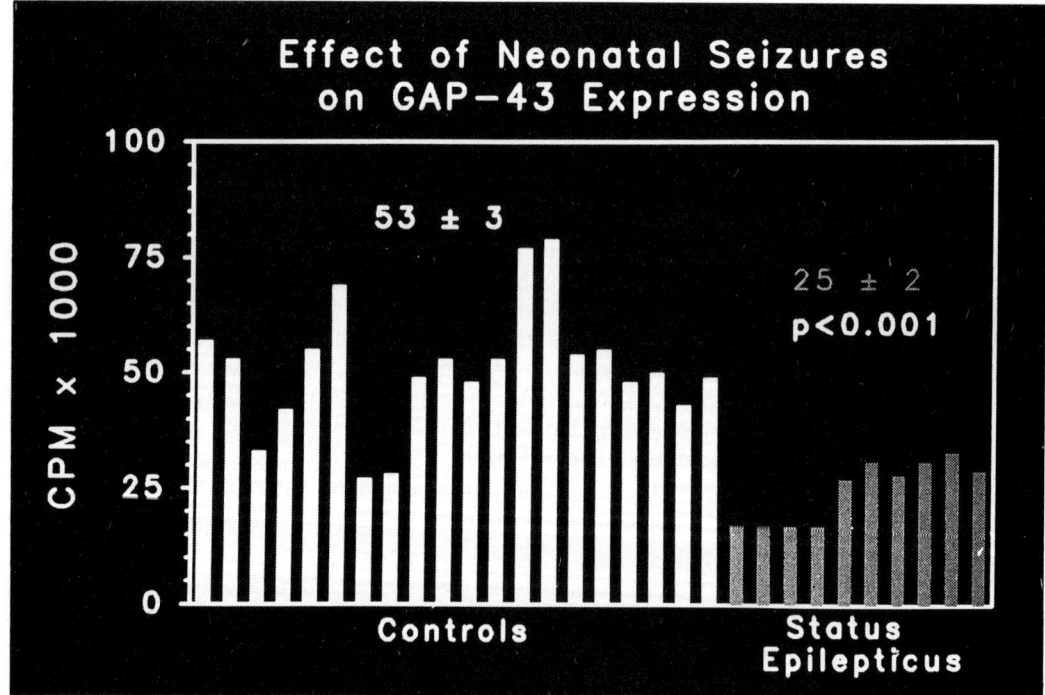

Fig. 8. *Effect of neonatal seizures on the expression of the axonal growth cone marker protein GAP–43. A 4-day-old rat was subjected to 2 h of flurothyl seizures or to sham handling and was sacrificed 2 days later. Proteins from forebrain homogenates were separated by SDS-PAGE, transblotted onto nitrocellulose paper, incubated with a monoclonal antibody to GAP–43, a secondary antibody, and conjugated with ^{125}I-protein A (Thompson et al., 1992).*

Clinical correlation

The correlation of laboratory data with clinical experience is made difficult by the fact that the presently available laboratory models of epilepsy do not simulate the human situation satisfactorily. This is especially true of many of the developmental epileptic syndromes in childhood. Clinical experience suggests that there are human epileptic syndromes with posterior foci that have very different long-term prognoses.

Available clinical data suggests that the outcome of seizures/epilepsy attributable to posterior foci in children is determined by the presence vs absence of structural lesions as well as the developmental stage during which seizures intervene. It appears likely that the two factors are related – it seems that epilepsies resulting from identifiable posterior structural lesions generally result in seizures at an early stage and tend to have a catastrophic outcome while familial syndromes without known structural abnormalities associated with their electrographic foci generally present in older children and tend to have a benign prognosis.

A clinical syndrome with extremely benign prognosis was described by Gastaut (1985) in which occipital rhythmic spike waves occur frequently after eye closure. These children experience visual ictal symptoms associated with the spike waves, but have no known structural lesion. An autosomal dominant pattern for the EEG abnormalities with age-dependent expression and variable penetrance of the seizure disorder has been proposed (Kuzniecky & Rosenblatt, 1987). The mean age of onset of this syndrome is around 6 years (Gastaut, 1982).

On the other hand, posterior structural lesions, whether they be a presentation of phakomatoses such as Sturge–Weber syndrome or tuberous sclerosis, or cortical dysplasias marking aberrant migration of neuroblasts, result in a severe epileptic syndrome of infancy known as infantile spasms (IS), also known as West syndrome. The onset of seizures associated with IS occurs around or before 6 months of age in the vast majority of patients and approximately 90 per cent of IS begin before 12 months of age (Holmes, 1987). The prognosis for these children is generally considered catastrophic, with evolution to further seizure types and progressive mental retardation. It is also of interest to note that the small minority of infants who tend to have a better outcome after suffering from West syndrome generally come from cryptogenic cases and have no identifiable structural lesion nor a metabolic abnormality. This group generally responds early to treatment and does not endure a sustained epileptic condition during what may be a critical period in neurodevelopment.

Huttenlocher's classic study (1979) of the developmental changes in synaptic density of the human cortex suggested a sharp increase in synaptic density from birth to about 6 months of age, a period of stable synaptic density followed by a decline from about 7 years to 16 years, reaching a second plateau, which is stable until the late decline associated with senescence. He also reported that the synapses gradually took on adult morphological characteristics between ages 6 and 24 months. More recent data (Kornhuber et al., 1988) on the human cortex demonstrate that the ontogenic curve plotting binding densities (pmol/mg protein) for glutamate binding against age parallels the Huttenlocher curve. There is a sharp increase in binding densities during the early postnatal period, with a transient peak between age 1 and 2 years that is reminiscent of the transient overexpression of NMDA receptors in the immature brain of rats.

Thus, available laboratory evidence and clinical data seem to be converging on a consistent pattern of age-dependent susceptibility to seizures and to seizure-induced brain damage affecting development. The clinical syndromes differ in both the aetiology and the timing of the seizures, thus placing a limitation on our ability to draw clear conclusions. However, the timing seems to be related to the aetiology. Improved understanding of these processes will emerge as animal models that better mimic the human condition become available.

References

Adler, J., Erba, G., Winston, K.R., Welch, K. & Lombroso, C.T. (1991): Results of surgery for extratemporal partial epilepsy that began in childhood. *Arch. Neurol.* **48**, 133–140.

Akira, T., Baldwin, R.A. & Wasterlain, C.G. (1992): Nitric oxide is responsible for continued synaptic transduction following hypoxic and excitotoxic events. *Abstr. Soc. Neurosci.* (in press).

Baxter, C.F., Wasterlain, C.G., Oh, C.C. & Baldwin, R.A. (1991): Post–ictal changes in GABA metabolism in the substantia nigra. *Abstr. Soc. Neurosci.* **17**, 596.

Bredt, D.S., Hwang, P.M., Glatt, C.E., Lowenstein, C., Reed, R.R. & Snyder, S.H. (1991): Cloned and expressed nitric oxide synthase structurally resembles cytochrome P-450 reductase. *Nature* **351**, 714–718.

Campochiaro, P. & Coyle, J.T. (1978): Ontogenic development of kainate neurotoxicity: correlates with glutamatergic innervation. *Proc. Natl. Acad. Sci. USA* **75**, 2025–2029.

Cherubini, E., Rovira, C., Gaiarsa, J.L., Corradetti, R. & Ben-Ari, Y. (1990): GABA mediated excitation in immature rat CA3 hippocampal neurons. *Int. J. Dev. Neurosci.* **8**, 481–490.

Choi, D.W. (1985): Glutamate toxicity in cortical cell culture is calcium-dependent. *Neurosci. Lett.* **58**, 293–297.

Choi, D.W., Koh, J.Y. & Peters, S. (1988): Pharmacology of glutamate neurotoxicity in cortical cell cultures: attenuation by NMDA antagonists. *J. Neurosci.* **8**, 185–196.

Connors, B.W., Bernardo, L.S. & Prince, D.A. (1983): Coupling between neurons of the developing rat neocortex. *J. Neurosci.* **3**, 773–782.

Dawson, T.M., Bredt, D.S., Fotushi, M., Hwang, P.M. & Snyder, S.H. (1991): Nitric oxide synthase and neuronal NADPH diaphorase are identical in brain and peripheral tissues. *Proc. Natl. Acad. Sci. USA* **18**, 7797–7801.

Dudek, F.E., Obenhaus, A. & Tasker, J.G. (1990): Osmolality-induced changes in extracellular volume alter epileptiform bursts independent of chemical synapses in the rat: importance of non-synaptic mechanisms in hippocampal epileptogenesis. *Neurosci. Lett.* **120**, 267–270.

Dwyer, B.E. & Wasterlain, C.G. (1982): Electroconvulsive seizures in the immature rat adversely affect myelin accumulation. *Exp. Neurol.* **78**, 616–628.

Dwyer, B.E. & Wasterlain, C.G. (1985): Neonatal seizures in monkeys and rabbits: brain glucose depletion in the face of normoglycemia, prevention by glucose loads. *Pediatr. Res.* **19**, 992–995.

Engel, J. Jr. & Shewmon, D.A. (1991): Impact of the kindling phenomenon on clinical epileptology. In: *Kindling and synaptic plasticity. The legacy of Graham Goddard*, ed. F. Morrell. Boston: Birkhauser.

Gale, K. (1985): Mechanism of seizure control mediated by γ-aminobutyric acid: role of the substantia nigra. *Fed. Proc.* **44**, 2414–2424.

Gastaut, H. (1982): A new type of epilepsy: benign partial epilepsy of childhood with occipital spike-waves. *Clin. Electroencephalogr.* **13**, 13–22.

Gastaut, H. (1985): Benign epilepsy of childhood with occipital paroxysms. In: *Epileptic syndromes in infancy, childhood and adolescence*, eds. J. Roger, C. Dravet, M. Bureau, F.E. Dreifuss & P. Wolf. London: John Libbey.

Goldberg, M.P., Weiss, J.H., Pham, P.C. & Choi, D.W. (1987): N-methyl-D-aspartate receptors mediate hypoxic neuronal injury in cortical culture. *J. Pharmacol. Exp. Ther.* **243**, 784–791.

Hablitz, J.J. & Heinemann, U. (1987): Extracellular K^+ and Ca^{2+} changes during epileptiform discharges in the immature rat cortex. *Dev. Brain. Res.* **36**, 299–303.

Holmes, G.H. (1987): Infantile spasms. In: *Diagnosis and management of seizures in children*, pp. 212–225. Philadelphia: Saunders.

Huttenlocher, P.R. (1979): Synaptic density in human frontal cortex – developmental changes and effects of aging. *Brain Res.* **163**, 195–205.

Jorgensen, O.S., Dwyer, B.E. & Wasterlain, C.G. (1980): Synaptic proteins after electroconvulsive seizures in immature rats. *J. Neurochem.* **35**, 1235–1237.

Kornhuber, J., Retz, W., Riederer, P., Heinsen, H. & Fritze, J. (1988): Effect of antemortem and postmortem factors on [^{3}H]glutamate binding in the human brain. *Neurosci. Lett.* **93**, 312–317.

Kuzniecky, R. & Rosenblatt, B. (1987): Benign occipital epilepsy: a family study. *Epilepsia* **28**, 346–350.

Lipton, S.A. & Kater, S.D. (1989): Neurotransmitter regulation of neuronal outgrowth, plasticity and survival. *Trends Neurosci.* **12**, 265–270.

McDonald, J.W., Silverstein, F.S. & Johnston, M.V. (1988): Neurotoxicity of N-methyl-D-aspartate is markedly enhanced in developing rat central nervous system. *Brain Res.* **459**, 200–203.

McDonald, J.W. & Johnston, M.V. (1990): Physiological and pathophysiological roles of excitatory amino acids during central nervous system development. *Brain Res. Rev.* **15**, 41–70.

Morin, A.M., Dwyer, B.E., Fujikawa, D.G. & Wasterlain, C.G. (1988): Low [^{3}H]-cytochalasin B binding in the cerebral cortex of newborn rat. *J. Neurochem.* **51**, 206–211.

Moshe, S.L. (1987): Epileptogenesis and the immature brain. *Epilepsia* **28**, S3–S15.

Olney, J.W. (1978): Neurotoxicity of excitatory amino acids. In: *Kainic acid as a tool in neurobiology*, eds. E.G. McGeer, J.W. Olney & P.L. McGeer, pp. 96–107. New York: Raven Press.

Reynolds, E.H. (1981): Biological factors in psychological disorders associated with epilepsy. In: *Epilepsy and psychiatry*, eds. E.H. Reynolds & M.R. Trimble. Edinburgh: Churchill Livingstone.

Rothman, S. (1984): Synaptic release of excitatory amino acid neurotransmitter mediates anoxic neuronal death. *J. Neurosci.* **4**, 1884–1891.

Sloviter, R.S. (1987): Decreased hippocampal inhibition and a selective loss of interneurons in experimental epilepsy. *Science* **235**, 73–76.

Sloviter, R.S. (1991): Permanently altered hippocampal structure, excitability and inhibition after experimental status epilepticus in the rat: the 'dormant basket cell' hypothesis and its possible relevance to temporal lobe epilepsy. *Hippocampus* **1**, 41–66.

Sperber, E.F., Haas, K.Z., Stanton, P.K. & Moshe, S.L. (1991): Resistance of the immature hippocampus to seizure-induced synaptic reorganization. *Dev. Brain Res.* **60**, 88–93.

Suga, S. & Wasterlain, C.G. (1980): Effects of neonatal seizures or anoxia on cerebellar mitotic activity in the rat. *Exp. Neurol.* **67**, 573–580.

Sutula, T.P., Cascino, G., Cavazos, J., Parada, I. & Ramirez, L. (1989): Mossy fiber synaptic reorganization in the epileptic human temporal lobe. *Ann. Neurol.* **26**, 321–330.

Sutula, T.P. (1990): Experimental models of temporal lobe epilepsy: new insights from the study of kindling and synaptic reorganization. *Epilepsia* **31** (suppl. 3), S45–S54.

Swann, J.W., Brady, R.J., Smith, K.L. & Pierson, M.G. (1988): Synaptic mechanisms of focal epileptogenesis in the immature nervous system. In: *Disorders of the developing nervous system: changing views on their origins, diagnoses and treatments*, eds. J.W. Swann & A. Messer, pp. 19–49. New York: Alan R. Liss, Inc.

Swann, J.W., Smith, K.L. & Brady, R.J. (1991): Age-dependent alterations in the operations of hippocampal neural networks. *Ann. N.Y. Acad. Sci.* **627**, 264–276.

Thompson, K., Wasterlain, C.G. & Penix, L. (1992): Perforant path stimulation in immature brain. *Neurology* **42**, 961S.

Tremblay, E., Roisin, M.P., Represa, A., Charriaut-Marlangue, C. & Ben-Ari, Y. (1988): Transient increased density of NMDA binding sites in the developing rat hippocampus. *Brain Res.* **461**, 393–396.

Wallis, R.A., Panizzon, K.L. & Wasterlain, C.G. (1992): Nitric oxide synthase antagonism provides protection against hypoxia in the hippocampal slice. *Neurology* **42**, 755S.

Wasterlain, C.G. (1976): Effects of neonatal status epilepticus on rat brain development. *Neurology* **33**, 821–827.

Wasterlain, C.G., Fujikawa, D.G., Dwyer, B.E. *et al.* (1990): Brain damage in the neonate: multiple periods of selective vulnerability each reflect discrete molecular events resulting from normal brain development. In: *Neonatal seizures*, eds. C.G. Wasterlain & P. Vert. New York: Raven Press.

Wasterlain, C.G., Baxter, C.F. & Baldwin, R.A. (1991): Failure of GABA synthesis in substantia nigra in experimental status epilepticus. *Epilepsia* **32**, 46.

Yang, C.X., Morin, A.M., Fujikawa, D.G., Schwartz, P.H., Hattori, H. & Wasterlain, C.G. (1989): Ontogenesis of NMDA-mediated excitotoxicity. *Neurology* **39** (Suppl. 1), 373.

Chapter 4

Structures and functions of the occipital lobe

Giuliano Avanzini

Department of Neurophysiology, Istituto Nazionale Neurologico 'Carlo Besta', via Celoria 11, 20133 Milan, Italy

Summary

In describing the occipital lobe, morphological criteria should be completed by the information on functional representation and connectivity patterns. According to this approach, it is appropriate to state that: (1) of the three classical cytotectonic areas 17, 18 and 19, only area 17 is structurally and functionally homogeneous; (2) the boundaries between visual occipital cortex and parietal/temporal cortices are still undefined; (3) the visual representation extends beyond the occipital lobe in parietal, temporal and frontal cortices. No less than 20 areas in primates have been identified as visual and shown to be hierarchically organized in visual subsystems specialized in processing different submodalities. The abstracted information is then fed into inferotemporal and parietal regions, where complex processing, related to the qualities and the relations of objects in visual space, is carried out. The available data of visual cortical representation in humans are drawn from the analysis of visual defects caused by cerebral injuries and of the effects of cortical stimulation performed during surgery or in blind patients implanted with intracranial stimulation prostheses. Additional information is provided by PET and RM studies and by the analysis of ictal epileptic phenomenology. Out of the many putative visual areas only V1 has been confidently identified as corresponding to Brodmann's area 17. The visual field representation extends 5° into the ipsilateral hemisphere: this accounts for macular sparing in unilateral injuries. Both lesion and stimulation studies localize the foveal representation in the occipital pole. The more peripheral areas of the visual field are progressively represented more anteriorly. The horizontal meridian of each half field lies along the depth of the calcarine sulcus. On the ground of available information, elementary visual hallucinations reported as symptoms of partial seizures indicate the site of origin of epileptic discharges (according to the visuotopic map) only if the focus is located in V1. The visual representation is in fact more and more irregular as one moves to higher order areas. The apparent movement of visual epileptic hallucinations may be accounted for by the associated eye deviation. Complex visual hallucinations may result from a spread of the epileptic discharge along the cortical channels resulting from serial interareal connections. Ocular movements reported as tonic deviation clonic jerks or 'epileptic nystagmus' frequently occurring in occipital seizures are by no means specific to the occipital lobe. The fact that the traditional definition of the occipital lobe does not account for the complexity of visual cortical organization, raises the question of how appropriate is the current definition of partial visual seizures as occipital seizures, until more details of the anatomo-functional organization of the human occipital lobe are available.

Anatomical definition of the occipital lobe

According to gross anatomical criteria the occipital lobe is separated from parietal and temporal lobes by the conventional boundaries reported in Fig. 1. Only on its mesial aspect is the boundary with the parietal lobe marked by a natural sulcus, the parieto-occipital fissure. These boundaries correspond to those of area 19 defined according to Brodmann's cyto-

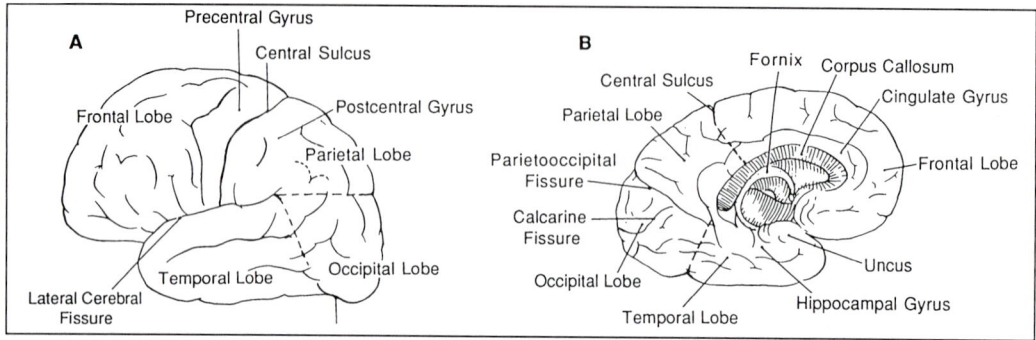

Fig. 1. Schematic representation of the lateral and medial surfaces of the cerebral hemispheres showing the division into four main lobes. From Shepherd (1988), with permission.

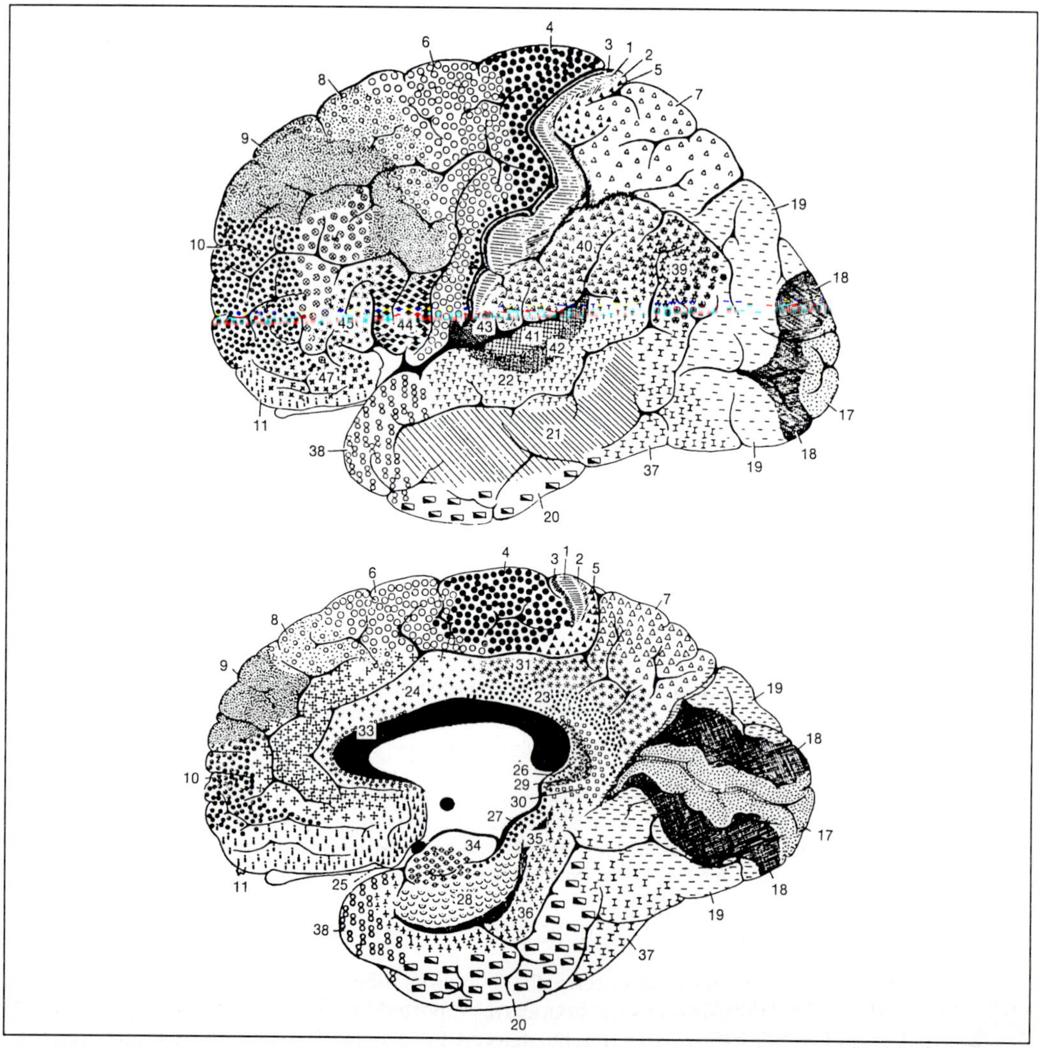

Fig. 2. Brodmann's (1909) cytoarchitectural map of the human brain. From Brodal (1969), with permission.

architectonic maps (Fig. 2). However, the cytoarchitectural criterion is by no means an absolute one, due to the existence of transitional zones between different cortical areas, and it must be realized that the traditional division into four main cerebral lobes has only a descriptive value and is meaningless in operational terms.

The old notion that cerebral functions are organized in terms of lobes is in fact giving way to the new idea that cerebral functions are organized in terms of distributed systems. There is increasing experimental evidence that pathways connecting different lobes form distributed systems, so that there are maximal opportunities for areas located in different lobes to interact. Within a given lobe, each area contributes with its specific operational properties to process the incoming inputs, the centres being connected through both a serial and a parallel arrangement. In describing the organization of the cerebral cortex, the cytoarchitectural criterion should therefore be integrated by information on functional representation and connectivity patterns. Such an approach leads, for the occipital cortex, to the following statements:

1. Out of the three occipital areas: 17, 18, 19, classically identified on cytoarchitectonic ground, only the area 17 appears to be structurally and functionally homogeneous, while the 18 and 19 areas can be further divided into sub-areas with different functional significance;
2. The boundaries between visual occipital cortex and parietal/temporal cortices cannot be sharply defined due to the insufficient information on the organization of the bordering fields;
3. The visual representation extends beyond the occipital lobe in parietal, temporal and frontal cortices.

Visual representation on the cerebral cortex

Thanks to the systematic studies of vision physiology, carried out by David Hubel and Torsten Wiesel, who were awarded the Nobel Prize in 1981, we know the processing sequence of visual signals taking place in different categories of cortical neurons defined as simple, complex and hypercomplex, and organized according to serial patterns of connectivity (Hubel & Wiesel, 1962, 1965, 1972).

Simple cells respond selectively to a bar or edge of light with a specific orientation in a particular position in the visual field. Their properties are due to the convergence of inputs from neurons with centre-surround antagonism located in different laminae of the lateral geniculate thalamic nucleus.

Complex cells are specifically sensitive to a bar or edge with a specific orientation but placed anywhere in the visual field. It was logically assumed and experimentally demonstrated that they receive inputs from different simple cells tuned on the same orientation.

Hypercomplex cells respond to bars of specific length or width depending again on the interaction of inputs from the other cell categories. Simple and complex cells are mainly located in the primary visual area (V1) which approximately corresponds to area 17 of the cytoarchitectural map. The hypercomplex cells are more numerous in the other visual areas organized in strips adjoining V1.

According to Van Essen (1985), 20 areas are candidates for being largely or exclusively visual in function in the macaque; 11 of these are demonstrably visual and have been identified with some degree of certainty (Fig. 3). The following description is based on Van Essen (1985). V1 is anatomically identified by a heavily myelinated layer 4B (stria of Gennari). It has an orderly and complete representation of the contralateral visual hemifield, its constituent neurons have well-defined receptive field properties and its lesion produces virtually complete scotomas or perceptual blindness over the corresponding portion of the visual field.

The adjacent visual area 2 (V2) has a long common border with V1 and a visual representation which is a mirror image of that of V1; it is not coextensive with the area 18.

Visual area 3 (V3) and the ventral posterior area (VP) occupy a narrow strip adjoining the dorsal

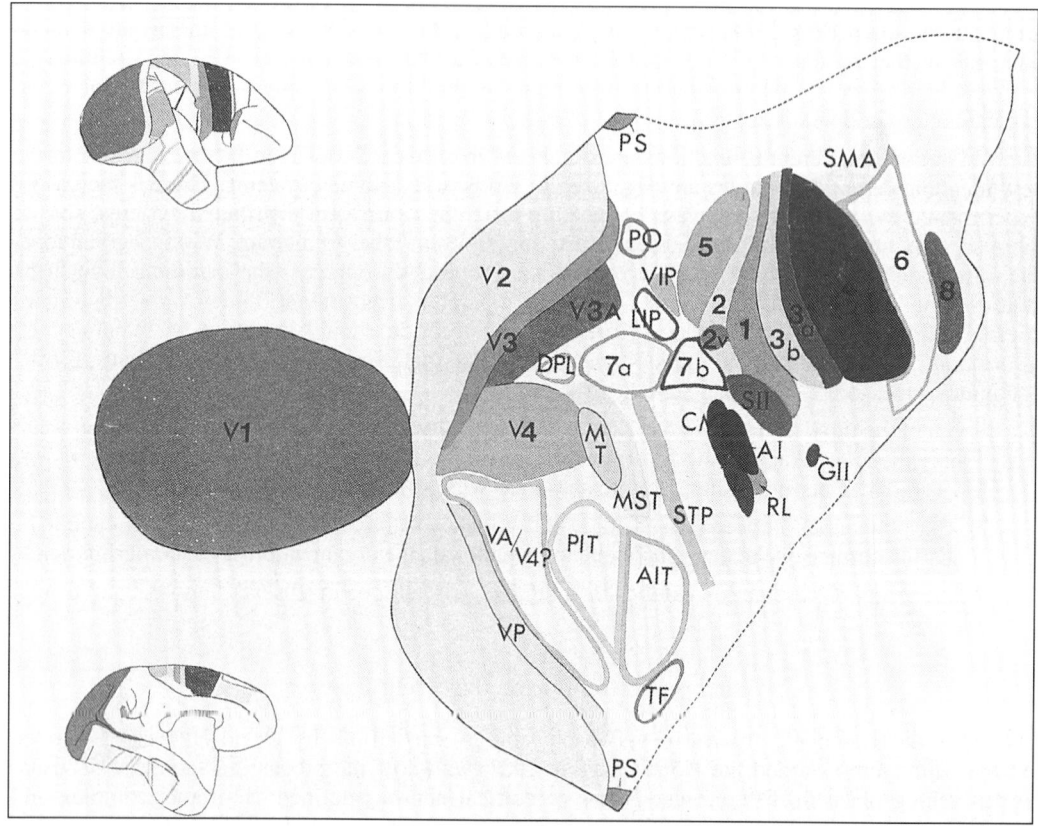

Fig. 3. Cortical areas in the macaque monkey as represented on lateral and medial views (insets), and on an unfolded, two-dimensional map of the entire hemisphere. Areas which have been identified with reasonable confidence are shown in various shades of solid grey; those whose identification is less certain are shown only in outline. The following abbreviations designate visual and vision-related areas. V1, V2, V3, V4: visual 1-4; V3A: visual 3 anterior; VP: ventral posterior; VA: ventral anterior; MT: medial temporal; PO: parieto occipital; VIP: ventral intraparietal; PIT: posterior infero-temporal; AIT: anterior infero-temporal; 7a: parietal 7a; LIP: lateral intraparietal; STP: superior temporal polysensorial; PS: prostriate; TF: temporal field; 8: frontal 8. Reproduced in grey from the van Essen (1985) colour plate, with permission.

(V3) and ventral (VP) parts of V2. They receive projections from V1. V3 seems to be mainly concerned with visuospatial analysis, and VP with colour vision and/or pattern recognition.

The contiguous area is also subdivided in the fourth dorsal visual area (V4) and ventral anterior (VA/V4) parts on the ground of its connectivity patterns with V2. Medial temporal (MT) is a small V1-recipient area located on the posterior edge of the superior temporal sulcus.

In addition to the above-mentioned visual areas, lying mainly within the occipital lobe, one can recognize three occipito-visual areas, V3A, PO and prelunate dorsal (DPL), one medial superior temporal (MST) and one ventral intraparietal (VIP) area, two inferotemporal posterior (PIT) and anterior (AIT) areas, and a group of visuomotor or polysensory areas: 7a, lateral intraparietal (LIP), superior temporal polysensorial (STP), TF, prostriate (PS) and 8.

A schematic representation of the interconnections between these different visual areas is presented in Fig. 4, stressing the concept of a hierarchical organization, although transverse connections between areas belonging to the same hierarchical stage are also indicated.

This scheme does not include subcortical connections, which cannot fit into the concept of cortical

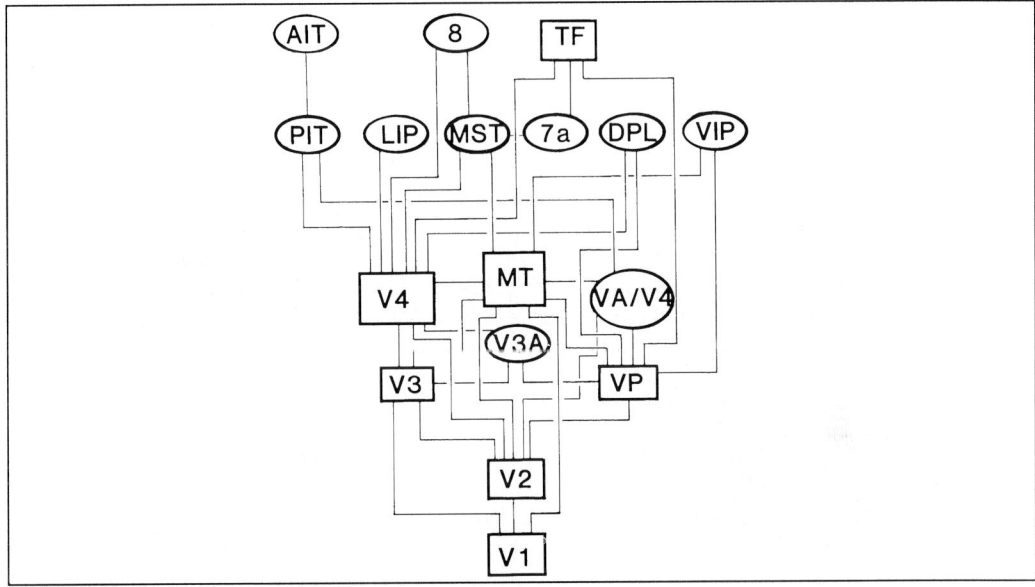

Fig. 4. Diagram of hierarchy of visual areas in the macaque, based on the pattern of cortico-cortical connections. For abbreviations see text. From Van Essen (1985), with permission.

hierarchy until other criteria are developed to fit cortical-subcortical loops into a broader hierarchical pattern. It has to be borne in mind, however, that the visual input can reach visual areas not only through the intracortical serial pathways, but also through subcortical, namely thalamo-cortical, connections. Their cortical distribution, according to the functionally identified visual areas, has not yet been defined satisfactorily. The most specific thalamo-cortical visual projection system connects the lateral geniculate nucleus (LGN) with V1, although modern techniques have revealed an additional, albeit weak, projection to other visual areas (Tigges & Tigges, 1985). On the other hand, the pulvinar-lateralis posterior (Pul-LP) complex sends projections to virtually all of the photically responsive occipital, parietal and temporal areas (Tigges & Tigges, 1985). Intralaminar thalamic nuclei (ILN), namely the centralis lateralis (CL), paracentralis (Pc) and centralis medialis (CeM) nuclei project widely to visual cortical areas (Macchi & Bentivoglio, 1982). They are viewed as relays transferring activity from mesencephalic reticular formation to the cortex and may therefore be involved in saccadic eye movements, gaze control and visual attention. The functional significance of serial hierarchically organized visual cortical subsystems can be referred to their specialization in processing different visual submodalities. According to Van Essen (1985), colour information arrives from parvocellular LGN and is processed through V1 and V2 to V4. Stimulus orientation arrives in V1 from both parvo and magnocellular LGN and is processed through V2, V3 to V4 and MT. A similar sequence applies to binocular disparity information. Information about direction of movement arrives in V1 from magnocellular LGN and is transferred directly, and also through V2, to MT. This parallel array of abstracted information is then fed into the higher visual centres, namely the inferotemporal and parietal regions, where complex processing related to the qualities and the spatial relations of objects in visual space is carried out.

Human visual cortex

The full extent of the visual cortex in humans has yet to be accurately mapped. Out of the many putative visual areas, only V1 has been confidently identified in human cortex and corresponds approximately to Broadmann's area 17.

The available functional information is drawn from the analysis of visual defects caused by cerebral injuries and from reports of the effects of cortical stimulations performed during surgery or in blind patients implanted with intracranial stimulation prosthesis. Additional information is provided by PET and RM studies and by the analysis of the ictal phenomenology associated with epileptic discharges arising in the visual cortex.

A brief historical account of the identification and mapping of the visual cortex in humans with cerebral lesions has recently been published by Glickstein & Whitteridge (1987). The first comprehensive pathological study by Henschen (1890), on patients in which hemianopsia had been produced by brain lesions, demonstrated that the critical focus of the lesion was in the occipital lobe, specifically in the striate cortex which, in the human brain, lies on the lips, banks and depths of the calcarine fissure. Some years later, an important contribution came from the largely unrecognized work of a Japanese ophthalmologist, Tatsuji Inouye, on 29 Japanese soldiers hit by bullets that had had a relatively straight course through the brain.

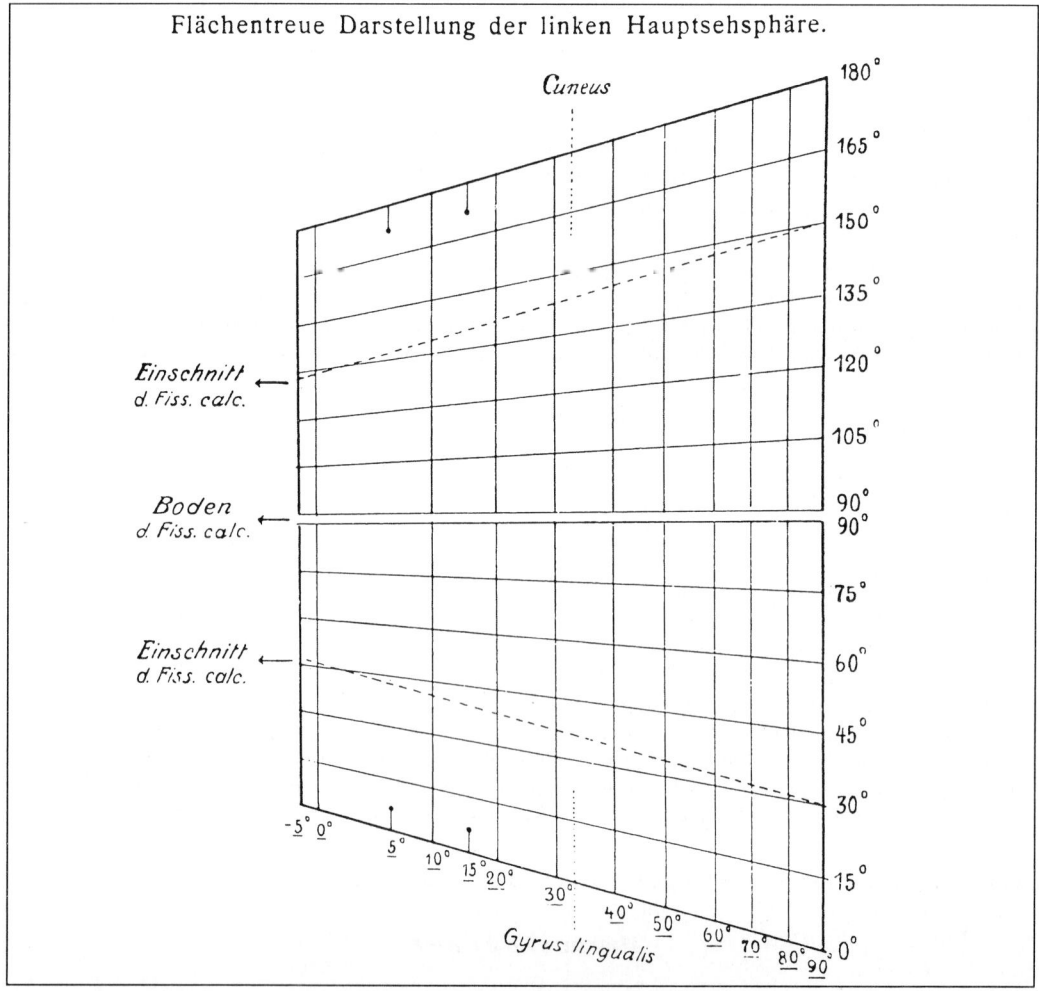

Fig. 5. Inouye's (1909) scheme for the projection of the visual fields on the human striate cortex. From Glickstein & Whitteridge (1987) with permission.

In order to define the actual brain lesion caused by the bullet, Inouye devised a special instrument, the cranio-cordinometer, to locate precisely the coordinates of the entry and exit wounds, with respect to the major cortical fissure. The results, published in Leipzig in 1909 (Inouye, 1909) are summarized in the map shown in Fig. 5 which shows the centre of the visual field to be on the posterior part, and the extreme periphery to be at the anterior extremity of the calcarine fissure. In addition, Inouye was able to demonstrate that more cortex is devoted to the representation of the centre of the visual field than to the periphery, and that the field representation extends 5° into the ipsilateral visual field, which accounts for macular sparing in unilateral injuries. Holmes & Lister's (1916) careful analysis of field defects in British soldiers injured in the First World War confirmed the validity of Inouye's conclusion except for the ipsilateral representation which was wrongly interpreted as an artifact. Holmes' map (Fig. 6) shows, in a more immediate display, the representation of the contralateral half-field on the striate cortex. The fovea is represented at the occipital pole, and more peripheral areas of the visual field are progressively represented more anteriorly within the sagittal fissure. The horizontal meridian of each half-field is represented along the depth of the contralateral calcarine sulcus, with the upper quadrant of the field represented in the cortex immediately below, and the lower quadrant immediately above. The upper border of the striate representation is formed by the vertical meridian of the contralateral lower quadrant, and the lower border by the vertical meridian of the contralateral upper quadrant. Although the representation of visual field in non-striate visual areas has not systematically been studied in man, it is likely that it is represented twice in mirror-image fashion in the cortex beyond the upper and lower limits of V1, as demonstrated in cats and monkeys (Halliday & Michael, 1972).

Another important source of information on the visual cortex in man is provided by the analysis of phosphenes elicited by cortical stimulation during surgical operations. The stimulation of the occipital pole has been reported by Löwenstein & Borchardt (1918) to cause a patient to see flickering in the opposite half of the visual field. Cortical electrical phosphenes (bright coloured balls, stars and flames) were discovered in single patients by Krause (1924) and Foerster (1929) to vary systematically with the point stimulated according to Inouye's and Holmes' maps.

Penfield & Rasmussen (1952) and Penfield & Jasper (1954) give general summaries of the visual consequences of stimulating the occipital cortex during neurosurgical operations in about 27 patients. The phosphenes were described as stars, wheels, discs, spots or, occasionally, as streaks or lines. They might be single or multiple for stimulation of a single point. Phosphenes were often said to be moving and often to be coloured red, blue, green, yellow, brown, pink or gold. Colours were more often reported in calcarine phosphenes than in those produced from secondary visual areas. Except for this character the description of phosphenes differs very little between area 17 and secondary areas in all but two patients, with complex visual hallucinations similar to those occurring in their spontaneous epileptic seizures.

A privileged opportunity to examine the properties of cortical electrical phosphenes without the limitations imposed by working during surgical operations was provided by visual prosthetic implants devised by Brindley & Lewin (1968). In two blind patients implanted in 1967 and 1972, Brindley carried out a detailed analysis of cortical electrical phosphenes (Brindley & Lewin, 1968; Brindley, 1973). The implants consisted of arrays of 80 and 76 platinum electrodes, closely apposed, respectively, to the occipital pole and the posterior part of the medial surface of the right hemisphere.

Typically, during a train of short pulses applied through a single electrode, the patient saw a very small flickering spot of white or light yellow described as stars or grains of sago at a fixed position in the left half of the visual field. Position variations from one day to another did not exceed 1° for phosphenes within 10° of the point of regard, and 5° for any phosphenes.

A few electrodes gave phosphenes consisting of two, three or more spots, all with the same threshold. In many other cases a weak stimulus gave a single phosphene, while a stronger stimulus added an additional spot in the opposite quadrant confirming the idea that there may be two maps

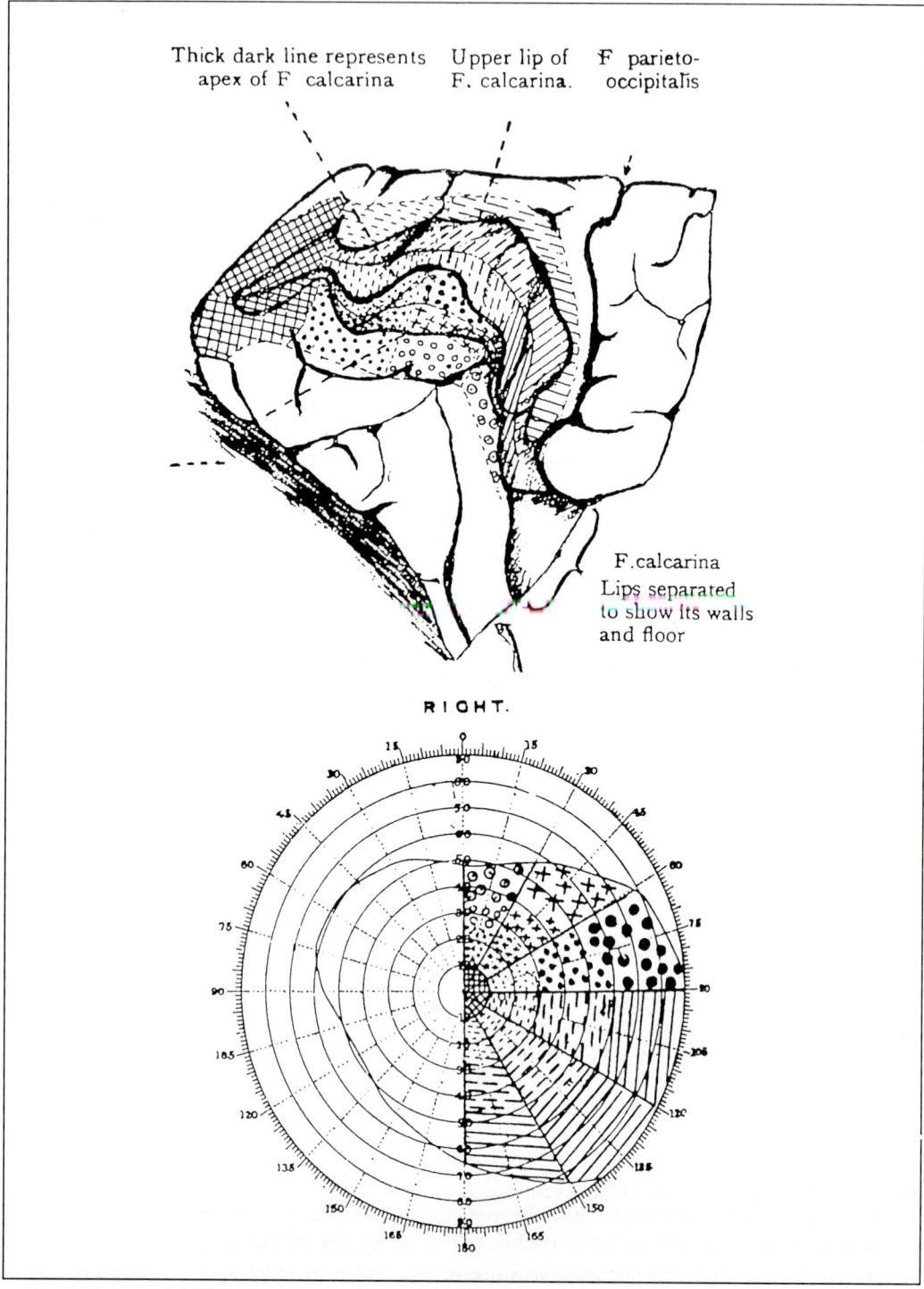

Fig. 6. Holmes' (1918) map of the contralateral half-field on the striate cortex of one hemisphere in man. From Halliday & Michael (1972), with permission.

of visual fields in mirror-image fashion on the occipital cortex. The position of the phosphenes within the visual field was plotted by the patients in a bowl perimeter with the left hand, while they held the fixation knob of the perimeter with the right hand so as to direct the gaze towards it. The map so obtained agreed roughly with the classical maps of Inouye (1909) and Holmes (1918) (Fig. 7).

A very interesting finding was the demonstration that during voluntary eye movements the phosphenes moved with the eyes.

Brindley (1973) was unable to find any difference in phosphene properties between the primary visual area and the surrounding cortex that he felt corresponded to area 18.

Recently, a new promising approach to the analysis of functional location of the human visual cortex has been proposed based on combined use of positron emission tomography (PET) and magnetic resonance imaging (MRI) (Mora *et al.*, 1989). By converting PET measurements of cerebral blood flow in MRI coordinates, Mora *et al.* (1989) succeeded in mapping stimulus-evoked changes with reference to specific striate and extrastriate visual areas.

Relevance of anatomo-functional information to the pathophysiology of occipital seizures and epilepsies

The results summarized above raise a provocative question: is it still appropriate to speak of occipital seizures at all? It is clear, in fact, that the traditional definition of the occipital lobe including three main visual areas does not account for the complexity of visual cortical organization. On one hand, the occipital region has been shown to include several visual subsystems interacting in a very complex way and processing specific visual submodalities. On the other hand, the cortical integration of visual information involves areas lying outside the conventional boundaries of the occipital lobe. It may be replied that similar reservations can also apply to the other cerebral lobes. However, the fact that they are composite entities has indeed been long recognized even with reference to partial seizures arising in their context. It is usual in fact to define a seizure

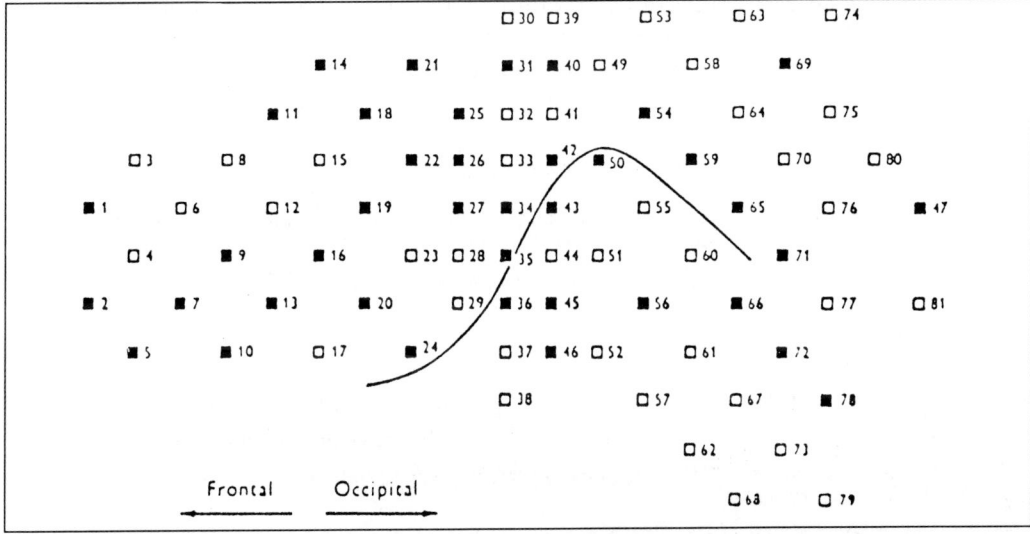

Fig. 7. The arrangement of cortical-stimulating electrodes implanted on a blind patient according to Brindley's technique (see text). The 39 electrodes that have given phosphenes are shown as filled squares. The heavy line shows the conjectured position of the calcarine fissure in relation to the electrodes. From Brindley & Lewin (1968), with permission.

as rolandic or supplementary motor or orbitofrontal, rather than simply frontal; and auditory, olfactory or somatosensory seizures are more suitably defined as such than as temporal or parietal lobe seizures. So, it would be advisable to define the so-called occipital seizures as seizures with visual symptomatology and the so-called occipital epilepsies as epilepsies with visual seizures.

The aim of this chapter is to provide a basis for anatomo-clinical correlations leading to recognition of the site of origin and the way of propagation of epileptogenic discharges responsible for seizures with visual symptomatology. On the grounds of the available information, this is possible only to a very limited extent. Elementary visual hallucinations, such as bright stars or spots, are often reported by patients as early symptoms of partial supposedly occipital seizures. According to the visual cortical map, their location within the visual field may be taken as an indication of the site of origin of the epileptic discharge in the contralateral occipital lobe only if the focus is located in V1. The visuotopic representation is in fact more and more irregular as one moves from V1 to higher order areas. Visual epileptic hallucinations are frequently reported to move, in contrast with Brindley's (1973) observation that electrical visual phosphenes were always fixed and were perceived to move only during ocular movement. It must be noted, however, that the eye deviation which occurs frequently during visual seizures, may readily account for the apparent movement of visual images.

Since complex hallucinations were never elicited by electrical stimulation of V1 and V2 areas (Brindley, 1973), it is generally assumed that their ictal occurrence locates the origin of the discharge in high order visual areas. This assumption must be regarded with caution for two reasons. First of all, the local effect of a very small stimulating electrode may be compared to that of punching a small hole in an opaque screen covering a picture. The observer will only see a small spot, no matter how complex is the scene covered by the screen. Second, if an epileptic discharge arising in V1 or V2 spreads immediately along one of the visual channels, processing specific submodalities (see above), it may instantly result in a very complex hallucination.

The ocular movements which are reported to occur frequently in occipital seizures, such as tonic deviation, clonic jerks, 'epileptic nystagmus', are by no means specific to this (nor to any other) lobe. Oculomotor areas have in fact been described in all cerebral lobes, as may be expected from the important part that they play in every kind of orientation reaction.

More subtle clinical and instrumental tests should be developed to identify specific visual dysfunctions associated with ictal discharges affecting specific visual subsystems.

References

Brindley, G.S. (1973): Sensory effects of electrical stimulation of the visual and paravisual cortex in man. In: *Handbook of sensory physiology*, Vol. VII/3, *Visual centers in the brain*. ed. R. Jung, pp. 583–594. Berlin: Springer-Verlag.

Brindley, G.S. & Lewin, W.S. (1968): The sensations produced by electrical stimulation of the visual cortex. *J. Physiol.* **196**, 479–493.

Brodal, A. (1969): *Neurological anatomy in relation to clinical medicine*. 2nd edition. New York: Oxford University Press.

Brodmann, K. (1909): *Vergleichende Lokalizationslehre der Grosshirnrinde*. Leipzig: J.A. Barth.

Foerster, O. (1929): Beträge zur Pathophysiologie der Sehsphäre. *J. Psychol. Neurol.* (Leipz) **39**, 463–485.

Glickstein, M. & Whitteridge, D. (1987): Tatsuji Inouye and the mapping of the visual fields on the human cerebral cortex. *Trends Neurosci.* **10**, 350–353.

Halliday, A.M. & Michael, W.F. (1972): Pattern-evoked potentials and the cortical representation of the visual field. In: *Neurophysiology studied in man*, ed. G.G. Somjen, pp. 250–259. Amsterdam: Excerpta Medica.

Henschen, S.E. (1890): *Klinische und anatomische Beitrage zur Pathologie des Gehirns* (Pt 1). Uppsala: Almquist and Wiksel.

Holmes, G. (1918): Disturbances of vision by cerebral lesions. *Brit. J. Ophthalmol.* **2**, 353–384.

Holmes, G. & Lister, W.T. (1916): Disturbances of vision from cerebral lesions with special reference to the cortical representation of the macula. *Brain* **39**, 34–73.

Hubel, D.H. & Wiesel, T.N. (1962): Receptive fields, binocular interaction and functional architecture in the cat's visual cortex. *J. Physiol. (Lond.)* **160**, 106–154.

Hubel, D.H. & Wiesel, T.N. (1965): Binocular interaction in striate cortex of kittens reared with artificial squint. *J. Neurophysiol.* **28**, 1041–1059.

Hubel, D.H. & Wiesel, T.N. (1972): Laminar and columnar distribution of geniculo-cortical fibers in the macaque monkey. *J. Comp. Neurol.* **146**, 421–450.

Inouye, T. (1909): *Die Sehstörungen bei Schussverletzungen der kortikalen Sehsphäre nach Beobachtungen an Versundeten der letzten Japanische Kriege.* Leipzig: W. Engelmann.

Krause, F. (1924): Die Sehbahnen in chirurgischer Beziehung und die faradische Reizung des Sehzentrums. *Klin. Wochenschr.* **3**, 1260–1265.

Löwenstein, K. & Borchardt, M. (1918): Symptomatologie und elektrische Reizung bei einer Schußverletzung des Hinterhauptlappens. *Dtsch. Z. Nervenheilk.* **58**, 264–292.

Macchi, G. & Bentivoglio, M. (1982): The organization of the efferent projections of the thalamic intralaminar nuclei: past, present and future of the anatomical approach. *Ital. J. Neurol. Sci.* **2**, 83–96.

Mora, B.N., Carman, G.J. & Allman, J.M. (1989): *In vivo* functional localization of the human visual cortex using positron emission tomography and magnetic resonance imaging. *Trends Neurosci.* **12**, 282–284.

Penfield, W. & Jasper, H. (1954): *Epilepsy and the functional anatomy of the human brain.* Boston: Little Brown and Co.

Penfield, W. & Rasmussen, T. (1952): *The cerebral cortex of man.* New York: Macmillan.

Shepherd, G.M. (1988): *Neurobiology*, 2nd edition. New York: Oxford University Press.

Tigges, J. & Tigges, M. (1985): Subcortical sources of direct projections to visual cortex. In: *Cerebral cortex*, Vol. 3, eds. A. Peters & E.G. Jones, pp. 351–378. New York, London: Plenum Press.

Van Essen, D.C. (1985): Functional organization of primate visual cortex. In: *Cerebral cortex*, Vol. 3, eds. A. Peters & E.G. Jones, pp. 259–329. New York, London: Plenum Press.

Chapter 5

Visual testing in the first 2 years of life

Lieven Lagae and Paul Casaer

Catholic University Leuven, Faculty of Medicine, Department of Paediatrics and Paediatric Neurology; University Hospital Gasthuisberg, Herestraat 49, B-3000 Leuven, Belgium

Summary

This paper reviews some developmental aspects of vision in infants. In visual development, two main questions are addressed: first, is the child able to discriminate different visual stimuli, and second, can it shift its attention to a new visual stimulus? Different modalities of a visual stimulus can be tested for discrimination. Most commonly, acuity ('size discrimination') is measured with age-adapted preferential looking methods. With age, acuity increases almost uniformly, with adult acuity reached between 3 and 4 years. In contrast, the development of orientation discrimination shows a step function around the age of 6 weeks as demonstrated in the VEP studies of Braddick *et al.* (1986). A similar step function was found for other visual modalities like binocularity and colour vision.

The study of eye movements is one approach to studying attention mechanisms in infants. Here too, a step function in the development of different modalities (smooth pursuit, disappearance of asymmetric OKN) around the age of 3 months is a striking finding.

It is argued that these step functions in visual development indicate a reorganization in the visual cortex, with cortical areas starting to inhibit subcortical centres. Interestingly, this coincides with the appearance of the visual smile around the age of 6 to 10 weeks.

Introduction

The assessment of visual functions in infants is an important part of the clinical neurological examination, not only to evaluate vision and to prevent visual deficits but also to test sensory information processing in the brain in general. Indeed, human behaviour is often based on the analysis of visual information, stored in the memory or present in the outside world.

Various research lines have examined the visual development: behavioural and clinical studies, electrophysiology and neuro-imaging, including PET-scan nowadays. The majority of these studies focus on two important aspects of visual behaviour: first, is the child able to discriminate and second, can it shift its attention to a new visual stimulus? In general, discrimination implies that a behavioural or electrophysiological response is elicited when a visual stimulus is presented. For instance, a 2-month-old infant is able to discriminate a drawing of a regular human face from a scrambled version of the same pattern: it will preferentially look at the normal face (Maurer & Barrera, 1982). This indicates that the content of the visual stimulus (size, spatial frequency, contrast, wavelength etc.) is – in some way, and perhaps not at the perceptual level yet – analysed in the brain. For any visual stimulus, different modalities can be defined: size, spatial frequency, contrast, colour, rigidity, position, direction and speed of motion. In primates, neurophysiological and anatomical studies have shown different visual areas in the occipital pole, giving rise to two major information streams, both starting in the primary visual cortex or V1 (De Yoe & Van Essen, 1988; Mishkin *et al.*, 1983). The ventral stream leads to the inferotemporal cortex and is involved in the analysis of object identification (size, colour etc.). The dorsal stream leads to the posterior parietal cortex and is mainly involved in the analysis of object localization (position, disparity, motion). These two streams with different specialized visual areas are now also being recognized in humans (Zeki *et al.*, 1991). Therefore, testing the discrimination of different modalities is one approach to examine different processing streams in the visual cortex.

Shifting attention from one stimulus to another usually implies an eye movement to that new stimulus in order to fixate it (overt attention). In this respect, the study of eye movements in infants indirectly assesses attention mechanisms. Another limiting factor for attention mechanisms is the development of the visual field extent. Recent PET-scan studies in humans have shown at least three attention centres in the brain: a posterior parietal system is involved in directing attention to a new stimulus, while an anterior (cingulate) system makes a selection between different new stimuli. Another system is a 'general alertness' system, located in the right hemisphere (Posner, 1990; Corbetta *et al.*, 1990). Again, different testing strategies in the assessment of attention can uncover the activity of different brain areas.

These – mostly experimental – data have made it clear that the visual assessment in infants should not be restricted to an acuity measurement; other important visual functions like colour vision, binocular vision, orientation discrimination, motion perception, should also be examined in order to get a more complete view on visual functioning. In the next paragraphs, we will review some important developmental aspects in the assessment of these different visual functions.

Acuity measurement

Acuity measurement is a key test in the assessment of spatial vision. In general, acuity reflects the smallest stimulus (size) that still can be discriminated from another stimulus. Other stimulus-related properties like contrast and colour will also influence the acuity measurement. Therefore, stimuli have been standardized and are well known as optotypes (for instance Snellen optotype E). However, testing acuity with optotypes can only be done in older, verbal, children. In infants, other techniques have been introduced such as the preferential looking test (Dobson *et al.*, 1978). This latter test is based on the innate behaviour of infants to preferentially fixate a patterned stimulus (Fantz, 1958). In this test, the child is confronted with two simultaneously presented stimuli, a homogeneous non-patterned stimulus and a patterned stimulus. The patterned stimulus usually is a grating, consisting of alternating light and dark stripes. If the spatial frequency of the patterned stimulus is low enough, that is if the width of the stripes is large enough, the child will preferentially look at the patterned stimulus. The pattern with the highest spatial frequency that still can elicit preferential looking gives an estimate of acuity. This test has been standardized and is commercially available ('acuity cards'). Testing acuity in this way takes about 10 to 15 min. It is important to realize that preferential looking is based on a visuomotor response: an independent observer, hidden behind the screen on which the stimuli are presented and unaware of the position of the patterned stimulus, has to judge, observing the visuomotor responses of the infant (eye movements, head and trunk turning) on what side the patterned stimulus is presented. When his judgement is correct in a majority of presentations, then it is concluded that the child can discriminate the presented grating. In older children, operant techniques are necessary to keep the attention of the child.

Different research groups have shown that preferential looking is a reliable tool to measure acuity. With age, acuity increases almost uniformly at a rate of about 0.75 to 1 cycle/deg per month. Adult acuity (on average 30 cycles/deg. corresponding to a Snellen E optotype of 0.9 cm in overall height at 6 m) is reached between the third and the fourth year of life.

The spatial vision function can be fully characterized by the contrast sensitivity curve. This gives the contrast sensitivity for each spatial frequency and can be constructed by measuring (with for instance the preferential looking paradigm) the minimum contrast that is needed for each spatial frequency to elicit a preferential looking response. Typically, in adults, this gives an upside-down 'U' curve, with the maximum sensitivity between 1 and 10 cycles/deg. This means that for these optimum spatial frequencies, less contrast is needed for the preferential looking response than for higher or lower spatial frequencies. The highest spatial frequency that still can be detected, although a high contrast is needed, refers to the acuity. In infants and children, three major differences in the contrast sensitivity curves are observed (Atkinson et al., 1977; Wilson, 1988): (1) the higher upper cut-off (acuity) is lower; (2) overall sensitivity is lower; and (3) there is no lower cut-off. This latter difference indicates that, in infants, less contrast is needed than in older children and adults to detect the lower spatial frequency range. Different physiological mechanisms underlie these developmental changes. At the retinal level, it has been shown that the inward foveal migration of cones, together with the growth of the foveal cone outer segment and the decrease of the cone diameter can explain the acuity and sensitivity increase with age (Yuodelis & Hendrickson, 1986). However, the lower acuities in infants should not be reduced to a pure retinal bottle-neck. For instance, the appearance of the lower cut-off in older children is probably caused by a cortical inhibitory mechanism. The excessive proliferation of inhibitory GABA receptors in the visual cortex during the first years of life can underlie this inhibition (Huttenlocher & de Courten, 1987).

Acuity can also be measured with visual evoked potentials (VEP), although this approach is not commonly used in clinical practice. It requires less cooperation from the infant, but fixation of the stimulus is still needed. Steady state evoked potentials are elicited with a patterned stimulus (most commonly a checkerboard), appearing and disappearing at a fixed temporal frequency. This stimulation will give rise to a sinusoidal evoked response following the temporal stimulation frequency. The amplitude of the response is positively correlated with the check size (= spatial frequency): the larger the checks, the larger the response amplitude. The checkerboard with the smallest checks that still gives a substantial response can be used as a measurement of acuity (Marg et al., 1976; Sokol & Dobson, 1976).

In the majority of the studies, VEP acuity shows a more rapid developmental course than preferential looking acuity. Part of this discrepancy can be explained by methodological and statistical differences, but it is clear that the two methods also test different neural functions. With VEPs, only pure sensory information processing is tested, while in preferential looking, a behavioural response is required in addition.

Orientation discrimination

It has been shown in numerous animal studies that orientation selectivity is a pure cortical property (Hubel & Wiesel, 1977). The activity (measured as action potentials/s) of a cortical visual cell will change with the orientation of the visual stimulus. In subcortical areas, orientation differences will not influence the cellular response. Therefore, testing orientation discrimination is a direct approach to examine (visual) cortical activity. However, only a few experimental studies have been devoted to orientation discrimination in infants and no 'easy', standardized test has been introduced in clinical practice yet.

Interestingly, orientation discrimination shows a completely different developmental course than acuity. Maurer & Martello showed in a habituation paradigm study that 5- to 6-week-old infants are able to discriminate orientation. After habituation to a familiar stimulus orientation, 5- to 6-week-old infants will fixate a novel orientation for a significantly longer time. This indicates orientation processing and thus cortical processing (Maurer & Martello, 1980). This has been confirmed in a longitudinal VEP study by Braddick *et al.* (1986). Their stimulus consisted of a grating pattern that changed its orientation at a fixed temporal frequency. A VEP response that is time-locked to the orientation change indicates a cortical response specific to the orientation change. This study showed that such an orientation response could only be obtained in infants older than 5 to 6 weeks. It thus appears that there is a step function in the development of orientation discrimination. A possible explanation is that the cortical visual areas start to dominate (= inhibit) subcortical brain centres (Atkinson, 1984). In agreement with this hypothesis, the visual behaviour of monkeys in which the visual cortex has been removed resembles in many respects the behaviour of infant monkeys (Humphrey, 1974).

A similar developmental step function has been found for several other visual functions. For instance, binocular vision can be tested with a pair of stereograms, in which a disparity signal is built in. This gives rise to a depth perception in trained subjects. From 3 months on, this disparity signal can be shown on evoked potential recordings, indicating disparity processing (Braddick & Atkinson, 1983). However, depth perception is only observable from 5 months on: it underlies the reaching behaviour and the avoidance responses observed at that age.

Attention

Attention should be considered as a selection mechanism: it selects which particular stimulus in the rich visual environment will be chosen for further processing. For the visual system, paying attention commonly involves an eye movement towards this stimulus in order to fixate it (overt attention). Fixation makes a much more detailed analysis of the stimulus possible; for instance, acuity and colour vision are best developed in the fovea and its projection streams.

In agreement with other visual functions, the development of eye movements shows a turning point around the age of 2 to 3 months. Before that age, the infant can fixate over an accommodation range of 20 to 75 cm and is able to catch a peripheral visual stimulus by a series of hypometric saccades and small head movements. Eye scanning studies showed that for large objects, the border of the object was especially fixated (externality effect; Maurer & Salapatek, 1976). Beyond the age of 3 months, smooth pursuit eye movements can be elicited for the first time; the externality effect disappears and there is less influence of other sensory stimuli in the generation of eye movements.

Eliciting the optokinetic nystagmus reflex still remains an elegant way to study eye movements in infants, especially when combined with electro-oculography. The optokinetic nystagmus (OKN) can be induced by any global pattern and consists of the two major eye movements types: a slow smooth pursuit phase, and a rapid saccadic phase. It is a reflex that serves to stabilize the image on the fovea. When tested binocularly in infants, the OKN is symmetric, i.e. moving the stimulus temporonasal or nasotemporal will induce a similar response. However, when tested monocularly, there exists a clear asymmetry in infants below the age of 3 months: temporonasal motion will induce a larger response than nasotemporal motion. This asymmetry disappears around the age of 3 months. A well-developed binocular visual cortical pathway is needed for a response to nasotemporal motion (Atkinson & Braddick, 1981). As already illustrated above, binocularity develops around the age of 3 months, thus explaining the asymmetry in the OKN before that age.

The other limiting factor for the attention mechanism is the extent of the visual field. Mohn & Van Hof-van Duin (1986) studied the development of the visual field in infants by means of kinetic perimetry. The extent of the visual field was estimated using a behavioural (visuomotor) response to an approaching stimulus. They showed that there is a gradual increase of the visual field in all directions. Since the peripheral retina appears to be mature at birth, the increase must be due to (sub)cortical mechanisms. They hypothesize that an increase in the connectivity between different visual areas is a possible determining factor in the development of the visual field. Confirming previous examples, the development of the binocular visual field showed a rapid increase beyond the age of 2 to 3 months.

Conclusions

As illustrated in this paper, the development of many visual functions (orientation, binocularity, smooth pursuit, but also colour, motion, perceptual constancy) shows a 'step function' around the age of 2 to 3 months. There is experimental evidence that at that time cortical functioning becomes apparent (see 'Orientation discrimination'), probably with the inhibition of lower subcortical areas and increased connectivity between cortical visual areas. Interestingly, this coincides with the appearance of the visual smile at the age of 6 to 10 weeks. Therefore, the appearance of the visual smile in infants represents an important developmental milestone. Indeed, the incidence of delayed visual maturation (late appearance of the visual smile) is higher in infants with a suboptimal neurological condition (birth asphyxia, intraventricular haemorrhage). Moreover, infants in which delayed visual maturation is the only symptom often show neurological abnormalities like epilepsy and learning disorders in later years (Casaer & Lagae, 1991).

Different new clinical tests have become available to assess the visual functions in infants. It is now possible to get a more complete view of the visual capacities of an infant. It is logical that testing a variety of visual functions will increase the sensitivity of the assessment. Undoubtedly, this will lead to a more detailed description of more subtle deficits in visual functioning and brain functioning in general.

References

Atkinson, J. (1984): Human visual development over the first 6 months of life: a review and a hypothesis. *Hum. Neurobiol.* **3**, 61–74.

Atkinson, J. & Braddick, O. (1981): Development of optokinetic nystagmus in infants: an indicator of cortical binocularity? In: *Eye movements: cognition and visual perception*, eds. D.F. Fisher, R.A. Monty & J.W. Senders, pp. 53–64. Hillsdale, New Jersey: Lawrence Erlbaum.

Atkinson, J., Braddick, O. & Moar, K. (1977): Development of contrast sensitivity over the first 3 months of life in the human infant. *Vision Res.* **17**, 1037–1044.

Braddick, O. & Atkinson, J. (1983): Some recent findings on the development of binocularity: a review. *Behav. Brain Res.* **10**, 133–141.

Braddick, O.J., Wattan-Bell, J. & Atkinson, J. (1986): Orientation-specific cortical responses develop in early infancy. *Nature* **320**, 617–619.

Casaer, P. & Lagae, L. (1991): Age-specific approach to neurological assessment in the first year of life. *Acta Paed. Jpn.* **33**, 125–138.

Corbetta, M., Miezin, F.M., Dobmeyer, S., Shulman, G.L. & Petersen, S.E. (1990): Attentional modulation of neural processing of shape, colour and velocity in humans. *Science* **248**, 1556–1559.

De Yoe, E.A. & Van Essen, D.C. (1988): Concurrent processing streams in monkey visual cortex. *Trends Neurosci.* **11**, 219–226.

Dobson, V., Teller, D.Y. & Lee, C.J. (1978): A behavioural method for efficient screening of visual acuity in young infants: I. Preliminary laboratory development. *Invest. Ophthalmol. Vis. Sci.* **17**, 1142–1150.

Fantz, R.L. (1958): Pattern vision in young infants. *Psychol. Rev.* **8**, 43–47.

Hubel, D.H. & Wiesel, T.N. (1977): Functional architecture of macaque monkey visual cortex. *Proc. R. Soc. Lond. (Biol.)* **198**, 1–59.

Humphrey, N.K. (1974): Vision in a monkey without striate cortex: a case study. *Perception* **3**, 324–337.

Huttenlocher, P.R. & de Courten, C. (1987): The development of synapses in striate cortex in man. *Hum. Neurobiol.* **6**, 1–9.

Marg, E., Freeman, D.N., Peltzman, P. et al. (1976): Visual acuity development in human infants: evoked potential measurements. *Invest. Ophthalmol. Vis. Sci.* **15**, 150–153.

Maurer, D. & Salapatek, P. (1976): Developmental changes in the scanning of faces by young infants. *Child Develop.* **47**, 523–527.

Maurer, D. & Martello, M. (1980): The discrimination of orientation by young infants. *Vision Res.* **20**, 201–204.

Maurer, D. & Barrera, M.E. (1982): Infants' perception of natural and distorted arrangements of a schematic face. *Child Develop.* **52**, 196–202.

Mishkin, M., Ungerleider, L.G. & Macko, K.A. (1983): Object vision and spatial vision: two cortical pathways. *Trends Neurosci.* **6**, 414–417.

Mohn, G. & Van Hof-van Duin, J. (1986): Development of the binocular and monocular visual fields during the first year of life. *Clin. Vision Sci.* **1**, 51–64.

Posner, M.I. (1990): The attention system of the human brain. *Annu. Rev. Neurosci.* **13**, 25–42.

Sokol, S. & Dobson, V. (1976): Pattern reversal visually evoked potentials in infants. *Invest. Ophthalmol. Vis. Sci.* **15**, 58–62.

Wilson, H.R. (1988): Development of spatiotemporal mechanisms in infant vision. *Vision Res.* **28**, 611–628.

Yuodelis, C. & Hendrickson A. (1986): A qualitative and quantitative analysis of the human fovea during development. *Vision Res.* **26**, 847–855.

Zeki, S., Watson, J.D.G., Lueck, C.J., Friston, K.J., Kennard, C. & Frackowiak, R.S.J. (1991): A direct demonstration of functional specialization in human visual cortex. *J. Neurosci.* **11**, 641–649.

Chapter 6

Neurophysiological examinations of visual function in the development of the infant

Samuel Sokol

New England Eye Center Box 820, Tufts University School of Medicine, New England Medical Center, 750 Washington Street, Boston, MA 02111, USA

Summary

A number of different methods have been used to study the development of visual function in human infants. These include optokinetic nystagmus (OKN), preferential looking (PL) and the pattern visually evoked cortical potential (VEP), an electrophysiological technique.

Two parameters of the pattern VEP have been used to monitor visual development: amplitude and latency. Studies of the development of infant VEP acuity, based on amplitude measures, have shown that the newborn infant's acuity is between 20/200 and 20/400 Snellen. By 6 months of age, VEP acuity has reached adult levels and is in the range of 20/20–20/40 Snellen. In contrast to the amplitude measures of acuity, studies of the VEP using the peak latency have shown that the visual pathways continue to develop up to 5 years of age, particularly when VEPs are elicited by small checkerboard pattern stimuli.

The development of lateral inhibitory interactions in the infant visual system as reflected by the visual evoked potential amplitude has been studied using a radial, asymmetrical windmill-dartboard stimulus. These studies have shown that the long-range lateral interactions (large receptive fields) are adult-like by 2 months of age while the short range lateral interactions (small receptive fields) are not adult-like until 5–6 months of age. In contrast, corresponding phase data indicated significant immaturities at 5–6 months of age for both the large and small receptive fields.

Thus, both VEP amplitude and latency can be used to monitor infant visual development. However, each component reflects a different developmental time course.

Introduction

Several different evoked potential methodologies have been used to study visual development in infants. One method, used primarily with flash stimuli, follows specific changes in VEP morphology, amplitude, peak latency or phase and has little relationship to the development of pattern vision. Studies using this method will not be discussed here but reviews of the results can be found in Ellingson (1967, 1970), Maurer (1975) and Kurtzberg & Vaughan (1985). A second methodology, using pattern stimuli, monitors suprathreshold changes in the waveform morphology, amplitude or latency of the VEP as an index of the visual maturation (Sokol & Jones, 1979; Moskowitz & Sokol, 1983; Spekreijse, 1978, 1983). A third approach uses VEP amplitude as a

49

threshold estimate (Sokol, 1978; Pirchio *et al.*, 1978; Sokol, 1982; Norcia & Tyler, 1985a; Sokol *et al.*, 1988). This method assumes a relationship between the electrical activity of the visual cortex and behaviour, an assumption that is supported by data obtained from adults (Campbell & Maffei, 1970). The purpose of this chapter will be to provide a brief overview of the developmental data obtained with these methodologies. More detailed reviews can be found in Sokol (1990a, b).

Suprathreshold spatial vision

Amplitude-response functions

The suprathreshold development of spatial vision in infants and young children has been followed by determining the check size which produces the largest VEP amplitude (Harter & Suitt, 1970; Sokol & Dobson, 1976; Harter *et al.*, 1977; Sokol, 1978; Spekreijse, 1978; DeVries-Khoe & Spekreijse, 1982). Harter *et al.* (1977) using stationary patterns, back illuminated with a photo-stimulator, found that young infants (1–4 weeks) showed the largest amplitude response for checks between 16 and 24 minutes of arc which disappeared by 6 weeks; the largest response was then obtained for 50 minutes of arc checks and then shifted to smaller check sizes, reaching adult levels (20 minutes of arc) by 6 months.

Sokol & Dobson (1976) and Sokol (1978), using pattern reversal stimuli and Spekreijse (1978) and DeVries-Khoe & Spekreijse (1982) using on-off stimuli found that the largest amplitude signal was

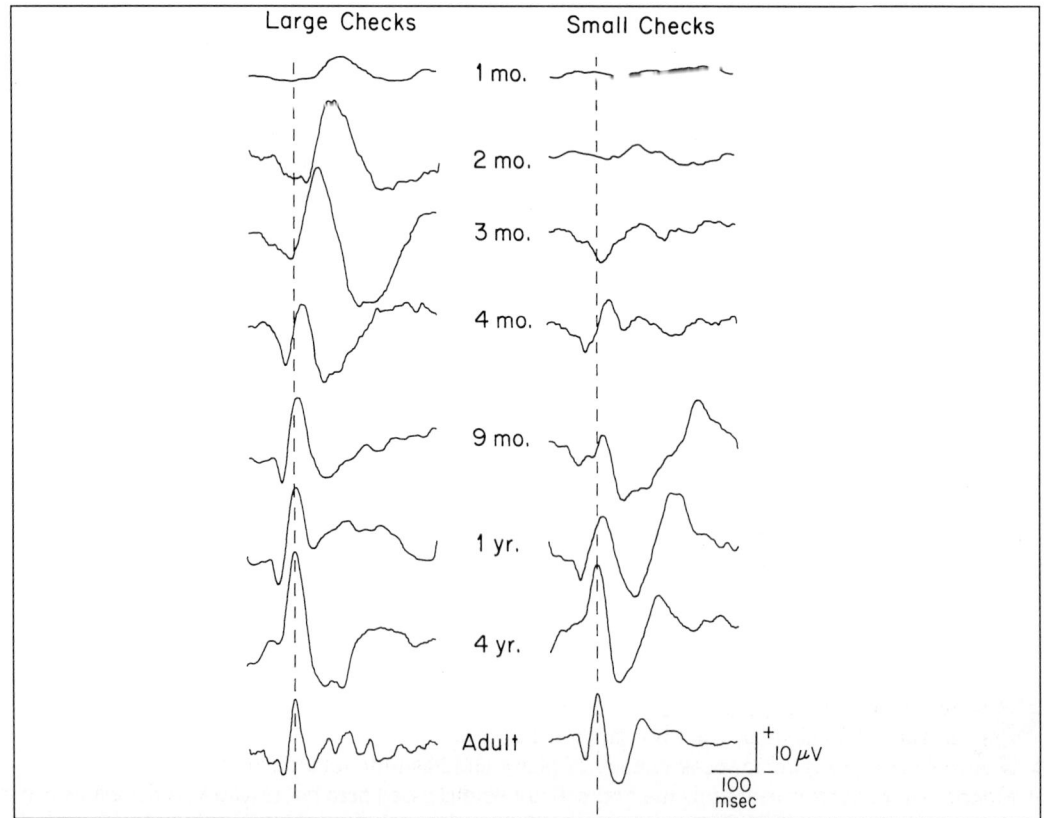

Fig. 1. Pattern-reversal transient VEPs obtained from visually normal infants, children, and an adult in response to large (60 minute of arc) and small (15 minute of arc) checks (Moskowitz & Sokol, 1983).

obtained with 30–40 minute of arc checks for 2–3 month-old infants. By 6 months of age the largest amplitude signal was obtained with 10–20 minute of arc checks which is the same check size that elicits the largest response in adults.

Changes in waveform morphology and latency

Instead of measuring the amplitude of the VEP, Sokol & Jones (1979) and Moskowitz & Sokol (1983) monitored changes in waveform morphology and peak latency in over 400 infants and children. Figure 1 shows representative VEP waveforms from individual infants of several different ages, ranging from 1 month to 4 years, and from an adult in response to large (60 minute of arc) and small (15 minute of arc) checks.

The adult responses for both large and small checks show an initial negative component at 85 to 95 ms (N1) and a prominent positive component at 100 to 120 ms (P1). The adult response to small checks also shows a second negative component at 140 to 160 ms (N2) and a second positive component (P2) at approximately 200 ms. The records obtained from infants and young children show that the latency of all components of the pattern-reversal VEP, and most notably P1, decreases with increasing age. At 1 month of age, the VEP to large checks has a simpler wave form than that in an adult, consisting of only a slowly rising positive wave (P1). No measurable response is obtained for small checks. At 2 months, the larger positive wave in response to large checks is

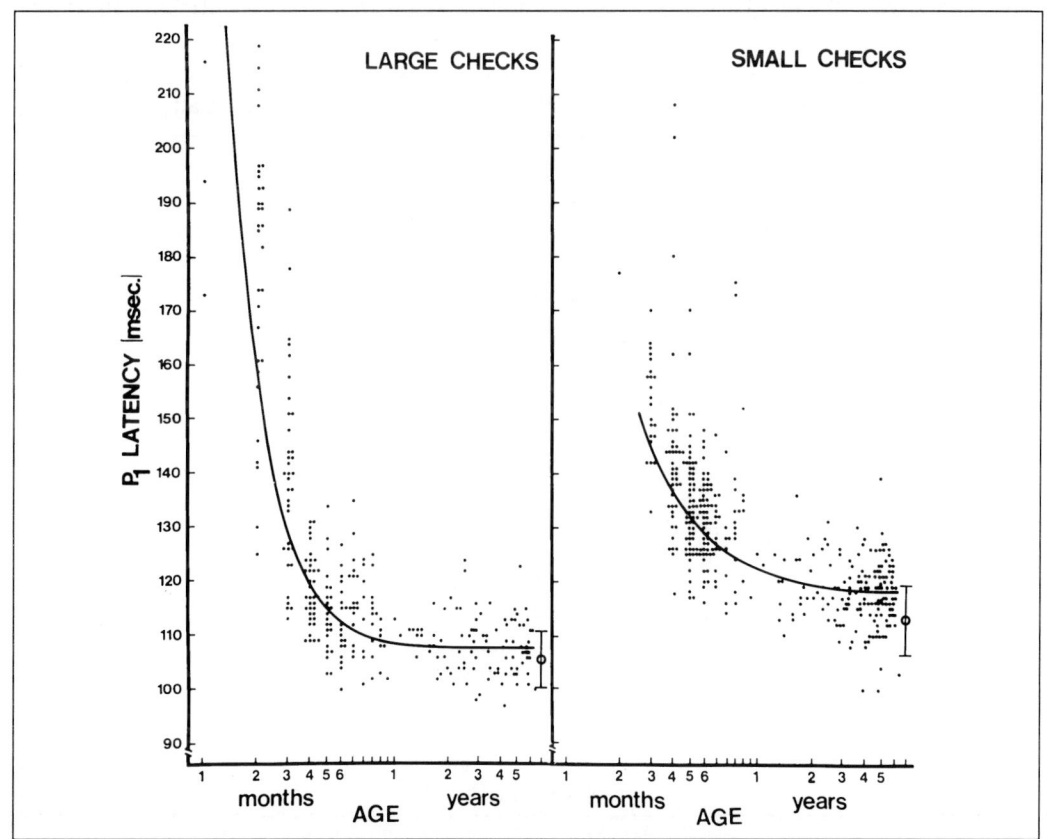

Fig. 2. P_1 latency as a function of log age for large checks (48 and 60 minutes of arc, left) and small checks (12 and 15 minutes of arc, right). Open circles show the mean adult latency ± 1 s.d. Hyperbolic curves were fit to the data by the procedure of least squares (Moskowitz & Sokol, 1983).

preceded and followed by negative potentials (N1 and N2), and P1 has appeared in response to small checks. At 3 months, a late positive wave has emerged in the response to large checks; between 9 months and 4 years, the latency of this late positive component in response to small checks shortens dramatically. By 4 years of age, the VEP is very similar to that obtained from adults.

Thus with increasing age there is an increase in the complexity of the VEP waveform and a shortening of latency. As seen in Fig. 2 this temporal evolution proceeds at a faster rate for VEPs elicited by large checks than by small checks. It is important to keep this differential rate of change as a function of check size in mind when using latency as a clinical parameter of visual development.

Threshold spatial vision: acuity

Direct methods of monitoring acuity development in infants are based on a variant of an extrapolation technique introduced by Campbell & Maffei (1970). They found good agreement in adult subjects between psychophysical contrast threshold and VEP contrast threshold using a 0 μV criterion. This principle has been used to estimate visual acuity in infants by extrapolating the peak of the transient or steady state VEP response function to 0 μV (Sokol, 1978; Norcia & Tyler, 1985a, b) or by estimating the highest spatial frequency grating that produces an identifiable VEP (Marg et al. 1976).

Figure 3 summarizes the development of VEP acuity as reported by various investigators. VEP acuity increases linearly during the first 6 months of age and more slowly thereafter. Marg et al.

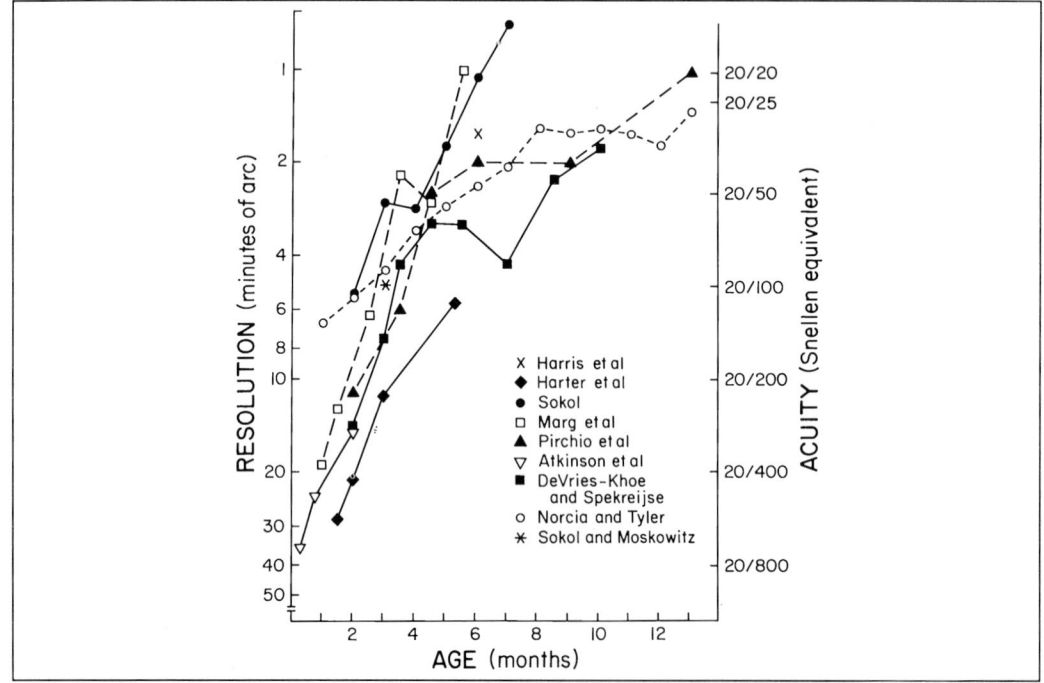

Fig. 3. Acuity development measured with the visually evoked potential. The acuity data from Sokol (1978), Harter & Suitt (1970) and DeVries-Khoe & Spekreijse (1982) have been corrected to account for the fact that the fundamental frequency of a checkerboard stimulus is higher than the fundamental frequency of a grating by a factor of 1.4 (Sokol et al., 1988).

(1976) and Sokol (1978) found adult-like acuity between 5 and 6 months of age, while DeVries-Khoe & Spekreijse (1982) and Norcia & Tyler (1985a) found that it occurs later.

Development of lateral interaction in the infant visual system

The human visual system comprises lateral and direct pathways which carry inhibitory and excitatory information respectively (Ratliff, 1965; Schiller, 1986). The lateral inhibitory mechanisms have been studied in adults using VEP recordings obtained with a radial 'windmill-dartboard' stimulus (Zemon & Ratliff, 1982; Ratliff, 1982). The windmill-dartboard stimulus is a radial pattern comprising concentric contrast reversing zones with contiguous static zones (see Fig. 4, right). Temporal contrast-reversal of only some of the spatial regions in the pattern, while keeping contrast in the remaining regions static, results in an asymmetrical stimulus. The asymmetry occurs during one cycle of contrast-reversal, when the perception of the stimulus changes from that of a windmill to a dartboard. Because of the asymmetry of the windmill-dartboard stimulus, sinusoidal modulation of the pattern produces two distinct processes: a strong intermodulation response at the fundamental frequency and an attenuation of the normally dominant component at twice the stimulus

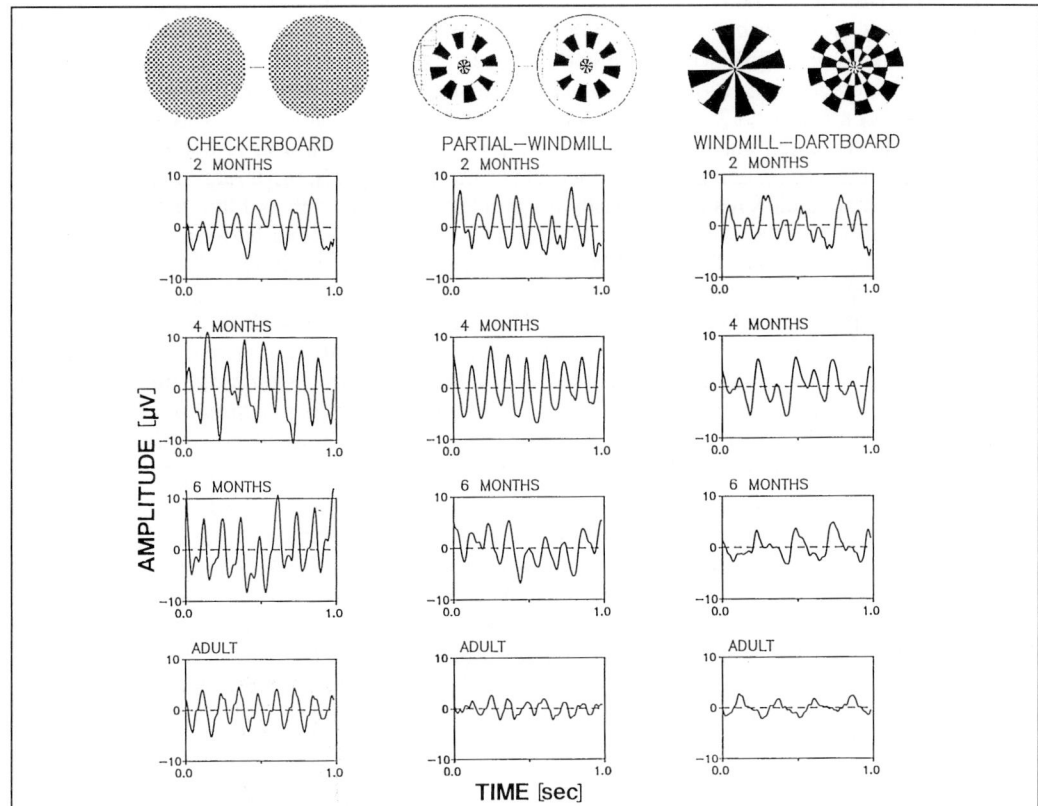

Fig. 4. VEP waveforms from 2-, 4- and 6-month-old infants and an adult obtained with checkerboard, partial windmill, and windmill-dartboard stimuli at 100 per cent contrast. The contrast of the dynamic regions of the asymmetric windmill-dartboard stimuli and the contrast of the symmetric partial windmill and checkerboard stimuli were reversed sinusoidally at 4 Hz. The responses were averaged over a 1 s period. A waveform of 4 cycles indicates a dominant fundamental component; a waveform of 8 cycles indicates a dominant second harmonic component (Sokol et al., 1992).

frequency (Zemon & Ratliff, 1982; Ratliff & Zemon, 1982). On the other hand, contrast reversal of a partial windmill stimulus (Fig. 4, middle) as well as checkerboard and grating stimuli, (Fig. 4, left) produces only a major component at twice the frequency of the modulation.

There are several lines of evidence in adults demonstrating that the generation of the fundamental component and attenuation of the second harmonic component reflect independent processes. First, when the contrast of the static regions of the stimulus is increased and the contrast of the dynamic regions is held constant at 30 per cent, the amplitude of the fundamental response increases and then decreases beyond 30 per cent contrast while the amplitude of the second harmonic decreases monotonically with increasing static contrast (Zemon & Ratliff, 1982). Second, patients with seizure disorders, who are thought to have deficits in GABA (γ-aminobutyric acid) mediated inhibition, have abnormalities of only the fundamental component (Ratliff & Zemon, 1982; Zemon et al., 1986). Finally, the amplitudes of the two components vary independently as a function of the separation of the static and dynamic zones of the stimulus patterns; the amplitude of the fundamental component decreases sharply with increasing spatial separation while the amplitude of the second harmonic increases gradually. This piece of evidence further suggests that the fundamental component reflects short-range processes, whereas attenuation of the second harmonic component reflects long-range processes.

In a recent study Sokol et al. (1992) monitored the development of these short- and long-range lateral mechanisms in a group of 42 infants between 2 and 6 months of age. Figure 4 shows representative averaged waveforms (sweep duration of 1 s) obtained with the three types of stimuli at 100 per cent contrast for a 2-, 4- and 6-month-old infant and one adult. A waveform of 4 cycles per second indicates a dominant fundamental component and a waveform of 8 cycles indicates a dominant second harmonic component. Under all stimulus conditions, the infants' VEP amplitudes were larger than the adult's responses. Also, as expected, both the adult and the infants' responses to checkerboard and partial windmill stimuli exhibit a dominant second harmonic component (8 Hz). In contrast, inspection of the adult's responses to the windmill-dartboard stimulus show a dominant fundamental component, while the 2-month-old infant's responses suggest a relatively equal contribution from fundamental and second harmonic components. With increasing age, the infant's responses show a systematic shift to a dominant first harmonic response so that by 6 months the infant's response, like the adults, consists of four cycles. The 6-month-old infant's and the adult's second harmonic responses elicited by the windmill-dartboard stimulus are attenuated relative to corresponding responses elicited by the partial windmill stimulus. Comparison of the windmill-dartboard responses of the 6-month-old infant and the adult shows a large phase shift.

Figure 5 (top) shows the magnitude of second harmonic attenuation, which reflects the strength of the long-range lateral interaction, expressed as the ratio of the amplitude of the 8 Hz component measured under the windmill-dartboard condition to the amplitude of the 8 Hz component measured under the partial windmill condition. Nearly all the ratios are less than one, indicating that the second harmonic attenuation effect is present in infants of all ages tested. Also, the ratios are relatively constant over this age range and similar to those of the adults, suggesting that for high contrast stimuli the strength of the long-range lateral interaction is fully developed at 8 weeks of age. Figure 5 (bottom) shows the phase of the 8 Hz components measured under the windmill-dartboard condition. The phase plots show a rapid lead up to 15 weeks of age followed by a relatively constant phase up to 26 weeks. The phase differences between the 25-week-old infants and the adults were significant ($t = 3.415$, $P < 0.005$).

Figure 6 (top) shows the strength of the short-range lateral interaction as a function of age as measured by the amplitude of the first harmonic response to the windmill-dartboard stimulus. Our primary interest in analysing these data was to compare the relative amounts of fundamental and attenuated second harmonic response components both within and between infant and adult subjects. Since infants generate larger amplitude responses than adults and their data is more variable, comparison of absolute amplitudes is not possible. In order to normalize the data, an amplitude ratio was calculated for each subject by subtracting the amplitude of the 8 Hz component from that of the 4 Hz component and dividing the difference by the larger of the two amplitudes. This transforms all the data to a scale of –1 to +1. A value of +1.0 indicates that the VEP signal contains only 4 Hz activity; a –1.0 indicates that the VEP signal contains only 8 Hz activity, and a ratio of 0 indicates equal amounts of activity at 4 and 8 Hz. The amplitude ratios for adults range from slightly less than 0 to 0.7, indicating larger amplitudes for the fundamental (4 Hz) than the second harmonic (8 Hz) component. Nearly half of the infants between 6 and 20 weeks had ratio values within the adult range. The amplitude ratios of the remaining half were less than 0, indicating larger amplitudes for the second harmonic than the fundamental component. By 20 weeks, amplitude ratios were consistently greater than 0 in all infants tested and in some cases were even larger than the adults.

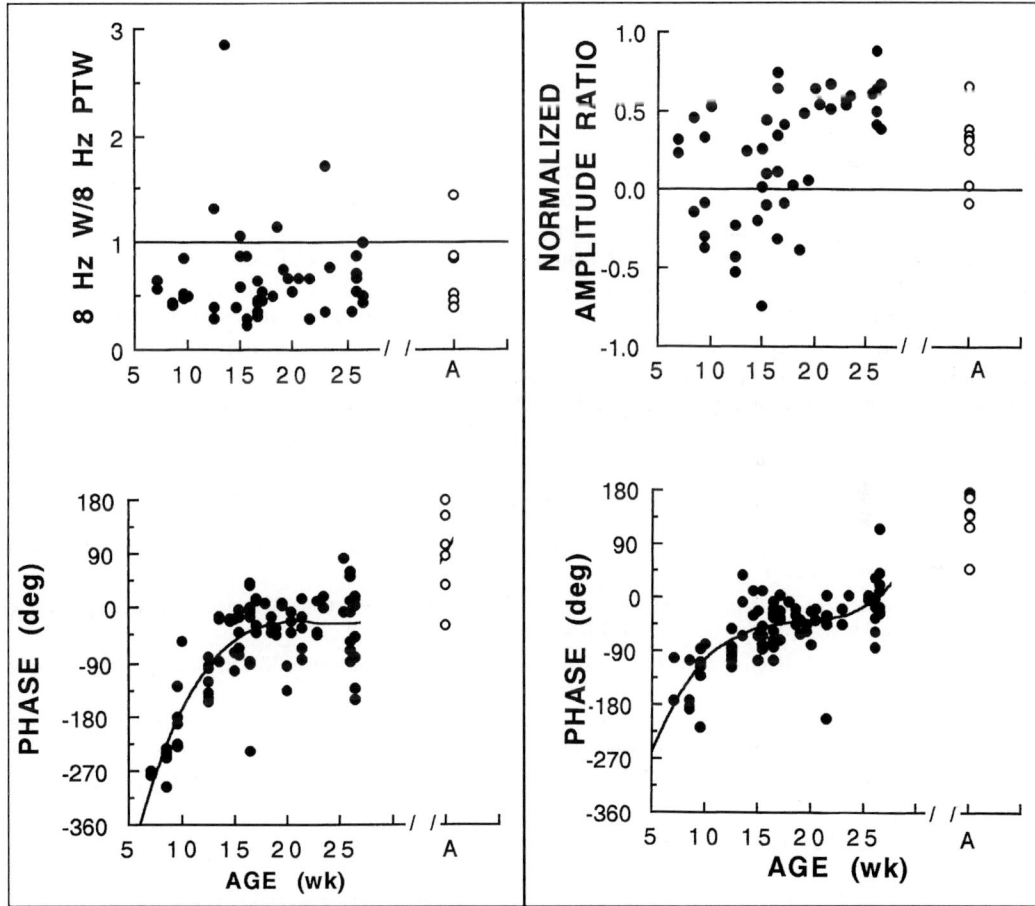

Fig. 5. (Top) Ratio of the amplitude of the 8 Hz component obtained with a windmill-dartboard stimulus and the amplitude of the 8 Hz component obtained with a partial windmill stimulus as a function of age; closed circles: infants; open circles: adults. (Bottom): phase of the 8 Hz component of the windmill-dartboard VEP as a function of age (Sokol et al., 1992).

Fig. 6. (Top) The normalized amplitude ratio of the 4 and 8 Hz components of the VEP obtained with a windmill-dartboard stimulus. A value of +1.0 indicates that the VEP signal contains only 4 Hz activity; a –1.0 indicates that the VEP signal contains 8 Hz, and 0 indicates equal amounts of activity at 4 and 8 Hz. (Bottom): Phase of the 4 Hz component of the windmill-dartboard VEP as a function of age (Sokol et al., 1992).

Figure 6 (bottom) shows the phase of the fundamental component of VEPs as a function of age for the windmill-dartboard stimuli. The 4 Hz phase data initially starts at $-180°$, advances dramatically between 7 and 20 weeks of age and is constant after 20 weeks. Adult phase is different from the 25-week-old infants' phase ($t = 7.119$, $P < 0.001$) demonstrating continuing immaturity in the visual system of infants as old as 6 months.

These data are compatible with a concept of different receptive field sizes of the mechanisms involved in generating the fundamental (Fig. 6) and attenuated second harmonic (Fig. 5).

For example, small receptive fields would be sensitive to small gaps between the dynamic and static regions which might be involved in generating fundamental short-range processes. Larger receptive fields, unaffected by small gaps, might underlie the attenuation of the second harmonic. This would explain why the long-range processes are present from an early age and are reflected in the low acuity of younger infants while the short-range processes may emerge later.

Lateral interactions in epilepsy

While there are no studies of evoked potentials in children with occipital seizures and epilepsy using the asymmetric stimuli described above, Ratliff & Zemon (1984) recorded windmill-dartboard and checkerboard VEPs from five epileptic adults. They found that the checkerboard pattern VEPs, which consist only of second harmonic components, were normal in these patients while the amplitude and phase of the fundamental harmonic component of the VEPs elicited by the windmill-dartboard stimulus were abnormal. Ratliff & Zemon concluded that the windmill-dartboard stimulus reveals an abnormality not seen with conventional checkerboard stimuli and suggest that, while not pathognomonic for epilepsy, there are abnormal lateral interactions in epilepsy. Future studies of windmill-dartboard evoked potentials in infants and children thought to have occipital seizures may provide useful diagnostic and prognostic information.

References

Atkinson, J., Braddick, O. & Moar, K. (1977): Development of contrast sensitivity over the first three months of life in the human infant. *Vision Res.* **17**, 1037–1044.

Campbell, F.W. & Maffei, L. (1970): Electrophysiological evidence for the existence of orientation and size detectors in the human visual system. *J. Physiol. (Lond.)* **207**, 635–652.

De Vries-Khoe, L.H. & Spekreijse, H. (1982): Maturation of luminance and pattern EPs in man. *Doc. Ophthalmol. Proc. Series* **31**, 461–475.

Dobson, V. & Teller, D.Y. (1978): Visual acuity in human infants: a review and comparison of behavioural and electrophysiological studies. *Vision Res.* **18**, 1469–1483.

Ellingson, R.J. (1967): The study of brain electrical activity in infants. In: *Advances in child development and behavior*, eds. L. Lipsitt & S. Spiker, pp. 162–173. New York: Academic.

Ellingson, R.J. (1970): Variability of evoked responses in the human newborn. *Electroencephalogr. Clin. Neurophysiol.* **29**, 10–19.

Harris, L., Atkinson, J. & Braddick, O. (1976): Visual contrast sensitivity of a 6-month-old infant measured by the evoked potential. *Nature* **264**, 570–571.

Harter, M.R. & Suitt, C.D. (1970): Visually evoked cortical responses and pattern vision in the infant: a longitudinal study. *Psychon Sci.* **18**, 235–237.

Harter, M.R., Deaton, F.K. & Odom, J.V. (1977): Pattern visual evoked potentials in infants. In: *Visual evoked potentials in man: new developments*, ed. J. Desmedt, pp. 332–352. Oxford: Clarendon.

Kurtzberg, D. & Vaughan, H.G. (1985): Electrophysiologic assessment of auditory and visual function in the newborn. *Clin. Perinatol.* **12**, 277–299.

Marg, E., Freeman, D.N., Peltzman, P. & Goldstein, P.J. (1976): Visual acuity development in human infants: evoked potential measurements. *Invest. Ophthalmol.* **15**, 150–153.

Maurer, D. (1975): Infant visual perception: methods of study. In: *Infant perception: from sensation to cognition*, Vol. 1, *Basic visual processes*, eds. L. Cohen & P. Salapatek, pp. 36–52. New York: Academic Press.

Moskowitz, A. & Sokol, S. (1983): Developmental changes in the human visual system as reflected by the latency of the pattern reversal VEP. *Electroencephalogr. Clin. Neurophysiol.* **56**, 1–15.

Norcia, A.M. & Tyler, C.W. (1985a): Spatial frequency sweep VEP: visual acuity during the first year of life. *Vision Res.* **25**, 1399–1408.

Norcia, A.M. & Tyler, C.W. (1985b): Infant VEP acuity measurements: analysis of individual differences in measurement error. *Electroencephalogr. Clin. Neurophysiol.* **61**, 359–369.

Pirchio, M., Spinelli, D., Fiorentini, A. & Maffei, L. (1978): Infant contrast sensitivity evaluated by evoked potentials. *Brain Res.* **141**, 179–184.

Ratliff, F. (1965): *Mach Bands: quantitative studies on neural networks in the retina*. San Francisco: Holden-Day, Inc.

Ratliff, F. (1982): Radial spatial patterns and multifrequency temporal patterns: possible clinical applications. *Ann. N. Y. Acad. Sci.* **388**, 651–656.

Ratliff, F. & Zemon, V. (1982): Some new methods for the analysis of lateral interactions that influence the visual evoked potential. *Ann. N. Y. Acad. Sci.* **388**, 113–124.

Ratliff, F. & Zemon, V. (1984): Visually evoked potentials elicited in normal subjects and in epileptic patients by windmill-dartboard stimuli. In: *Evoked potentials II*. eds. R. Nodar & C. Barber, pp. 251–259. Boston: Butterworth.

Schiller, P. H. (1986): The central visual system. *Vision Res.* **26**, 1351–1386.

Sokol, S. (1978): Measurement of infant visual acuity from pattern reversal evoked potentials. *Vision Res.* **18**, 33–39.

Sokol, S. (1982): Infant visual development: evoked potential estimates. *Ann. N. Y. Acad. Sci.* **388**, 514–525.

Sokol, S. (1990a): The visually evoked cortical potential in optic nerve and visual pathway disorders. In: *Electrophysiologic testing in disorders of the retina, optic nerve and visual pathway: ophthalmology monographs*, eds. G.A. Fishman & S. Sokol, pp. 105–141. American Academy of Ophthalmology.

Sokol, S. (1990b): Maturation of visual function studied by visual evoked potentials. In: *Visual evoked potentials: clinical neurophysiology updates*, Vol. 3, ed. J.E. Desmedt, pp. 35–44. Amsterdam: Elsevier.

Sokol, S. & Dobson, V. (1976): Pattern reversal visually evoked potentials in infants. *Invest. Ophthalmol.* **15**, 58–62.

Sokol, S. & Jones, K. (1979): Implicit time of pattern evoked potentials in infants: an index of maturation of spatial vision. *Vision Res.* **19**, 747–755.

Sokol, S. & Moskowitz, A. (1985): Comparison of pattern VEPs and preferential looking behavior in three-month-old infants. *Invest. Ophthalmol. Vis. Sci.* **26**, 359–365.

Sokol, S., Moskowitz, A., McCormack, G. & Augliere, R. (1988): Infant grating acuity is temporally tuned. *Vision Res.* **28**, 1357–1366.

Sokol, S., Zemon, V. & Moskowitz, A. (1992): Development of lateral interactions in the infant visual system. *Vis. Neurosci.* **8**, 3–8.

Spekreijse, H. (1978): Maturation of contrast EPs and development of visual resolution. *Arch. Ital. Biol.* **116**, 358–369.

Spekreijse, H. (1983): Comparison of acuity tests and pattern evoked potential criteria: two mechanisms underlying acuity maturation in man. *Behav. Brain Res.* **10**, 107–117.

Zemon, V. & Ratliff, F. (1982): Visual evoked potentials: evidence for lateral interactions. *Proc. Natl. Acad. Sci. USA* **79**, 5723–5726.

Zemon, V., Victor, J. D. & Ratliff, F. (1986): Functional subsystems in the visual pathways of humans characterized using evoked potentials. In: *Evoked potentials*, pp. 203–210. New York: Alan R. Liss Inc.

Chapter 7

VEP in children with damage of vision

Piernanda Vigliano, Giorgio Capizzi and Lorella Tornetta

Institute of Child Neuropsychiatry, University of Turin, Piazza Polonia 94, 10126 Turin, Italy

Summary

The maturation of visual pathways in children conditions the interpretation of visual evoked potentials (VEP). They are a useful means to evaluate visual function at an early age, in cases where visual responsiveness and capacity to follow objects is lacking or in which strabismus or opacity of the eye occurs. Thanks to particular techniques it is possible to examine the retina and the optical nerve separately, thus allowing diagnosis of different diseases, both hereditary and acquired. Normally, latency increase and VEP amplitude decrease indicate retinal dysfunction, axonal damage, demyelination or cortical damage. Other than in ocular practice, VEPs are used in neurology to study demyelinating diseases with optical pathway damage. VEPs also seem to give different information in various types of epilepsy in which the occipital lobe is concerned. A personal study carried out on epileptic patients shows no significant relationship between occipital irritative anomalies and VEP waves, photosensitivity influence on VEP amplitude (increased values) and some relationship between wave modification and systems of involved neurotransmitters.

Introduction

The development of the visual system in man begins earlier than in other mammals, but finishes later. The fovea is clearly identifiable at 22 weeks of gestational age, but still immature at birth, reaching adult-like morphology at around 45 months. The processes of maturation involve, above all, the cones. These migrate towards the centre of the fovea, progressively increasing in density and length, modifying the synaptic junctions with bipolar and horizontal cells (Yuodelis & Hendrickson, 1986). At birth rod maturity by contrast has almost reached adult stage. Contemporaneously in the first 2 years of life, there are also maturation changes of the lateral geniculate nucleus, optic nerve myelination and cortical cell synaptic junctions (Sokol, 1986).

For such reasons the electroretinogram (ERG), which reflects the response of the photosensitive receptors and of the cells of the internal layer of the retina, is formed by all the waves. These are of smaller amplitude and longer latency, reaching values quite near those of adulthood by 1 year of age. Already from birth, flash visual evoked potentials (VEP) are made up by all wave elements, which have a longer inter-peak latency. Pattern-VEPs generated by the occipital cortex show only early elements, increased in latency as compared to that of adulthood. Latency values of main and above all maximum positive deflection waves also progressively decrease in relation to pattern size used for stimulation: with 60 minutes of arc checks at 1 year of age, values obtained are the same as those for adults, whereas with 15 minutes of arc checks such values are obtained at 4 years

(Moskowitz & Sokol, 1983). Visual acuity, which depends on sensitivity to the contrast of foveal receptive fields, is severely limited at birth, reaching adult values by 5–6 months of age. A study carried out on children 1 month to 5 years old showed that stimulation with checks of different spatial frequencies gave amplitude variations of waves according to a curve whose state, around the age of 5–6 months, is similar to that found in adults (Sokol, 1978). For early visual acuity evaluation, such an examination could be used after 2 months of age, as infants are awake longer and are more attentive.

Clinical application

Even within these limitations of maturation, neurophysiological studies show more sensitivity than clinical examinations and behavioural methods in manifesting troubles in the visual system (Sokol et al., 1983). With these studies a differential exploration of the retina, by means of ERG, and optical pathways, using VEP, is possible. Both can be recorded in response to white light flashes or structured stimuli (stripes and checks) with the possibility of changing the spatial frequency and contrast. The illustration of these methodologies is not the aim of this paper, but it must be remembered that a correct analysis of results depends on the stimulus selected and that the evaluation of the ERG must be preliminary to the elucidation of the evoked cortical potentials (Sherman, 1986).

Whole field flash ERG stimulation reflects the functioning of the entire retina. 'a' waves come from photosensitive receptors and 'b' waves from internal nuclear layer cells; no elements are generated from ganglion cells. ERG are pathological in cases of retinal degeneration: they are reduced in amplitude and lengthened or even annulled according to functional damage, even if the fundus is normal. As can be seen in Table 1 (in Leber's amaurosis and retinitis pigmentosa) even VEPs show morphological anomalies of latency and amplitude, as a consequence. On the other hand, macula diseases can give normal ERG results, due to low percentage of foveal cells contributing to this response. In this condition many authors underline the validity of high spatial frequency pattern ERG use (5 cycles/deg) for selective stimulus of the foveal region.

In cases of geniculostriatal fibre and cortex damage, normal ERG and abnormal VEPs are obtained transiently in the so-called delayed maturation and permanently in cortical blindness. Hoyt et al. (1983) have reported VEP data in eight children with delayed maturation, seen in the first month of life, unable to stare and follow an object. The lack of visual responsiveness in infants over 1 month of age makes one suspect that there is serious visual handicap and therefore requires deeper study. All children in this study had immaturity and prematurity anamnesis, delay in motor development and absence of oculovestibular reflexes. VEP responses, at first pathological, later showed a progressive regaining of wave latency values. This improvement was parallel to the appearance of saccadic eye movements. The normalization of values was between 26 and 44 weeks from control. Hoyt ascribes the pathological phenomena both to a delay in myelination and to synaptic and dendritic development.

Patients with serious visual defects, normal pupillary reflexes, normal fundus and no evidence of nystagmus make one think of a diagnosis of cortical blindness, and show pathological VEP in serial controls (Sokol, 1986).

White light flash VEPs give more qualitative than quantitative information on the visual system and can be useful:
- in infants under 2 months of age, in which constant supervision is impossible;
- when evaluating the remaining function of the visual cortex in an opaque condition of the eye;
- as a preliminary test to surgery of the lens;
- in a follow up of high-risk newborns who cannot be subjected to structural stimuli. In the last case, as can be seen from Table 1, pathological data may be encountered even before the onset

Chapter 7 VEP in children with damage of vision

Table 1. Comparison between neuro-ophthalmological data and neurophysiological results

	Visual acuity	Fundus	Visual field	ERG	F-VEP	P-VEP
Retinitis pigmentosa	Decreased	Disorganization of retinal pigmentary pattern. Arteriolar attenuation	Loss of peripheral fields	Abnormal		Abnormal
Leber's congenital amaurosis	Decreased	Variable retinal changes	Normal peripheral fields?	Abnormal or extinguished		Abnormal
Amblyopia	Decreased, usually monocular	Normal	Displaced blind spot; eccentric fixation; normal peripheral fields	Normal		Abnormal to small checks or gratings; asymmetry
Maculopathy	Decreased	Variable features	Central scotoma	Normal		Abnormal to small checks or gratings
Retrobulbar optic neuritis	Decreased, usually monocular	Normal	Central scotoma to large field defect	Normal		Abnormal, usually delayed
CNS degeneration	Normal or decreased	Variable features	Variable features	Normal		Abnormal, usually delayed
Ocular motor apraxia	Normal	Normal	Normal	Normal		Normal
Developmental delay	Decreased	Normal	Normal	Normal		Latency decreases coincidental with maturation of the visual pathways and cortex
Cortical blindness	Decreased or absent	Normal	Abnormal	Normal	Abnormal or absent, repeatedly	
High-risk newborns	?	Normal	?	Normal	Abnormal before development of handicap	
Hydrocephalus	Decreased	Normal	?	Normal	Delayed latency before surgery	

of neuromotor handicaps. In hydrocephalus patients, VEP pathological data does not mirror visual pathway functioning defects, but are a consequence of ischaemic damage, due to chronic hypoperfusion of the parieto-occipital lobes (Connolly et al., 1991). The repetition shows parameter normalization after surgery (Ehle & Sklar, 1979).

Pattern VEPs are the most useful in studying optical pathway pathology, which is caused by optic nerve inflammation and degeneration of the cerebral nervous system (leucodystrophy, spinocerebellar degeneration, lack of vitamin B_{12}). Wave latency increase, an expression of inflammatory or clastic demyelination, is considered pathognomonic (Markand et al., 1982).

Amblyopia evaluation is another important application, at an early age, of pattern VEPs thanks to the possibility of an interocular comparison of wave amplitude and latency (Wilcox & Sokol, 1980). VEP control during occlusal therapy is useful both in evaluating the recovery of the amblyopic eye and the visual loss in the healthy eye due to the occlusion (Odom et al., 1981). Another situation in which VEPs are indispensable is excluding the possibility of damage to the optic nerve in congenital ocular motor apraxia; in this case VEPs confirm the sensory pathways' integrity (Gittinger & Sokol, 1982).

VEP latency and amplitude anomalies can also be found in other pathologies such as epilepsy, where optical pathway integrity is not disputed, unlike cortical functioning. There are few articles in literature dedicated to this topic, and moreover they are not homogeneous in their choice of cases, anticonvulsant drugs and methods of stimulus. There is, however some agreement on principal positive wave amplitude increases in cases of photosensitive epilepsy, with flash and pattern VEP stimulations (Broughton et al., 1969; Lücking et al., 1970; Faught & Lee, 1984). Faught & Lee (1984) also found a VEP normalization tendency after VPA therapy. More controversial data are reported on the measure of latency, both for principal and later waves (Faught & Lee, 1984; Mervaala et al., 1985; Farnarier et al., 1988). Farnarier et al. (1988) noted a latency increase, not significant, in occipital partial idiopathic epilepsy.

We have studied 11 patients (six male and five female, age range 6–19 years) suffering from epilepsy, with the purpose of verifying if and in what way cortical hyperexcitability influences different VEP elements (morphology, latency and amplitude). All these subjects show no refraction flaws, no crises for 6 months to 8 years, and negative neuroradiological studies. They were patients with idiopathic epilepsy, occipital partial or generalized, which show occipital spikes and diffused spike and wave discharges, when resting or during intermittent photic stimulation (IPS). VEPs have been studied using 0.9 and 2.3 cycles/deg pattern reversal with 60 per cent contrast and an average luminance of 130 cd/m^2, and were obtained under monocular conditions. VEP responses were compared to those of an age- and sex-matched normal group. Responses were considered pathological if they exceeded 3 s.d. Data showed delayed latencies in 1/5 subjects with occipital spikes. An increase in N1 and P1 wave amplitude was encountered in 2/4 cases with photoparoxysmal response, and in one patient with diffused spike and wave discharges, without photosensitivity (Fig. 1), who had an apparently generalized seizure in front of the computer (Table 2 and Table 3).

Table 2. Number of patients with epileptic anomalies and VEP results

	Occipital anomalies	Occipital anomalies + photoconvulsive response	Photoconvulsive response	Generalized S-W discharges
P-VEP	5	1	4	1
P-VEP: increased P100 amplitude			2	1
P-VEP: increased P100 latency	1			

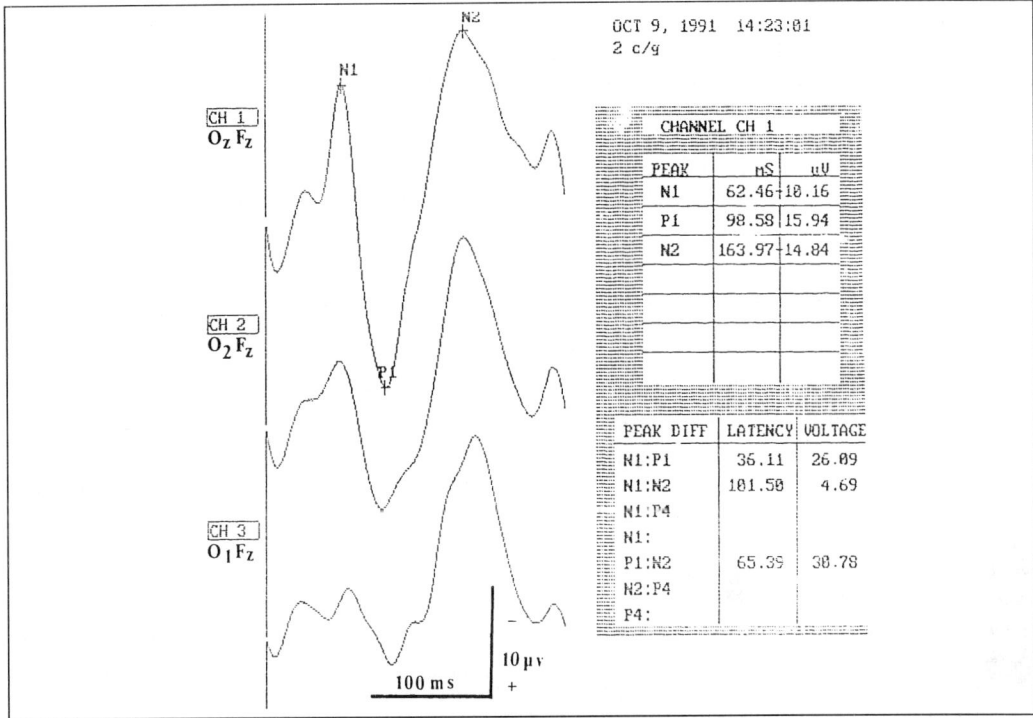

Fig. 1. Patient with diffuse S-W discharges, who had an apparently generalized seizure in front of the computer. Increased P100 amplitude in P-VEP recording.

Table 3. Data of patients with VEP anomalies

P-VEP: increased P100 amplitude (n.v. 13 ± 5.27 µV)					
M.E.	F	10 years	Photoconvulsive response	CBZ	23.8–29 µV
L.F.	M	10 years	Photoconvulsive response	CBZ	25–44 µV
C.M.	M	13 years	Generalized S-W discharges	–	25–33.6 µV
P-VEP: increased P100 latency (n.v. 88 ± 4.11 ms)					
C.P.	M	8 years	Occipital anomalies	VPA	102.5–108.3 ms

Conclusions

From what can be seen, it appears evident that VEPs allow us to discover visual pathway defects in infants that cannot verbally express themselves or who are uncooperative. They are therefore of valid help in ophthalmic practice.

In spite of the limitations of their interpretation, due to the nature of the disease, VEPs provide two important indications in paediatric neurology. The first is evaluating, at an early age, visual damage in high risk neonates or cerebropathic patients. In these subjects, who do not show any search behaviour and visual orientation, motor damage and mental deficiency are often associated. Visual pathological study is important so as to have an early therapeutic and prognostic evaluation. As regards the second indication, many authors believe that VEPs are able to individualize myelinic damage in degenerative pathologies in the absence of other positive parameters.

If the evoked potential study does not add any important contributions to the diagnosis of epilepsy, it may give indications of varied systems of neurotransmitters: GABAergic (Faught & Lee, 1984) and dopaminergic type (Quesney et al., 1981). This might be obtained with various stimulations of the visual sub-systems, in different clinical and therapeutic conditions. A stimulating, but as yet insufficiently supported, hypothesis is that the genesis of the amplitude increase of VEP waves is determined by characteristics of the retina itself and by neurotransmitters working in it. This suggests that ERG recording precedes VEP study, thus providing a more correct interpretation.

References

Broughton, R., Meier-Ewert, K.H. & Ebe, M. (1969): Evoked visual, somato-sensory and retinal potentials in photosensitive epilepsy. *Electroencephalogr. Clin. Neurophysiol.* **27**, 373–386.

Connolly, M.B., Jan, J.E. & Cochrane, D.D. (1991): Rapid recovery from cortical visual impairment following correction of prolonged shunt malfunction in congenital hydrocephalus. *Arch. Neurol.* **48(9)**, 956–957.

Ehle, A. & Sklar, F. (1979): Visual evoked potentials in infants with hydrocephalus. *Neurology* **29**, 1541–1544.

Farnarier, G., Bureau, M., Mancini, J. & Regis, H. (1988): Etude des potentiels évoqués multimodalitaires dans les épilepsies partielles de l'enfant. *Neurophysiol. Clin.* **18(3)**, 243–254.

Faught, E. & Lee, S.I. (1984): Pattern-reversal evoked potentials in photosensitive epilepsy. *Electroencephalogr. Clin. Neurophysiol.* **59**, 125–133.

Gittinger, J.W. & Sokol, S. (1982): The visual evoked potentials in the diagnosis of congenital ocular motor apraxia. *Am. J. Ophthalmol.* **93**, 700–703.

Hoyt, C.S., Jastrzebski, G. & Marg, E. (1983): Delayed visual maturation in infancy. *Br. J. Ophthalmol.* **67**, 127–130.

Lücking, C.H., Creutzfeld, O.D. & Heinemann, U. (1970): Visual evoked potentials of patients with epilepsy and of a control group. *Electroencephalogr. Clin. Neurophysiol.* **29**, 557–566.

Markand, O.M., Garg, B.P., DeMyer, W.E. & Warren, C. (1982): Brain stem auditory, visual and somatosensory evoked potentials in leukodystrophies. *Electroencephalogr. Clin. Neurophysiol.* **54**, 39–48.

Mervaala, E., Keränen, T., Penttilä, M., Partanen, J.V. & Riekkinen, P. (1985): Pattern-reversal VEP and cortical SEP latency prolongations in epilepsy. *Epilepsia.* **26(5)**, 441–445.

Moskowitz, A. & Sokol, S. (1983): Developmental changes in the human visual system as reflected by the latency of the pattern reversal VEP. *Electroencephalogr. Clin. Neurophysiol.* **56**, 1–15.

Odom, J.V., Hoyt, C.S. & Marg, E. (1981): Effect of natural deprivation and unilateral eye patching on visual acuity of infants and children. *Arch. Ophthalmol.* **99**, 1412–1416.

Quesney, L.F. (1981): Dopamine and generalized photosensitive epilepsy. In: *Neurotrasmitters, seizures and epilepsy*, eds. P.L. Morselli et al., pp. 263–272. New York: Raven Press.

Sherman, J. (1986): ERG and VEP as supplemental aids. In: *The differential diagnosis of retinal versus optic nerve disease*, eds. R.Q. Cracco & I. Bodis-Wollner, pp. 343–353. New York: Alan R. Liss, Inc.

Sokol, S. (1978): Measurement of infant visual acuity from pattern reversal evoked potentials. *Vision Res.* **18**, 33–39.

Sokol, S., Hansen, V.C., Moskowitz, A., Greenfield, P. & Towle, V.L. (1983): Evoked potential and preferential looking estimates of visual acuity in pediatric patients. *J. Ophthalmol.* **90**, 552–562.

Sokol, S. (1986): Clinical application of the ERG and VEP in the pediatric age group, In: *The differential diagnosis of retinal versus optic nerve disease.* eds. R.Q. Cracco & I. Bodis-Wollner, pp. 447–454. New York: Alan R. Liss, Inc.

Wilcox, L.M. & Sokol, S. (1980): Changes in the binocular fixation patterns and the visually evoked potentials in the treatment of esotropia with amblyopia. *J. Ophthalmol.* **87**, 1273–1281.

Yuodelis, C. & Hendrickson, A. (1986): A qualitative and quantitative analysis of the human fovea during development. *Vision Res.* **26**, 847–855.

Chapter 8

EEG in children with visual pathways damage

Laura Mira and Andrée Van Lierde

Servizio di Neurologia, Ospedale dei Bambini Vittore Buzzi, Via Castelvetro 32, Milan, Italy; and Istituto di Clinica Pediatrica dell'Università di Milano, Milan, Italy

Summary

EEG abnormalities with characteristic patterns have been described in the course of the maturational development in children affected with pathological conditions of the eye and visual pathways.

The visual systems of the human newborn is remarkably coarse with respect to other senses, mainly with regard to motility, visual search and exploration, prolonged fixation and stereoscopic vision. Yet at birth the human brain itself is far from perfect and is undergoing a progressive, continuous evolution.

Before discussing EEG in children with visual pathways impairment, we need to consider the stages of brain maturation as they manifest themselves in EEG recordings: we will take into account the evolution of posterior activity and reactivity and the evolution of activities evoked by visual stimulations. The EEG changes during brain maturation in children with damage to the visual system are investigated in relation to the relevant pathology. Interest is focused on basic activities in waking and sleeping conditions, on their reactivity, on evoked responses and also on irritative non-epileptic potentials.

The interaction between maturational processes of the visual system and of the cerebral cortex, as manifested in the EEG, calls for a deeper investigation into the conditions of maturational derangement in the hope of gaining a better understanding of the physiological mechanism of maturation.

EEG in children with visual pathways damage

During the 1950s and 1960s, the EEG patterns of the child with damage to the visual pathways were investigated with great interest and awareness of the underlying controversial issues. In the same years, neurophysiological research identified the characteristics of the normal EEG at different ages and the effect of the maturational process on the EEG. Gone was the time of 'curiosity' for the EEG, gone was the interest in verifying data from EEG in different pathological conditions, even those research trends concerned with EEG signs of damage to visual pathways were abandoned. Adrian & Matthews, as early as 1934, had provoked posterior rhythms of high frequency with light stimulation and had stated that in blind subjects alpha waves were absent due to the lack of light stimulation. Levinson *et al.* (1951), Stillerman *et al.* (1952), Kellaway *et al.* (1955), Gibbs *et al.* (1955), Lairy *et al.* (1962), Jeavons (1964), Lairy & Harrison (1968), Gibbs *et al.* (1968), Jeavons *et al.* (1970) and many others went on to analyse the various aspects of EEG in different conditions of blindness and visual defects; their contributions are still valuable today.

The interest in these research issues is almost concomitant with the study of the normal maturational evolution as manifested in the EEG. The stages of cerebral maturation and the parallel, complex evolution of the visual pathways and refinement of all complex mechanisms affording an adequate utilization of the whole visual system are factors of crucial relevance in understanding how EEG abnormalities set in and change over time in the child with visual pathways damage.

Thanks to fundamental studies by Dreyfus-Brisac & Fischgold (1957) and Monod & Tharp (1977) integrated with more recent data from Blume (1982), Niedermeyer (1987a) and Tharp (1990) it has been possible to reconstruct the maturational stages. Some parameters, like posterior activity differentiation, onset of specific anterior activity and sleep/wake differences represent the first signs of organization.

The EEG of the pre-term infant free from cerebral damaged shows some early signs of anteroposterior differentiation with the appearance, in the background of the discontinuous recording, of a slow posterior (posterior and central) activity, upon which fast frequencies are superimposed: starting from the 27th week of conceptional age, the first delta brushes become evident, first in all waking conditions then limited to sleep, then disappearing around birth or in the very first weeks of life.

A specifically anterior activity will differentiate only at the 34th week of conceptional age: these are the so-called frontal 'encoches', which appear early during sleep, are present also in the waking state and then persist during sleep up to 4–6 weeks after the end of gestation.

The recording is constantly discontinuous in the pre-term infant both in the waking and in the sleeping state up to the 34th week of conceptional age: then discontinuity will be limited to sleep and to some stages of sleep, to disappear completely, in the normal child, at about 1 month of life. On the basis of the discontinuity/continuity it is possible to point out the first characteristics of sleeping-waking differentiation (Fig. 1).

We cannot speak of posterior activity similar to the alpha rhythm of the mature subject before 3 months of real age (Pampiglione, 1977). This is the first posteriorly located activity evoked by 'passive' closure of the eyes. The initially low frequencies quickly proceed to frequencies similar to those of the adult (Fig. 2). This age, 3 months, seems very untimely considering the long maturational course of the visual system. At age 3 months a blocking response is also elicitable (Curzi-Dascalova, 1977).

Among evoked responses we will take into account only the lambda waves: they appear on eye opening and are related to visual exploration. They are present in the newborn (Ellingson, 1960; Moussalli & Arfel, 1977) as expression of a complex phenomenon in which different components are involved: Billings (1989a, b) offers a physiological interpretation, according to which they are dependent on a rather advanced maturation and on a balance between different mechanisms (two types of lambda: recovery of normal visual sensitivity in the peripheral visual field and release from suppression of central visual field).

The evolution of the response to intermittent photic stimulation follows a particular maturational course, but seems independent from the maturation of the alpha rhythm, which, after 3 months of age, appears regular and continuous. The response to intermittent photic stimulation, on the contrary, is discontinuous, there being a period with marked reactivity, although with peculiar properties like latency; then it is possible demonstrate a peak of 'resonance' at 7 months, which seems to diminish at about 1 year; on the other hand, response to low frequencies is maintained. The response to the intermittent photic stimulation matures rapidly starting from 5–6 years of age with responses to frequencies similar to those of the adult (Stofft, 1961; Niedermeyer, 1987a).

The subtle modulation of physiological processes is much richer than suggested by this brief review, which merely takes into account some fundamental activities and those activities more strictly related to the visual pathways and visual cortex, and dependent on visual behaviour.

Nothing is found in the literature about the EEG maturation in the premature, blind infant before

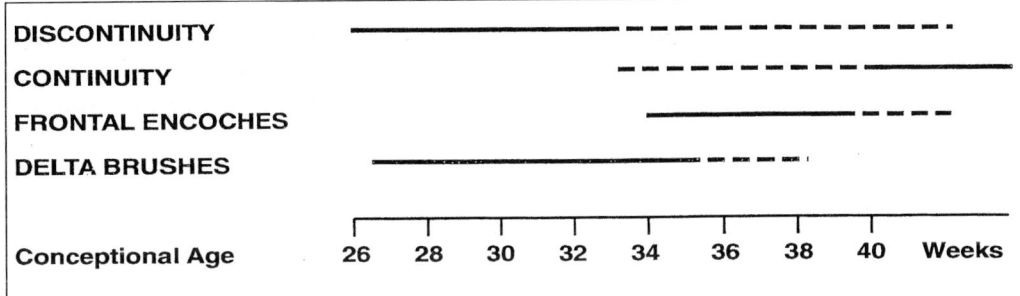

Fig. 1. EEG evolution in preterm and newborn infant.

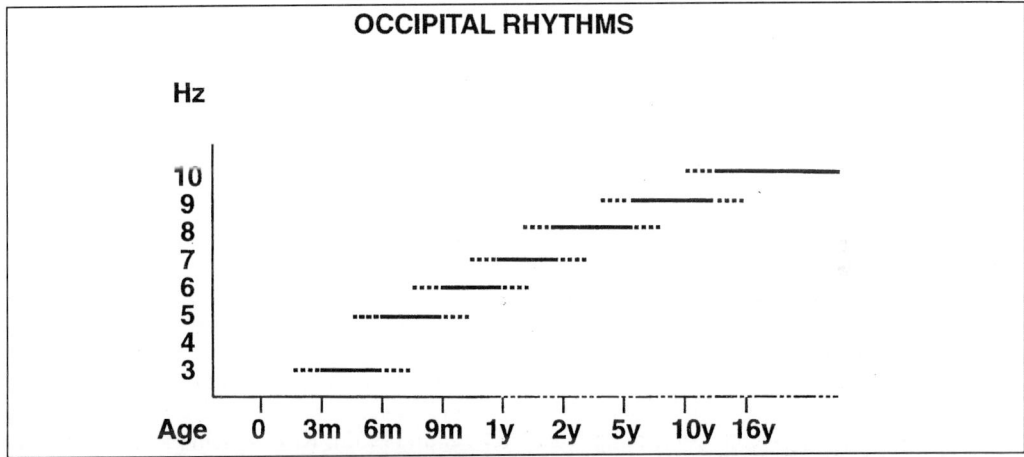

Fig. 2. Occipital rhythms in infancy and childhood.

the 40th week of conceptional age. The fundamental activities in the child with visual impairment are often deranged, depending on the severity of the visual defect and its age of onset: Jeavons (1964) and Enge *et al.* (1973) maintain that the adequate development of the alpha rhythm would need visual stimulation at some time early in life. Lairy *et al.* (1962) and Lairy & Harrison (1968) speak of the extreme scarcity of the alpha rhythm and of poor spatial differentiation, and find a correlation between these data and severity of visual impairment: some hypotheses concerning a relationship with neuropsychological functions, such as dyspraxia, hint at an inadequate spatial differentiation. Cohen *et al.* (1961) confirm the absence or scarcity of alpha rhythm, the abnormal topography and the difficulty in getting responses to intermittent photic stimulation, when, on the other hand, the alpha rhythm is present. These authors identify a minimal visual acuity compatible with a normal alpha rhythm (20/200). Jeavons (1964) reports the absence of alpha rhythm in 60 per cent of totally blind and partially sighted subjects: percentages are higher and significant when the visual damage occurs early and is associated with a global cerebral impairment. Enge *et al.* (1973) confirm that the impairment of the alpha rhythm (absent or poorly structured) occurs in 100 per cent of blind subjects and in 45 per cent of partially sighted subjects; the latter show a blocking response in only 25 per cent of cases and the response to intermittent photic stimulation is even lower.

These objective observations seems to reinforce a relationship between visual stimulation and alpha rhythm maturation, between information coming from the periphery and visual cortex development. Faced with these data, it is necessary to remember that the question of alpha rhythm generators is still open to discussion, with, on one hand, the advocates of their cortical origin (Lopes da Silva *et al.*, 1973; Lopes da Silva & Storm van Leewen, 1978; Hess, 1980) and, on the other, the advocates of their thalamic origin (Andersen & Andersson, 1974). At present no theory can be considered sufficiently proven (Niedermeyer, 1987b).

The most specific pathological activity of the EEG in children with visual pathways defects is represented by focal spikes in the occipital region: they were first described in 1951 by Levinson *et al.* and by Stillerman *et al.* (1952). These authors find foci of spikes exclusively with occipital location in squint-eyed children (30 per cent *vs* 0.5 per cent in normal children); they find foci of occipital spikes in 74 per cent of brain-damaged squinters against 38 per cent of brain-damaged non-squinters, who, on the other hand, present focal spikes with different topograhy. They report similar activities also in cortical blindness (92 per cent), not confirmed in subsequent studies.

Kellaway *et al.* (1955), in a sample population of 61 children affected with retrolental fibroplasia, add that early occurrence of the retinal damage (and of visual damage in general) and severe and bilateral visual impairment are crucial factors in the production of these foci of occipital spikes (uni- or bilateral). The same authors are the first to mention the age-dependency: foci are difficult to point out before 10 months, with a peak of onset after 2 years and a half and with a tendency to abate and disappear around 10 years. Studies by Metcalf (1959) and Cohen *et al.* (1961), again on retrolental fibroplasia, lead to similar conclusions. As far as retinitis pigmentosa is concerned, Cordier *et al.* (1956), Krill & Stamps (1960) and Lesny (1961), find similar abnormalities in cases of early onset, before 5 years.

Foci of occipital spikes in children with anophthalmia are reported by Subirana & Oller-Daurella (1964) and Gibbs & Gibbs (1981). Lairy *et al.* (1962) and Lairy & Harrison (1968) recognize relationships between foci of occipital spikes and gnosic-praxic neuropsychological functions in blind subjects. Jeavons (1964), on the contrary, finds only 15 per cent of foci of spikes in 129 cases, and only a minor part with occipital location, but stresses the abnormalities of the alpha rhythm. Jeannerod & Courjon (1964), analysing 35 EEGs of children with focal functional, non-epileptic spikes in the occipital region, find visual disturbances in five cases only: they also report that sleep is a strongly activating factor, confirming what Gibbs *et al.* (1955), Krill & Stamps (1960), Cohen *et al.* (1961) and Salzarulo (1975) had already pointed out.

In 1981 Beaumanoir *et al.* summed up the common properties of the foci of functional spikes with occipital topography. they are frequent in the population with visual disturbances and even with visuospatial neuropsychological defects; are superimposed on a recording which can be normal (except for the abnormalities in the occipital region) or poorly structured in space; are represented by spikes or spikes and waves characterized by great amplitude and stereotyped morphology; are activated by slow sleep and persist, attenuated, in the paradoxical stage; in the waking state they appear with closed eyes; are exaggerated by drugs; can be variable (in location and presence); are related to age (never seen before 10 months; peak from 2 to 5 years; disappearance at 10 years); they are inhibited or exaggerated by stimulation involving visual perception and visuospatial integration.

This definition by Beaumanoir *et al.* (1981) is still valuable and comprehensive and constitutes an excellent study protocol of the EEG abnormalities in children with damage to the visual pathways. The interaction between the maturational processes of the visual system and those of the cerebral cortex, investigated as expressed in the EEG, calls for a deeper investigation into the conditions of maturational derangement in the hope of gaining a better understanding of the physiological mechanisms of maturation.

Imbert (1992) suggests that in the long period of maturation of the visual brain, the primitive and coarse organization, genetically determined, changes into a final organization, adequate for high level functioning. The nervous activity plays an important role in the organization of connections and is modulated by experience.

We can therefore hypothesize that inadequate or deranged experiences can inappropriately mould the immature brain and that the damage to the visual pathways interferes with the maturational process of the visual brain. The organizational disorder affects the EEG with different modalities according to age: in the child it hinders the maturation of fundamental activities and facilitates the onset of foci of functional spikes. They are probably signs of inadequate afferentation, signs of the derangement of a physiological process during infancy.

Acknowledgements

We are very grateful to Carlo and Pietro Zerbi for their generous help.

References

Adrian, E.D. & Matthews, B.H.C. (1934): The Berger rhythm, potential changes form the occipital lobe in man. *Brain* **57**, 345-359.

Andersen, P. & Andersson, S.A. (1974): Thalamic origin of cortical rhythmic activity. In: *Handbook of electroencephalography and clinical neurophysiology*, Vol 2C, ed. A. Remond, pp. 90-118. Amsterdam: Elsevier.

Beaumanoir, A., Inderwildi, B. & Zagury, S. (1981): Paroxysmes EEG 'non épileptiques'. *Méd. Hyg.* **39**, 1911-1918.

Billings, R.J. (1989a): The origin of the initial negative component of the averaged lambda potential recorded from midline electrodes. *EEG Clin. Neurophysiol.* **13**, 914-922.

Billings, R.J. (1989b): The origin of the initial negative component of the averaged lambda potential recorded from midline electrodes. *EEG Clin. Neurophysiol.* **72**, 114-117.

Blume, W.T. (1982): *Atlas of paediatric electroencephalography*. New York: Raven Press.

Cohen, J., Boshes, L.D. & Snider, R.S. (1961): Electroencephalographic changes following retrolental fibroplasia. *EEG Clin. Neurophysiol.* **13**, 914-922.

Cordier, J., Dureux, J.B. & Barbier, J. (1956): L'électroencéphalogramme au cours des dégénérescences tapéto-rétiniennes: à propos de 50 cas. *Rev. Otoneuroophthalmol.* **28**, 193.

Curzi-Dascalova, L. (1977): EEG de veille et de sommeil du nourrisson normal avant 6 mois d'âge. *Rev. EEG Neurophysiol.* **7**, 316-326.

Dreyfus-Brisac, C. & Fischgold, H. (1957): Veille, sommeil, réactivité sensorielle chez le prématuré, le nouveau-né et le nourrisson. *EEG Clin. Neurophysiol.* **6S**, 417-424.

Ellingson, R.J. (1960): Cortical electrical responses to visual stimulation in the human infant. *EEG Clin. Neurophysiol.* **12**, 663-677.

Enge, S., Kaloud, H. & Lechner H. (1973): EEG-Untersuchungen bei blinden und sehschwachen Kindern. *Paediatrie und Paedologie* **8**, 175-180.

Gibbs, E.L., Fois, A. & Gibbs F. A. (1955): The EEG in retrolental fibroplasia. *N. Engl. Med. J.* **253**, 1, 1101-1108.

Gibbs, F.A. Gibbs, E.L., Gibbs E.L. & Gibbs, T.J. (1968): Relation between specific types of occipital dysrhythmia and visual defects. *The Johns Hopkins Med. J.* **122**, 343-349.

Gibbs, E.L. & Gibbs, F.A. (1981): Das Elektroenzephalogramm bei kongenitaler Anophthalmie. *EEG-EMG* **12**, 171-173.

Hess, R. (1980): The origin of alpha rhythm. *Electroencephalogr. Clin. Neurophysiol.* **49**, 110.

Imbert, M. (1993): Ontogenesis of the occipital lobe. In: *Occipital seizures and epilepsies in children*, eds. F. Andermann, A. Beaumanoir, L. Mira, J. Roger & C.A. Tassinari, pp. 3-8. London: John Libbey.

Jeannerod, E. & Courjon, J. (1964): Les pointes occipitales survenant pendant le sommeil chez l'enfant amblyope. *Rev. Neurol.* **111**, 346-350.

Jeavons, P.M. (1964): The electroencephalogram in blind children. *Br. J. Ophthalmol.* **48**, 83-100.

Jeavons, P.M., Harding, G.F.A., Ferries, G.W. & Thompson, C.R.S. (1970): Alpha rhythm in totally blind children. *Br. J. Ophthalmol.* **54**, 786-793.

Kellaway, P., Bloxsom, A. & MacGregor, M. (1955): Occipital spike foci associated with retrolental fibroplasia and other forms of retinal loss in children. *EEG Clin. Neurophysiol.* **7**, 469-470.

Krill, A.E. & Stamps, F.W. (1960): The electroencephalogram in retinitis pigmentosa. *Am. J. Ophthalmol.* **49**, 762-773.

Lairy, G.C., Netchine, S. & Neyraut, M.T. (1962): L'enfant déficient visuel. *Psychiat. Enf.* **5**/II, 357–440.

Lairy, G.C. & Harrison, A. (1968): Functional aspects of EEG foci in children. Clinical data and longitudinal studies. In: *Clinical electroencephalography of children*, eds. P. Kellaway & I. Petersen, pp. 197–212. New York, London: Grune & Stratton.

Lesny, I. (1961): EEG study in retinitis pigmentosa with specific reference to the slow waves blocked by eye opening. *EEG Clin. Neurophysiol.* **13**, 139.

Levinson, J.D., Gibbs, E.L. Stillerman, M.L. & Perlstein, M.A. (1951): Electroencephalogram and eye disorders. Clinical correlation. *Paediatrics* **7**, 422–427.

Lopes da Silva, F.H., Van Lierop, T.H.M.T., Schrijer, C.F. & Storm van Leeuwen, W. (1973): Organization of thalamic and cortical alpha rhythm: spectra and coherences. *Electroencephalogr. Clin. Neurophysiol.* **35**, 627–640.

Lopes da Silva, F.H. & Storm van Leeuwen, W. (1978): The cortical alpha rhythm in dog: the depth and surface profile of phase. In: *Architectonics of cerebral cortex*, eds. M.A. Brazier & H. Petsche. New York: Raven Press.

Metcalf, D.R. (1959): Electroencephalographic findings in ex-premature infants with partial and complete blindness due to retrolental fibroplasia. *EEG Clin. Neurophysiol.* **11**, 182.

Monod, N. & Tharp, B. (1977): Activité électro-encéphalographique normale du nouveau-né et du prématuré au cours des états de veille et de sommeil. *Rev. EEG Neurophysiol.* **7**, 302–315.

Moussalli, F. & Arfel, G. (1977): Ondes lambda chez le nouveau-né. *Rev. EEG Neurophysiol.* **7**, 361–364.

Niedermeyer, E. (1987a): Maturation of the EEG: development of waking and sleep patterns. In: *Electroencephalography*, eds. E. Niedermeyer & F. Lopes da Silva, pp. 133–157. Baltimore: Urban & Schwarzenberg.

Niedermeyer, E. (1987b): The normal EEG of the waking adult. In: *Electroencephalography*, eds. E. Niedermeyer & F. Lopes da Silva, pp. 97–117. Baltimore: Urban & Schwarzenberg.

Pampiglione, G. (1977): Development of rhythmic activities in infancy (waking state). *Rev. EEG Neurophysiol.* **7**, 327–334.

Salzarulo, P. (1975): Hypothèses et données préliminaires concernant la relation entre pointes occipitales et sommeil chez l'enfant avec déficit visuel. *Rev. EEG Neurophysiol. Clin.* **5**, 86–89.

Stillerman, M.L., Gibbs, E.L. & Perlstein M.A. (1952): Electroencephalographic changes in strabismus. *Am. J. Ophthalmol.* **35**, 54–63.

Stofft, P. (1961): Essai d'utilisation de la stimulation lumineuse intermittente pour l'appréciation du développement de la fonction visuelle chez le nourrisson. *Ann. Oculist.* **194**, 133–152.

Subirana, A. & Oller-Daurella, L. (1964): Etude EEG de deux cas d'anophthalmie. *Rev. Neur.* **111**, 350–351.

Tharp, B.R. (1990): Electrophysiological brain maturation in premature infant: an historical perspective. *J. Clin. Neurophysiol.* **7**, 302–314.

Chapter 9

Semiology of occipital seizures in infants and children

Anne Beaumanoir

Fondazione Pierfranco e Luisa Mariani, Neurologia infantile, Viale Bianca Maria 28, 20129 Milan, Italy

Summary

The long duration of maturation of the visual system in mammals and particularly in humans prompts us to look for differences in the semiology of occipital seizures according to the maturational stages of visual cortical areas and of their connections. According to the site of the initial discharge and its local or remote propagation, the seizure will be a partial sensory visual seizure with positive or negative symptomatology or an oculomotor seizure, sometimes followed by a versive tonic and hemiclonic seizure. The spreading of the discharge into neighbouring areas and rhinencephalic structures is quite frequent in the child, particularly during slow sleep. In infants it seems that a particular oculomotor symptomatology occurs, which can be the sign of a critical pathology in relation to the maturation of oculomotor systems. In children with age-related occipital epilepsy, seizures are revealed not only by visual symptoms, but also by autonomic disorders and headaches resembling, in some aspects, basilar migraine. The electroclinical study of the seizures shows, independent of the age of the child, that the critical discharges accompanying the positive sensory or motor signs are fast activities, while the negative signs, as well as the autonomic symptoms, with or without headaches, are accompanied by sharp wave discharges and monorhythmic slow waves.

Introduction

The long duration of maturation of the visual system in mammals and particularly in humans (Imbert, 1993; Lagae & Casaer, 1993; Sokol, 1993; Spreafico & Regondi, 1993), prompts us to look for differences in the semiology of occipital seizures according to the maturational stages of visual cortical areas and of their connections (Avanzini, 1992). Broadly, the 'visual cortex' is an area of reception and sensory integration as well as one of motor elaboration, strongly connected to neighbouring cortical areas and, by the inferior longitudinal fasciculus, to the ipsilateral temporal lobe, amygdala and hippocampus. Because of this, and according to the site of the initial discharge and of its local or remote propagation, the seizure will be a simple or partial sensory visual seizure or a motor oculogyric (or oculomotor) seizure or a sensorimotor one. It will easily and quickly imply a partial complex symptomatology and/or a motor or sensorimotor seizure, not limited to the eyes. However, in children with occipital partial epilepsy, seizures are revealed, besides visual symptoms, by autonomic disorders and headaches resembling, in certain aspects, basilar migraine (Beaumanoir, 1993; Lanzi & Balottin, 1993; Terzano et al., 1993). In infants and very young children it often happens that ictal EEG discharges confined to the occipital pole appear 'subclinical' to the observer. Indeed, before the acquisition of language the child cannot be aware of a seizure arising from an epileptic discharge in a cortical area devoid of motor or autonomic representation. The very young child very likely ignores his seizure, since, with his limited experience, he cannot recognize the strangeness of the situation. However, as in the older child, a gesture, a facial or vocal expression, may reveal a critical subjective event. The occipital ictal discharge arousing the sensory symptomatology spreads to other areas, provoking motor, automatic, autonomic symptoms that can be witnessed usually by the parents who are inclined to emphasize them.

Seizures are often nocturnal and occur with loss of consciousness, when prolonged. They can precede a secondarily generalized seizure; in these cases an initial sensory symptomatology cannot be identified. All these features together could explain why visual seizures are thought to be rare by some authors (for example 6 per cent of all seizures observed in 195 children with idiopathic partial or generalized epilepsy in the series of Deonna et al. (1984)). However, this is the same age group where spike, and spike and wave occipital foci are most frequent (Gibbs et al., 1954; Smith & Kellaway, 1963; Mira & Van Lierde, 1993) and where, as many papers reported (particularly the one of Delwaide et al. (1971)), occipital seizures are most frequent. This is exclusive to the child and is well demonstrated by the work of Cooper & Lee (1991) on the occipital reactive epileptiform activity. The age group of their study ranges from a few days to 71 years; however, the mean age is 7 years and 5 months, pointing to a clear predominance of epileptic occipital foci and of occipital epilepsies in childhood.

Semiology of partial seizures arising from a discharge in the visual cortex

Positive sensory symptomatology

This category includes elementary visual hallucinations, namely brightly coloured, moving phosphenes taking on geometrical shapes, circles, lines, lozenges, balls, etc. floating or often moving sideways in the visual field. Phosphenes can appear abruptly, or quickly move toward the face of the patient. These simple hallucinations are fleeting, lasting only a few seconds, and can precede complex hallucinations which may otherwise occur as the first sign. Micropsias, macropsias and metamorphopsias are more frequently described than dyschromatopsias: these are rarely isolated, and more often associated with a distortion of the object. A 10-year-old patient of ours, suffering for many years from occipital epilepsy with frequent sensory seizures said that during a seizure he saw the telephone changing shape and becoming pink, and added 'like the pink panther'. Questioned later, he described a dark red colour occupying the whole space. This modification in his story shows that the child is able to interpret the illusion. The same patient, who had frequent seizures during the morning, saw 'the left half of the library shrink in every dimension' until 'resembling a toy'. When he experienced phosphenes, he spoke of the rings of a jingle man, though stating that the rings moved sideways. Hallucinations can be more complex; a patient of Gastaut & Zifkin (1987) saw the image of number 57, another reported by Lerman & Kivity (1991) saw 'little elephants'. Seizures characterized by palinopsia are described, as well as modifications of stereoscopic vision. All these sensory symptoms occurred in the visual field contralateral to the ictal discharge (Ludwig & Ajmone Marsan, 1975; Munari et al., 1993).

When a patient speaks of 'blurred vision', careful questioning can reveal, as with one of our patients, that by this he means a fading of colours and a feeling of seeing objects at a distance rather than a blurring of vision. A proportion of occipital seizures, varying from 7 to 47 per cent, manifests these positive sensory symptoms. This wide range could be explained by the features, already mentioned, related to the age of the patients, who, in some cases, cannot describe their seizures. More than half of all diurnal seizures begin with, or are limited to, a sensory seizure. It is noteworthy that among the 18 cases of Panayiotopoulos (1989b) the only two patients with frequent diurnal seizures did not have visual hallucinations, whereas in the other 16 with nocturnal prolonged seizures a sensory symptomatology was never described. That obviously does not rule out the existence of sensory 'signal symptoms'.

Deficient sensory symptomatology

Deficient symptomatology includes scotomas, hemianopias, transient amaurosis. Scotomas are usually sparkling: this feature implies an association of deficient and positive symptoms. Ictal blindness is usually short lived. It is often described as a black veil passing with lightning speed before the eyes. However, some authors such as Gastaut & Zifkin (1987) describe deficient epileptic symptoms (amaurosis, hemianopia) of several minutes duration. Where the development of the seizure is known in full detail, amaurosis rarely occurs as the first sign. When blindness initiates the seizure, it must be assumed that the epileptic discharge arising from the primary visual cortex V1 on the border of the calcarine fissure blocks the reception of the sensory signal, provoking a transient cortical blindness. The blindness prevents an illusional symptomatology, but does not prevent hallucinatory or oculomotor symptoms.

Ictal blindness testifies the speed of the discharge spreading on the contralateral cortex. When amaurosis is brief and occurs, as is often the case, between sensory symptoms and deviation of the eyes, or any other ictal manifestation, it could not be the expression of postictal symptomatology. When, on the contrary, blindness occurs gradually and persists after the positive symptoms, postictal deficit can be assumed. An ictal deficient symptomatology is frequent in child and adolescent series: in that of Aso et al. (1987; 1988), seven of 19 patients; Nalin et al. (1989), five of 10 patients; Deonna et al. (1984), four of 12 patients; Gastaut & Zifkin (1984; 1987), 33/63, that is 52 per cent of patients; and of Terasaki et al. (1987), 71 per cent. It is more rare for ourselves (Beaumanoir, 1983), 2/18; for Herranz Tanarro et al. (1984), 2/18; for Aicardi & Newton (1987), 4/21; and for Panayiotopoulos (1989b), 1/18. These differences probably stem from a different nosological approach: some authors classify ictal symptoms which associate amaurosis, hemianopia, headache and autonomic disorders as migrainous attacks. The lack of ictal EEG or stereo EEG records makes diagnosis ambiguous, as Schaffler & Karbowski (1988) observed.

A normal movement of ocular pursuit towards the hallucination is possible. Some patients report that, during the seizure or before appearance of the first sensory symptoms, they feel compelled to focus on a point or an object in one visual field. However, deviation of the eyes is in most cases a consequence of ictal discharge in the oculogyric visual cortex (Avanzini, 1993).

Motor symptomatology

Oculomotor seizures have been induced in man by stimulation since 1951, by Penfield & Kristiansen. Since then, many authors have studied this phenomenon from a clinical point of view, with the help of EEG, stereo EEG and PET (Gastaut, 1960; Bancaud et al., 1961; Takeda et al., 1969; Huott et al., 1974; Engel et al., 1983; Rosenbaum et al., 1986; Munari et al., 1993). The motor seizure which follows subjective symptoms is characterized by a tonic conjugated adversion of the eyes, sometimes followed by an axial deviation of the head. The deviation is usually slow; ocular globes can remain fixed for some seconds in the corner of the eye, quickly reverting back to their initial position. This tonic seizure may be followed (one out of five times) by clonic movements of the ocular globes, which bring the eye back to their normal position. Seizure length ranges from 20–60 s to 2 min. On rare occasions, as in the case reported by Gastaut & Roger in 1954 under the unsuitable name of 'epileptic nystagmus', a few ocular jerks, increasingly rapid, can precede the forced deviation of the eyes. In all cases the cortical discharge is always contralateral to the slow lateral movement of the eyes. In the other seizures involving ocular movements, the clinical and anatomical diagnosis is more difficult. In the occipital visual cortex seizure, the deviation of the eyes precedes the deviation of the head and the occipital discharge is always contralateral to the side of the movement. On the other hand, in a frontal or amygdalo-hippocampal seizure with deviation of the eyes following forced deviation of the head, the ictal discharge may be occasionally ipsilateral.

Oculogyric and oculoclonic seizures are a frequent sign of idiopathic childhood epilepsy with occipital paroxysms (ICEOP). They are described in roughly the same proportions (from 25 to 35 per cent of occipital seizures) by Bancaud (1969), Ludwig & Ajmone Marsan (1975), Herranz Tanarro et al. (1984), Gastaut (1985), Cooper & Lee (1991) and Lerman & Kivity (1991). They are less frequent in the series of Beaumanoir (1983), Newton & Aicardi (1983), Terasaki et al. (1987) (from 12.5 to 20 per cent), though very frequent, 57 per cent, in the one of Panayiotopoulos (1989a). In the infant, eye deviation is often the only sign of an ictal occipital discharge. At this age, eye jerks and eyelid blinking may occur without a preceding ocular deviation: the polyspike and wave discharge is localized to the posterior areas of the scalp.

Fois et al. (1988) reported an ictal strabismus in two patients. They do not give full details of their observations, but this symptomatology appears to be exceptional.

Ocular jerks following eye adversion may last several seconds. The patient may complain of blurring of vision, sensations of disequilibrium or environment tipping, receding when ocular clonic movements stop, and may refer to it as vertigo.

Semiology of partial seizures arising from the involvement of the cortical area or anatomo-functional systems connected to visual areas

Epileptic discharges in structures connected to the visual cortex may provoke ictal events other than visual or oculomotor events. Adversion of the head can be followed by convulsive movements sometimes limited to the face. However, hemiconvulsions are more frequent: 50 per cent of the patients of Panayiotopoulos (1989a), 43 per cent of those of Gastaut & Zifkin (1984, 1987). These seizures are exceptional during daytime. A tonic axial deviation of the body together with an oculogyric seizure, experienced by the patient as vertigo, was reported by one of our patients. This tonic symptomatology was described in 11 per cent of patients of Ludwig & Ajmone Marsan (1975) but only in two of 63 patients of Gastaut (1985).

Gestural or oral automatisms accompanied or not by autonomic disorders may characterize the seizure. These signs are supposed to arise from the secondary ictal discharge of the basal limbic structures connected to the visual cortex V1.

Epileptic vomiting

This rare sign is reported mainly in frontal or frontotemporal epilepsies. Ricci et al. (1989), who were able to record this phenomenon four times (in two of the cases the ictal discharge was occipital) estimate it has no localizing value. On the other side, Panayiotopoulos (1993) states this is one of the fundamental symptoms of ICEOP. Vomiting is not the only sign; in fact, it can be the first manifestation of a prolonged seizure occurring during sleep. However, without an ictal EEG recording it is impossible to say if subjective symptoms did not precede vomiting. During daytime seizures, nausea is rare and may accompany the ictal visceral sensation.

Headaches

An epileptic cephalalgic seizure or an epileptic migraine is very rare; 1.3 per cent of the population of Blume & Young (1987). The cases explored by stereo-EEG show that the neocortex is not concerned in the discharge, which usually begins in the limbic area (Laplante et al., 1983; Isler et al., 1987). In children with ICEOP the cephalgic attack may be frequent: nine of the 63 patients of Lerman & Kivity (1986) complained of headache during the course of the seizure. Aso et al. (1987, 1988) show that in children headache is more frequently described in ICEOP than in symptomatic occipital epilepsy.

Duration of occipital seizures

Simple partial visual seizures are brief. Partial oculomotor seizures and seizures with automatisms can last from 1 to 2 min.

In children, nocturnal seizures with a complex autonomic symptomatology, often accompanied by loss of consciousness, can be prolonged and last several hours, as reported by Panayiotopoulos (1993) and by Vigevano & Ricci (1993). The loss of consciousness described only in prolonged seizures is never immediate.

Postictal symptomatology

Simple partial visual and oculomotor seizures end without postictal signs. After more prolonged seizures, headache, sometimes resembling a migrainous attack, is common enough (33 per cent of Gastaut & Zifkin's patients, 1987; Beaumanoir, 1993). As Deonna *et al.* (1986) or Lerman & Kivity (1991) point out, when the seizure is brief, it may be difficult to know whether the headache is ictal or postictal or both. The same applies to deficitary prolonged visual disturbances.

Activating and precipitating factors

Slow sleep is known to facilitate the prolongation and propagation of an occipital discharge, particularly in children. This explains why prolonged non-visual seizures of ICEOP are mainly nocturnal (Panayiotopoulos, 1993). Precipitating factors involve different ways of retinal stimulation. Occipital seizures occur in the same patient (one out of five times) when the light is suddenly switched on or when the patient steps into the light coming from a dark room (Lugaresi *et al.*, 1984; Beaumanoir *et al.*, 1989). Intermittent photic stimulation can equally be effective, as are, more rarely, saccadic eye movements of exploration.

The electroencephalogram

The total number of ictal EEGs reported until now does not allow an estimate of the possible difference between child and adult seizure discharges. Recorded seizures more often belong to a symptomatic occipital epilepsy in the adult, and to a benign occipital partial epilepsy in the child.

(a) Simple partial occipital seizures with positive signs are characterized by fast spike (S) activities which, when slowing down, can reach neighbouring regions of the scalp. While the amplitude of ictal activity increases, the frequency of repetition lessens. In oculoclonic seizures, spikes and spike and waves (S–W) are typical of the last part of the discharge. There are usually no postictal abnormalities. Phosphenes are related to the fast S activity, often quickly involving the two hemispheres; on the contrary, when the discharge is slower, complex hallucinations may take place.

In oculoclonic seizures, a localized occipital ictal fast S rhythm may be observed for a few seconds before the deviation of the eyes.

Case No. 1. A 10-year-old boy, suffering since the age of 6 from frequent sensory visual seizures. Neurological and psycho-intellectual features are normal. CT scan is normal (Fig. 1).

Case No. 2. Infant, real age 9 months. Born at 33 weeks, he suffered from a developmental dysharmonia, frequent daytime seizures with eye deviation, spasms and eyelid clonias during sleep (Fig. 2).

This case is similar to those described by Lortie *et al.* (1993). The observation (courtesy of Dr Laura Mira, Neurological Department, Ospedale dei Bambini 'Vittore Buzzi', Milan) of a provoked seizure in a premature infant at the crucial age for the maturation of oculomotor systems suggests to us a prospective study of electroclinical occipital seizures in the course of the development.

Case No. 4. A boy, 14 years old, presented frequent sensory visual seizures and rare ocular adversive seizures between the ages of 7 and 12. For some months he had been experiencing

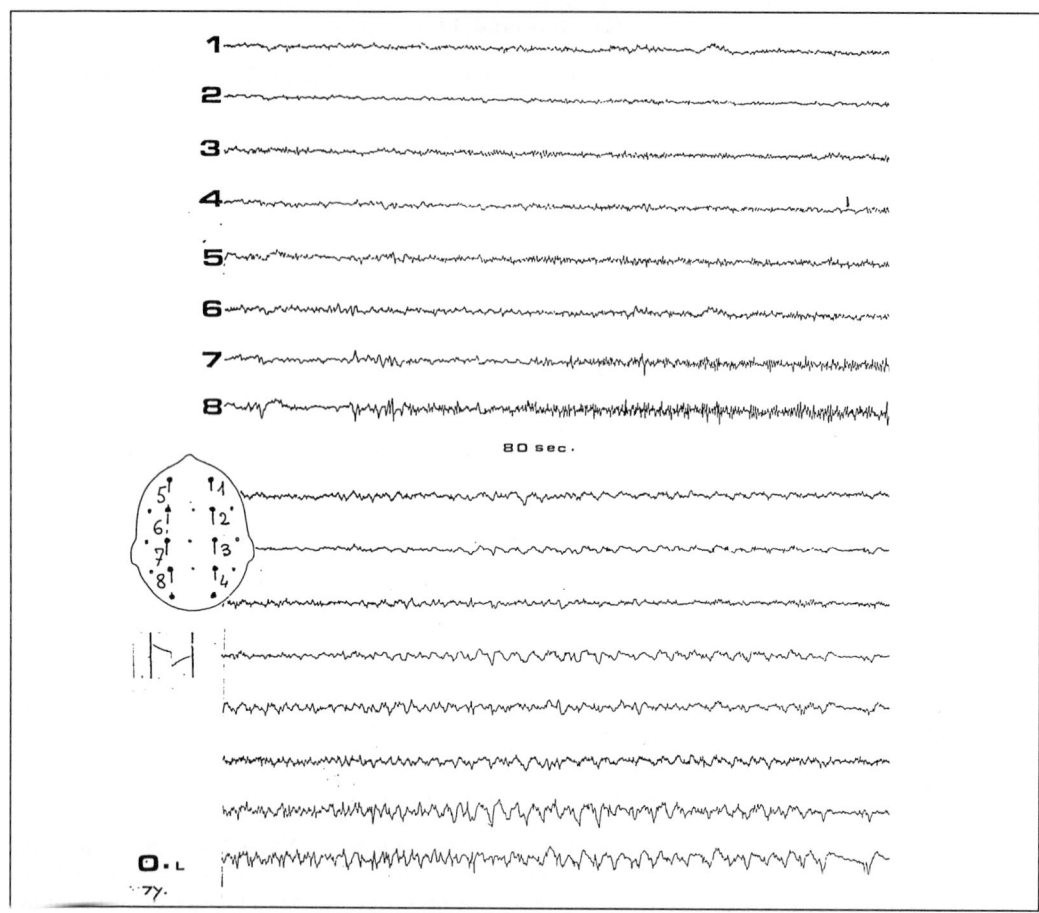

Fig. 1 (Case 1). In 8, parieto-occipital fast rhythms strictly localized on the occipital electrode. At this time, scintillating phosphenes. After 4 s the discharge reaches the parieto-occipital region; at this time the child sees a bundle of coloured balloons swinging in his right hemifield. This phase lasts 40 s. Then slow spikes appear, progressively slowing and spreading diffusely over the scalp. During this slow activity (bottom of figure) the patient complains of clouded vision.
A 6-year-old boy suffering since the age of three from visual seizures. At age 3 years he had a nocturnal left hemiconvulsion. The first EEG shows continuous S–W on the low occipital territories. It is a typical fixation off sensitivity spikes (FOSS) focus (Panayiotopoulos, 1983). Since age 4 years many brief sensory seizures (simple coloured hallucinations) are provoked by sudden darkness. This scotosensitive seizure often appears when the patient is in bed and the light is switched off (Fig. 3).

oculoclonic seizures preceded by visual symptomatology. This record depicts the EEG described by many authors during oculoclonic occipital seizures (Figs. 4a–c).

(b) Deficient epileptic occipital seizures with positive signs have rarely been recorded, with the exception of stereo EEG explorations. In Case No. 5 of Gastaut & Zifkin (1987) the record demonstrates that a progressive loss of vision occurs several seconds after the beginning of the ictal discharge, when the EEG shows bilateral delta slow waves.

In one of our cases, as in the one of Huott *et al.* (1974), or in Case No. 3 of Aso *et al.* (1987), or in one of the three cases of Jaffe & Roach (1988), and in the one of Aldrich *et al.* (1989), though

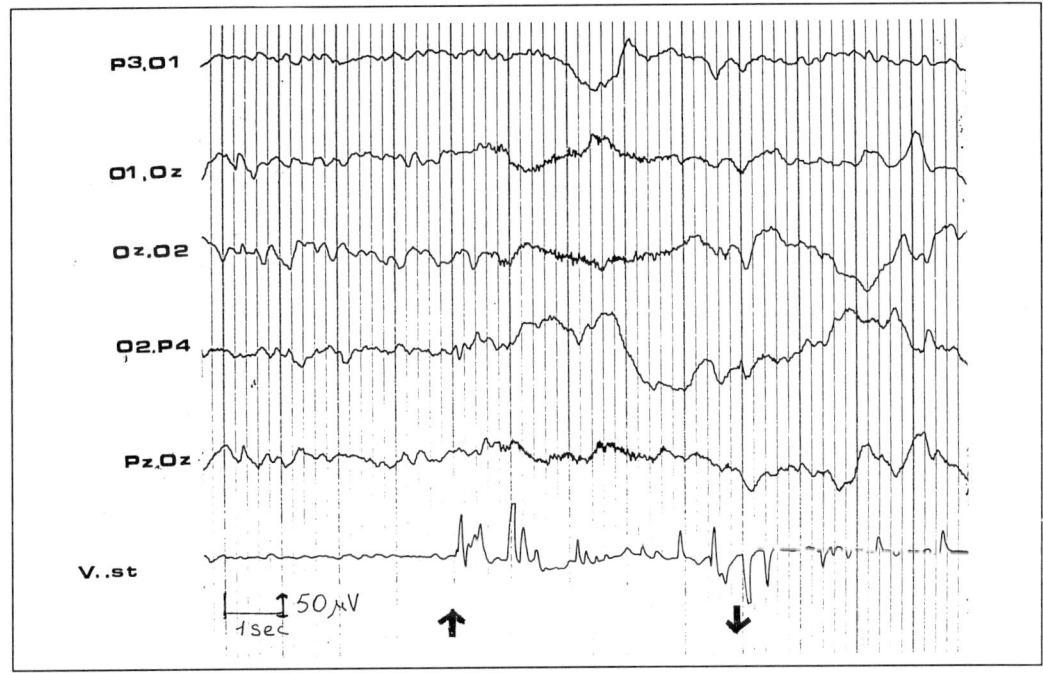

Fig. 2 (Case 2). Eye deviation to the right and lateral globus saccades. Then the eyes return to the front.

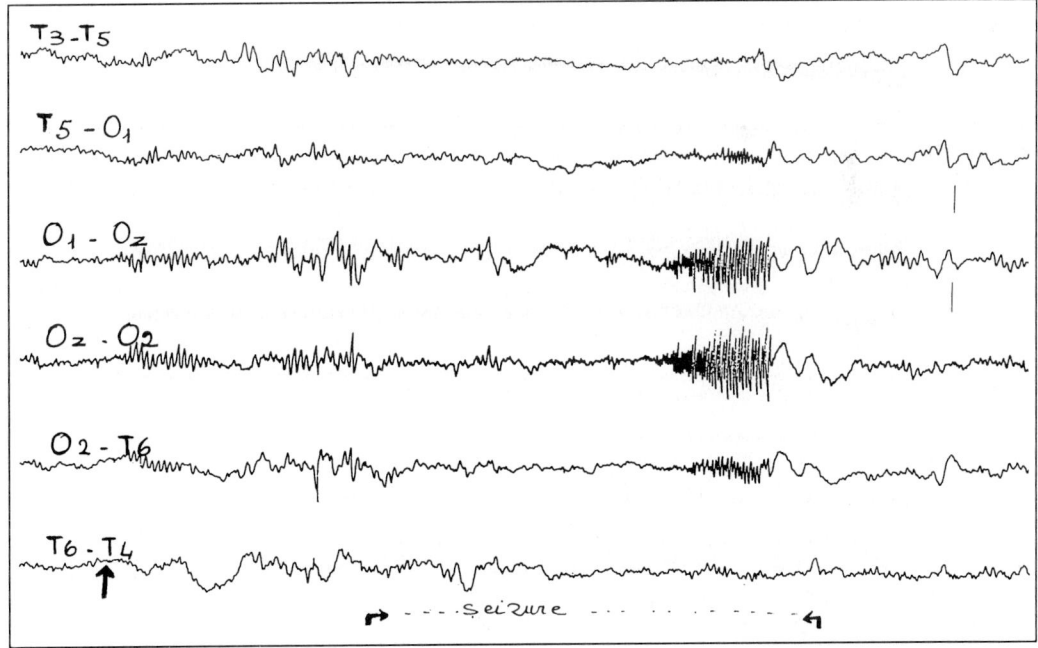

Fig. 3 (Case 3). This recording indicates the simple sensory seizure – see the fast spikes in the occipital discharges.

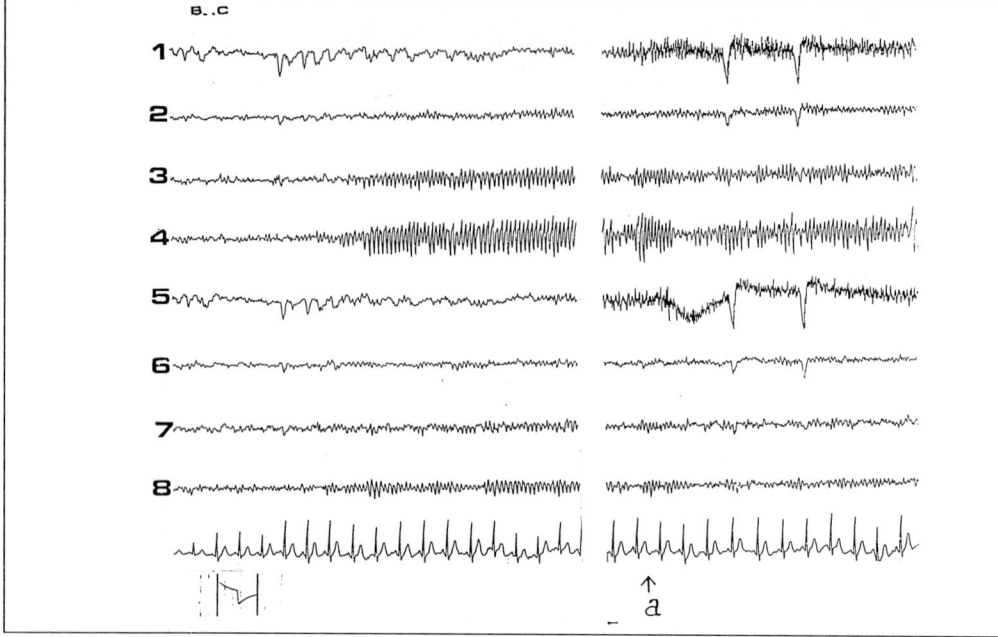

Fig. 4(a).

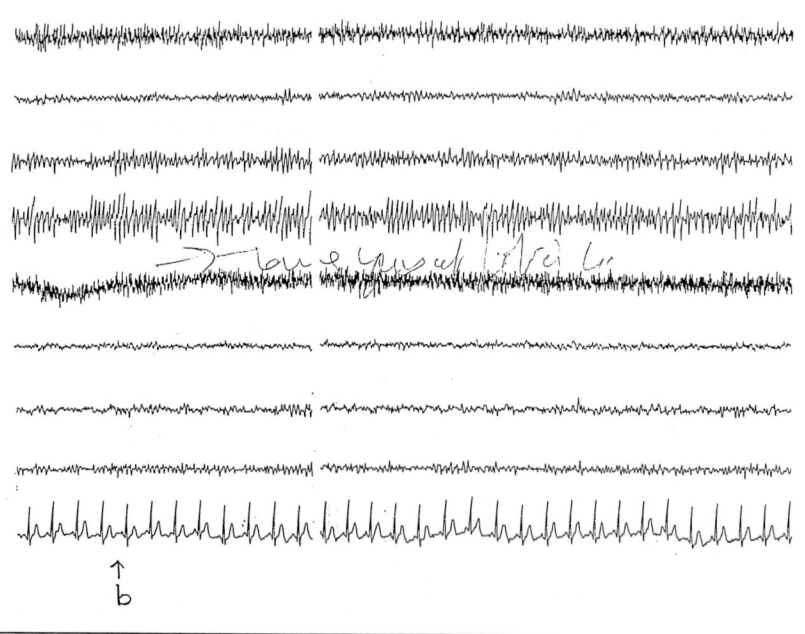

Fig. 4(b).

Chapter 9 Semiology of occipital seizures in infants and children

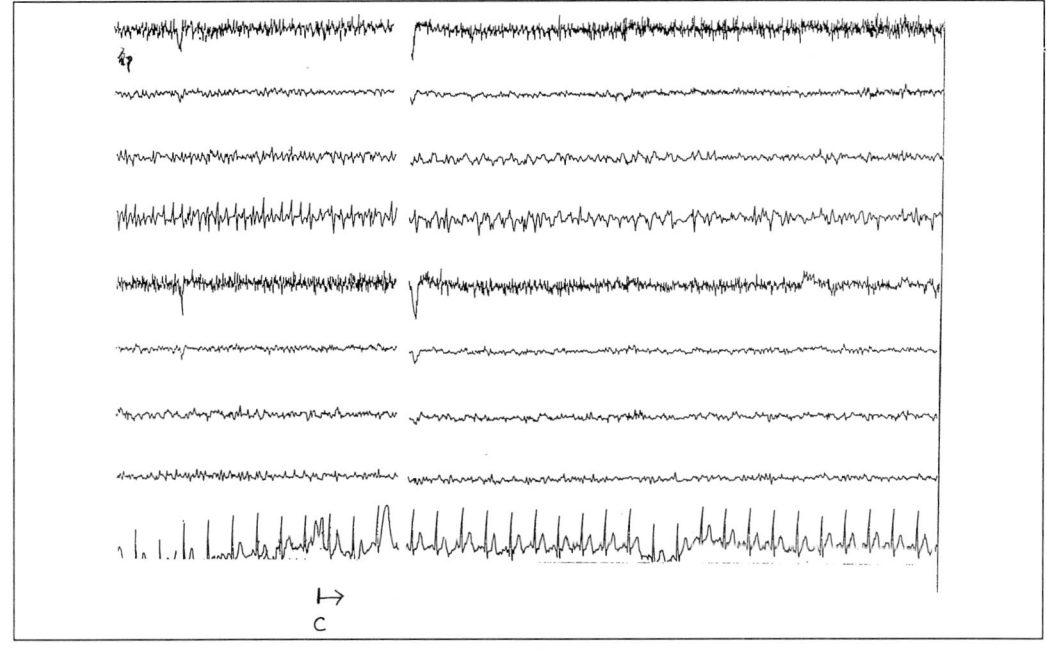

Fig. 4(c)

Fig. 4 (a, b, c): 1 = F2–F4; 2 = F4–C4; 3 = C4–P4; 4 = P4–O4; 5 = F1–F3; 5 = F3–C3; 7 = C3–P3; 8 = P3–O3; 1.5 cm = 1 s; 0.5 cm = 50 mV

The critical discharge starts in 4. After 1 s it is recorded in 3 as well as in 8 and 7. Thse bilateral higher discharges, starting on the right, last 18 s and are accompanied by coloured scintillating phosphenes. Then, in 'a', the eyes are deviated to the left; a brief and incomplete return to the normal position occurs twice. In 'b' of Fig. 4b the head starts to deviate tonically to the left. After 35 s the eyes return to the normal position with some saccades. The tonic deviation first of the eyes, then of the head, is over in 'c' of Fig. 4c.

these epilepsies are of different aetiology, the EEG during temporary blindness shows that the morphology of these abnormalities is different from that recorded during positive ictal signs.

Case No. 5. Concerns a 17-year-old girl presenting visual seizures with positive symptoms since the age of 9. She had undergone surgical correction of congenital squinting at 5 years. Her mother suffers from migraine. In 2 years, she has had two seizures (Fig. 5) with hemianopsia followed by headaches of short duration. CT scan was normal.

It is noteworthy that slow waves and pseudoperiodic sharp waves are seen in the only seizure with loss of vision and autonomic disorders among all the seizures recorded in Aso's patients, while in the other five patients with visual or motor symptoms the ictal record shows fast rhythms. Headaches have never been recorded during brief seizures; on the other hand, they have been documented by EEG records when associated with other symptoms, especially a visual deficit as in Case No. 4 of Aso et al. (1987) or autonomic symptomatology as in our Cases No. 5 and 6.

Case No. 6. An 8-year-old girl suffering from typical idiopathic partial epilepsy with FOS (fixation off sensitivity, see Fig. 6a). The first daytime sensory seizures occurred at 5 years of age. The first night-time seizures were noted at about 5 1/2 years. Her parents are warned by noises made by vomiting efforts. The child is awake, sometimes she is sitting in bed; her look is vague; she is not unconscious but appears clouded. She cannot answer questions because of vomiting efforts; sometimes she replies yes or no correctly. Her face is red, she cries. Her mother reports tachycardia. The girl complains about diffuse headache and after the seizures says that her vision was disturbed. The three seizures witnessed by her parents lasted 10–20 min (Figs. 6b–e).

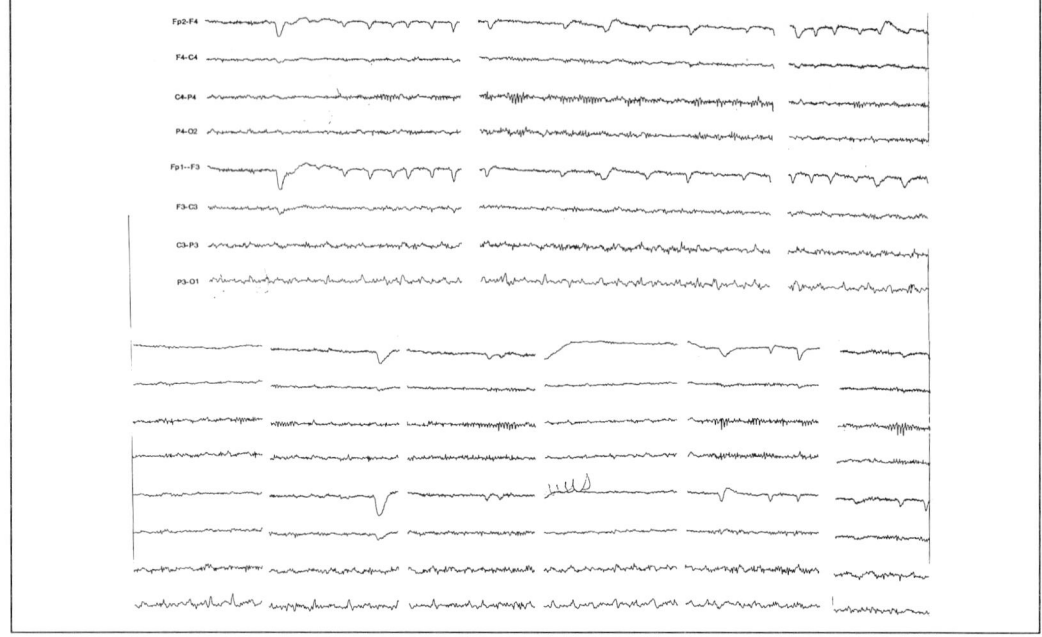

Fig. 5 (Case 5). Discharge duration: 7 minutes (any break corresponds to 45 s). See the pseudoperiodic sharp discharges on 01. During these slow sharp discharges the patient suffers from hemianopsia. The discharge is similar to those recorded during migraine (Beaumanoir, 1983).

In this case the seizure is revealed by slow waves which diffuse rapidly on both hemispheres and stop abruptly without lasting postictal abnormalities. In this respect it differs from migrainous attacks. However, the appearance of monomorphic diffuse slow waves, sometimes independent from the focal discharge (as in Case No. 21 of Aso), characterized by fast rhythms progressively slowing down, evokes an extracortical origin of the migrainous manifestations. This may express, as Beaumanoir & Jekiel (1987) already suggested and as also has been suggested by Gastaut & Zifkin (1987), the involvement of brainstem structures regulating cerebral vasomotricity in the course of the ictal discharge usually occurring in slow sleep.

These seizures could also be the consequence of kindling of basal limbic structures, though when the typical or oral and alimentary automatisms occur, ictal EEG abnormalities are characterized by slow waves, different in morphology, topography and frequency, as shown in Cases 1 and 2.

Electroclinical commentary

(a) Ictal discharges characterized by low amplitude fast spike activities confined to the occipital poles, of a few seconds duration, accompanying visual hallucinations or more rarely scotomas or very brief amaurosis sensation. It could correspond to the first seconds of critical EEG discharge on Fig. 1.

(b) Occipital fast spike discharge progressively slowing down while spreading to neighbouring areas, and sometimes to the other hemisphere. It can occasionally end with spikes and waves accompanying a simple partial seizure characterized by hallucinations and eye adversion followed or not by ocular jerks. This focal discharge can follow the discharge 'a' of Fig. 4.

(c) Occipital discharge of type 'a' or 'b', followed by motor, sensorimotor or temporal seizures. The rapidity of spreading of the occipital discharge is noteworthy (Figs. 4b, c).

Chapter 9 Semiology of occipital seizures in infants and children

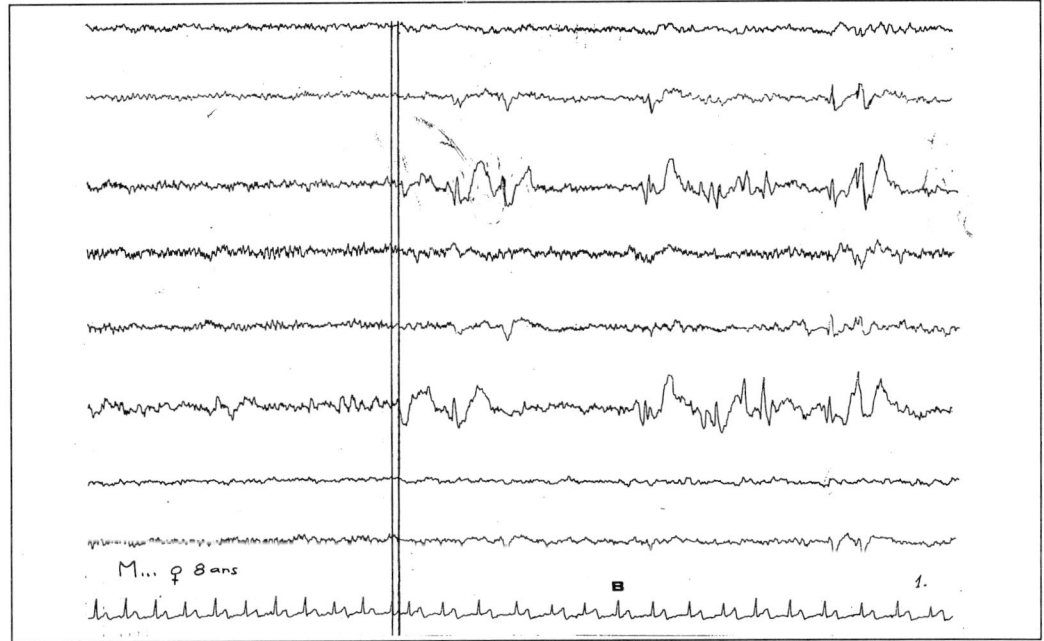

Fig. 6(a) (Case 6). Ambulatory continuous EEG recording. Observations:
$1 = F_{p1} - C_3$; $2 = C_3 - T_3$; $3 = T_3 - O_3$; $4, 5$ & $6 = 1, 2$ & 3 *on the left side*; $7 = F_Z - C_Z$; $8 = C_Z - P_Z$. *In B, eyes closed.*

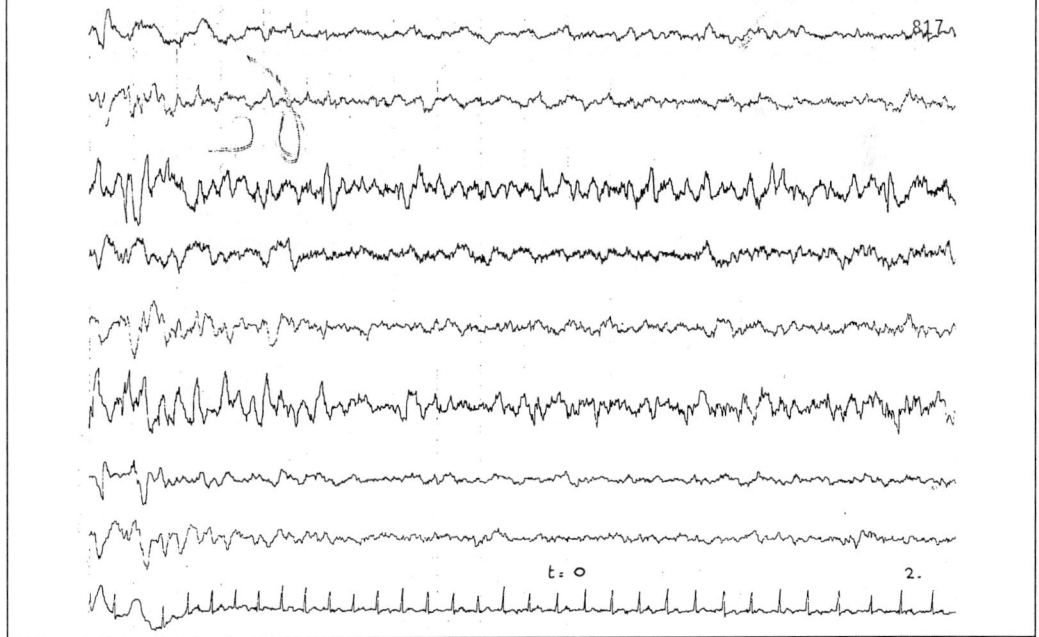

Fig. 6(b).

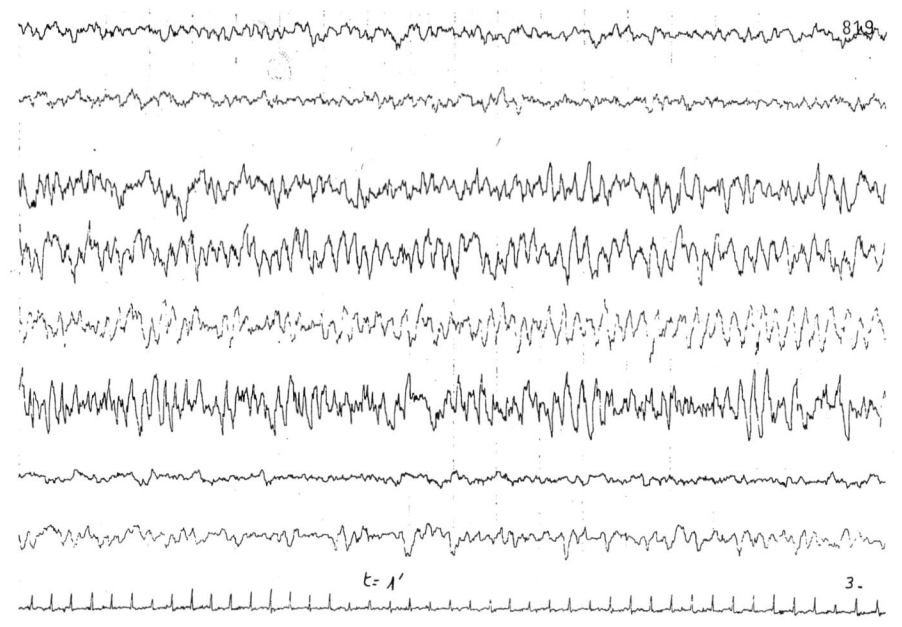

Fig. 6(c).

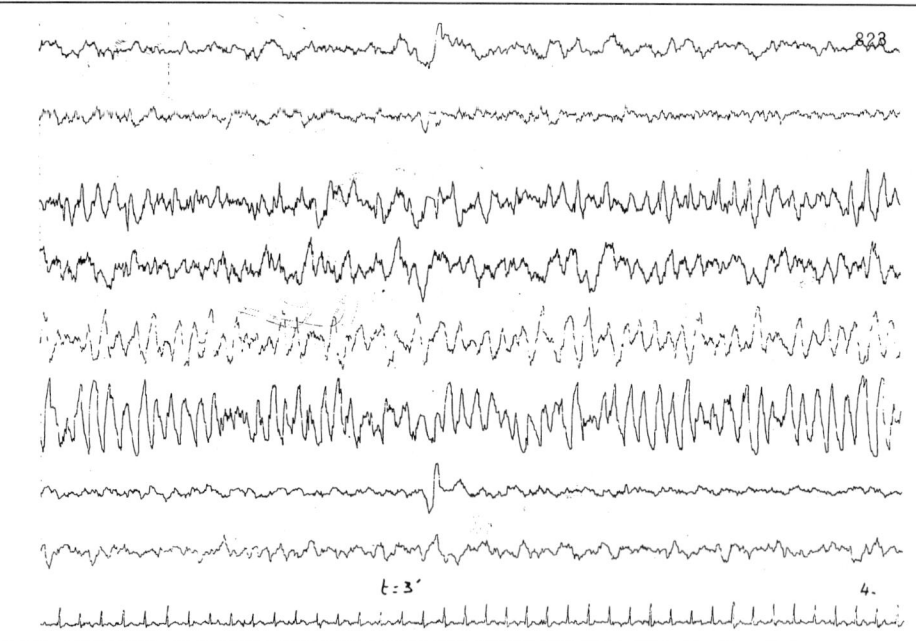

Fig. 6(d).

Chapter 9 Semiology of occipital seizures in infants and children

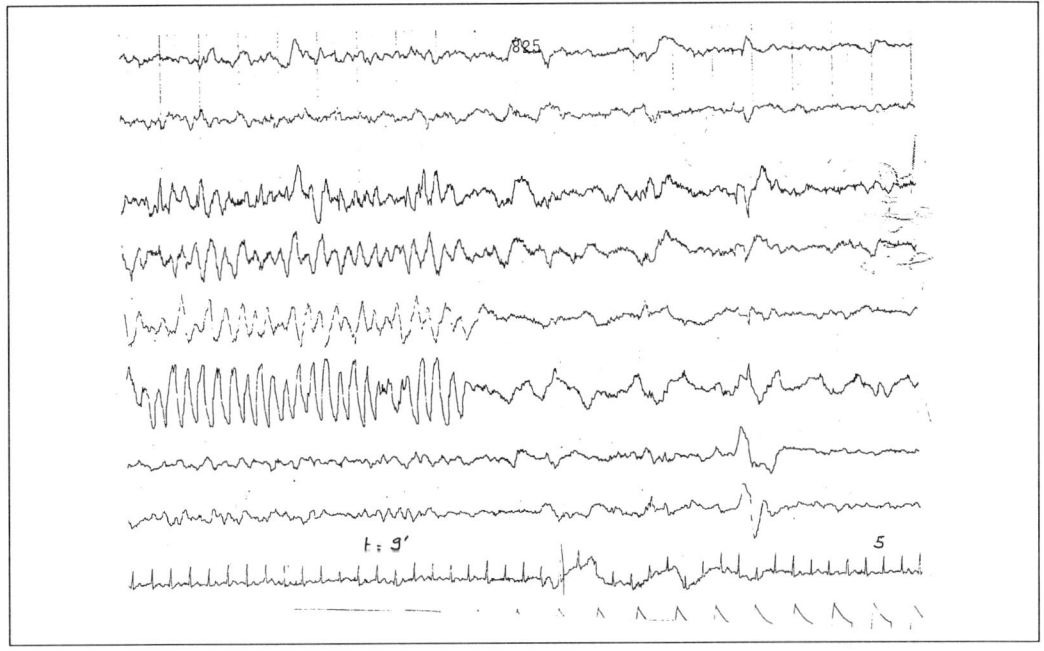

Fig. 6(e)
Figure 6a, b, c, d, e. Dynamic continuous recording (24 h).
During night-time sleep, at 12.45 a.m., second sequence of slow sleep (stage 2).
Critical discharge: 6b time 0, 6c time 1 min, 6d 3 min, 6e end.
The discharge lasted 9 min. The child was awake, with open eyes. She made frequent vomiting efforts, and complained about frontal headache.

(d) Occipital discharge of type 'a' or 'b' associated or quickly followed by ictal abnormalities as monomorphic delta waves in the bioccipital-temporal area. More often the abnormalities are diffuse, corresponding to autonomic symptoms which can evoke a basilar migraine (Fig. 6a).

Conclusion

The present data concerning electroclinical aspects of occipital seizures do not allow us to characterize different ictal patterns corresponding to developmental steps of visual pathways and functions. However, the child seems to be more likely than the adult to present seizures arising from an occipital focus. These seizures in the young child are more easily influenced by sleep than in the adult.

Some prolonged nocturnal seizures, with a symptomatology similar in some respects to basilar migraine (and which are fully described by Panayiotopoulos (1993) as well as by Vigevano & Ricci (1993)) are a prerogative of children with ICEOP.

Acknowledgement
The author thanks Drs. Laura Mira and Andrée Van Lierde for their help in revising the English version of this paper.

References

Aicardi, J. & Newton, R. (1987): Clinical findings in children with occipital wave complexes suppressed by eye opening. In: *Migraine and epilepsy*, eds. F. Andermann & E. Lugaresi, pp. 111–124. Boston, London: Butterworths.

Aldrich, M.S., Vanderzaut, C.W., Alessi, A.G., Aban-Khalil, B. & Sackellares, J. C. (1989): Ictal cortical blindness with permanent visual loss. *Epilepsia* **30**, 116–120.

Aso, K., Watanabe, K., Negro, T., Takaesu, E., Furune, E., Furune, A., Takahashi, I., Yamamoto, N. & Nomura, K. (1987): Visual seizures in children. *Epilepsy Res.* **1**, 246–253.

Aso, K., Watanabe, K., Takaesu, E., Furune, E., Takahashi, I., Yamamoto, N. & Nomura, K. (1988): Photosensitive partial seizures: the origin of abnormal discharges. *J. Epilepsy* **2**, 87–93.

Avanzini, G. (1993): Structures and functions of the occipital lobe. In: *Occipital seizures and epilepsies in children*, eds. F. Andermann, A. Beaumanoir, L. Mira, J. Roger & C.A. Tassinari, pp. 31–41. London: John Libbey.

Bancaud, J. (1969): Les crises épileptiques d'origine occipitale (étude stéréo-électroencéphalographique). *Rev. Otoneuroophthalmol.* **41**, 299.

Bancaud, J., Bonis, A., Morel, P., Talairach, J., Szikla, G. & Tournoux, P. (1961): Epilepsie occipitale à expression 'rhinencéphalique' prévalente. *Rev. Neurol. (Paris)* **121**, 297–305.

Beaumanoir A. (1983): Infantile epilepsy with occipital focus and good prognosis. *Eur. Neurol.* **22**, 43–52.

Beaumanoir, A. & Jekiel, M. (1987): Electrographic observations during attacks of classical migraine. In: *Migraine and epilepsy*, eds. F. Andermann & E. Lugaresi, pp. 163–180. Boston, London: Butterworths.

Beaumanoir, A., Capizzi, G., Nahory, A. & Yousfi, Y. (1989): Scotogenic seizures. In *Reflex seizures and reflex epilepsies*, eds. A. Beaumanoir, H. Gastaut & R. Naquet, pp. 203–217. Genève: Médecine et Hygiène.

Beaumanoir, A. (1993): An EEG contribution to the study of migraine and of the association of migraine and epilepsy in childhood. In: *Occipital seizures and epilepsies in children*, eds. F. Andermann, A. Beaumanoir, L. Mira, J. Roger & C.A. Tassinari, pp. 101–110. London: John Libbey.

Blume, W.T. & Young, G.B. (1987) Ictal pain: unilateral, cephalic and abdominal. In: *Migraine and epilepsy*, eds. F. Andermann & E. Lugaresi, pp. 235–247. Boston, London: Butterworths.

Cooper, G.W. & Lee, S.I. (1991): Reactive occipital epileptiform activity: is it benign? *Epilepsia* **32**, 63–68.

Delwaide, P. J., Barragan, M. & Gastaut, H. (1971): Remarques sur une épilepsie partielle: l'épilepsie occipitale. *Acta Neurol. Belg.* **71**, 383–391.

Deonna, T., Ziegler, H.L. & Despland P.A. (1984): Paroxysmal visual disturbance of epileptic origin and occipital epilepsy in children. *Neuropediatrics* **15**, 131–135.

Deonna, T., Ziegler, H.L., Despland P.A. & Van Melle G. (1986): Partial epilepsy in neurologically normal children: clinical syndromes and prognosis. *Epilepsia* **27**, 241–247.

Engel, J., Kuhl, D.E., Phelps, M.E., Rausch, R. & Nuwer, M. (1983): Local cerebral metabolism during partial seizures. *Neurology* **33**, 400–413.

Fois, A., Malandrini, F. & Tomaccini, D. (1988): Clinical findings in children with occipital paroxysmal discharges. *Epilepsia* **29**, 620–623.

Gastaut, H. & Roger, A. (1954): Formes inhabituelles de l'épilepsie: le nystagmus épileptique. *Rev. Neurol.* **90/2**, 130–132.

Gastaut, H. (1960): Un aspect méconnu des décharges neuroniques occipitales: la crise oculoclonique ou 'nystagmus épileptique'. In: *Les grandes activités du lobe occipital*, ed. T. Alajouanine, pp. 169–185. Paris: Masson.

Gastaut, H. & Zifkin, B.G. (1984): Ictal visual hallucinations of numerals. *Neurology* **34**, 950–953.

Gastaut, H. (1985): Benign epilepsy of childhood with occipital paroxysms. In: *Epileptic syndromes in infancy, childhood and adolescence*, eds. J. Roger, C. Dravet, M. Bureau, F.E. Dreifuss & P. Wolf, pp. 137–149. London: John Libbey.

Gastaut, H. & Zifkin, B.G. (1987) Benign epilepsy of childhood with occipital spike and wave complexes. In: *Migraine and epilepsy*, eds. F. Andermann & E. Lugaresi, pp. 47–81. Boston, London: Butterworths.

Gibbs, E.L., Gillen, H.W. & Gibbs, F.A. (1954): Disappearance and migration of epileptic foci in children. *Am. J. Dis. Child.* **88**, 596–603.

Herranz Tanarro, F.J., Lope, E.S. & Sassot, S.C. (1984): La pointe-onde occipitale avec et sans épilepsie bénigne chez l'enfant. *Rev. EEG Neurophysiol.* **14**, 1–7.

Huott, A. D., Madison, D.S & Niedermeyer, D. (1974): Occipital lobe epilepsy. A clinical and electroencephalographic study. *Eur. Neurol.* **11**, 325–39.

Imbert, M. (1993): Ontogenesis of the occipital lobe. In: *Occipital seizures and epilepsies in children*, eds. F. Andermann, A. Beaumanoir, L. Mira, J. Roger & C.A. Tassinari, pp. 3–8. London: John Libbey.

Isler, H., Wieser, H. G. & Egli, M. (1987): Hemicraniia epileptica: synchronous ipsilateral ictal headache with migraine features. In: *Migraine and epilepsy*, eds. F. Andermann & E. Lugaresi, pp. 249–263. Boston, London: Butterworths.

Jaffe, S. J. & Roach, E.S. (1988): Transient cortical blindness with occipital lobe epilepsy. *J. Clin. Neuroophthalmol.* **8**, 221–224.

Lagae, L. & Casaer, P. (1993): Visual testing in the first 2 years of life. In: *Occipital seizures and epilepsies in children*, eds. F. Andermann, A. Beaumanoir, L. Mira, J. Roger & C.A. Tassinari, pp. 43–48. London: John Libbey.

Lanzi, G. & Balottin, U. (1993): The semiology of migraine attacks in childhood. In: *Occipital seizures and epilepsies in children*, eds. F. Andermann, A. Beaumanoir, L. Mira, J. Roger & C.A. Tassinari, pp. 87–91. London: John Libbey.

Laplante, P., Saint Hilaire, J.M. & Bouvier, G. (1983): Headache as an epileptic manifestation. *Neurology* **33**, 1493–1495.

Lerman, P. & Kivity, S. (1986): Benign focal epilepsies of childhood. In: *Recent advances in epilepsy*, vol. 3, eds. T.A. Peddley & B.S. Meldrum, pp. 136–156. London: Churchill- Livingstone.

Lerman, K. & Kivity, S. (1991): The benign partial non-rolandic epilepsies. *J. Clin. Neurophysiol.* **8**, 275–287.

Lortie, A., Plouin, P., Pinard, J.M. & Dulac, O. (1993): Occipital epilepsy in neonates and infants. In: *Occipital seizures and epilepsies in children*, eds. F. Andermann, A. Beaumanoir, L. Mira, J. Roger & C.A. Tassinari, pp. 121–132. London: John Libbey.

Ludwig, B. & Ajmone-Marsan, C. (1975): Clinical ictal patterns in epileptic patients with occipital electroencephalographic foci. *Neurology* **25**, 463–471.

Lugaresi, E., Cirignotta, F. & Montagna, P. (1984): Occipital lobe epilepsy with scotosensitive seizures: the role of central vision. *Epilepsia* **25**, 115–120.

Kinast, M., Lauders, H., Rothner, D. & Erengerg, G. (1982): Benign local epileptiform discharges in childhood migraine (BFEDC). *Neurology* **32**, 1309–1311.

Mira, L. & Van Lierde, A. (1993): EEG in children with visual pathways damage. In: *Occipital seizures and epilepsies in children*, eds. F. Andermann, A. Beaumanoir, L. Mira, J. Roger & C.A. Tassinari, pp. 65–70. London: John Libbey.

Munari, C., Tassi, L., Francione, S., Kahane, P., Malapani, C., Lo Russo, G. & Hoffmann, D. (1993): Occipital seizures with childhood onset in severe partial epilepsy: a surgical perspective. In: *Occipital seizures and epilepsies in children*, eds. F. Andermann, A. Beaumanoir, L. Mira, J. Roger & C.A. Tassinari, pp. 203–211. London: John Libbey.

Nalin, A., Ruggerini, C., Ferrari, E., Galli, V., Ferrari, P. & Finelli, T. (1989): Clinique, diagnostic différentiel et évolution des crises épileptiques visuelles de l'enfant. *Neurophysiol. Clin.* **19**, 25–36.

Newton, R. & Aicardi, J. (1983): Clinical findings in children with occipital spike-wave complexes suppressed by eye-opening. *Neurology* **33**, 1526–1529.

Panayiotopoulos, C.P. (1989a): Benign nocturnal childhood occipital epilepsy: a new syndrome with nocturnal seizures, tonic deviation of the eyes and vomiting. *J. Child. Neurol.* **4**, 43–48.

Panayiotopoulos, C.P. (1989b): Benign childhood epilepsy with occipital paroxysms. A 15 year prospective study. *Ann. Neurol.* **26**, 51–56.

Panayiotopoulos, C.P. (1993): Benign childhood epilepsy with occipital paroxysms. In: *Occipital seizures and epilepsies in children*, eds. F. Andermann, A. Beaumanoir, L. Mira, J. Roger & C.A. Tassinari, pp. 151–164 London: John Libbey.

Penfield, W. & Kristiansen, K. (1951): Epileptic seizure patterns, pp. 22–33. Springfield, IL: Charles C. Thomas.

Ricci, S., Di Capua, M. & Fusco, L. (1989): Il vomito come sintomo critico. *Boll. Lega Ital. Epil.* **66**, 285–287.

Rosenbaum, D.H., Siegal, M. & Rowan, A.J. (1986): Contraversive seizures in occipital epilepsy: case report and review of the literature. *Neurology* **36**, 281–284.

Schaffler, L. & Karbowski, K. (1988): Zur Frage der epileptischen Aktivität des Okzipitallapens. *Fortschr. Neurol. Psychiatr.* **56/9**, 286–299.

Smith, I.M.B. & Kellaway, P., (1963): The natural history and clinical correlates of occipital foci in children. In: *Neurogical and electroencephalographic correlative studies in infancy*, eds. P. Kellaway & I. Petersen, pp. 230–249. New York: Grune & Stratton.

Sokol, S. (1993) Neurophysiological study of visual functions in the development of the infant. In: *Occipital seizures and epilepsies in children*, eds. F. Andermann, A. Beaumanoir, L. Mira, J. Roger & C.A. Tassinari, pp. 49–57. London: John Libbey.

Spreafico, R. & Regondi, M.C. (1993) Ontogenesis of the GABAergic system. In: *Occipital seizures and epilepsies in children*, eds. F. Andermann, A. Beaumanoir, L. Mira, J. Roger & C.A. Tassinari, pp. 9–13. London: John Libbey.

Takeda, A., Bancaud, J., Talairach, J., Bonis, H. & Bordas-Ferrer, M. (1969): A propos des accès épileptiques d'origine occipitale. *Rev. Neurol. (Paris)* **121**, 306–315.

Terasaki, T., Yamatogi, Y. & Ohtahara, S. (1987): Electroclinical delineation of occipital lobe epilepsy in childhood. In: *Migraine and epilepsy*, eds. F. Andermann & E. Lugaresi, pp. 125–137. Boston, London: Butterworths.

Terzano, M.G, Parrino, L., Pietrini, V. & Galli, L. (1993): Migraine-epilepsy syndrome: intercalated seizures in benign occipital epilepsy. In: *Occipital seizures and epilepsies in children*, eds. F. Andermann, A. Beaumanoir, L. Mira, J. Roger & C.A. Tassinari, pp. 93–99. London: John Libbey.

Vigevano, F. & Ricci, S. (1993): Benign occipital epilepsy of childhood with prolonged seizures and autonomic symptoms. In: *Occipital seizures and epilepsies in children*, eds. F. Andermann, A. Beaumanoir, L. Mira, J. Roger & C.A. Tassinari, pp. 133–140. London: John Libbey.

Chapter 10

The semiology of migraine attacks in childhood

Giovani Lanzi and Umberto Balottin

Chair of Child Neuropsychiatry, Mondino Neurological Institute Foundation, IRCCS, University of Pavia, Italy

Summary

The authors describe the various patterns of migraine with and without aura and of migraine equivalents in children, according to the classification of the International Headache Society. Particular attention is paid to diagnostic criteria and criteria for possible alternative diagnoses.

Introduction

Semiotics and semiology are the study of the signs and symptoms of disease and the ways they may be detected. In his preface to Rasario's book on medical semiotics (Rasario, 1972) Luigi Condorelli wrote that anyone who wants to teach semiotics must first of all instil in the student's mind the concept that the method of observing the patient is primarily a mental discipline and that the traditional clinical approach must be more important than instrumental methods of investigation.

Condorelli developed these concepts, and emphasized that semiotics cannot be reduced to a dry list of symptoms which should be the expression of a particular disease, and that there was the risk, all the more real today, that young doctors might adopt an excessively pragmatic approach, replacing clinical methods with scientific, and particularly instrumental, investigations. Although this method of diagnosis may allow a name to be given to the disease, it does not give a clinical diagnosis in the sense Condorelli intended.

The opinion of this great clinician seems to fit the approach to the semiology of migraine attacks in children perfectly. Years after the first classification by the Ad Hoc Committee on Classification in 1962, and now the introduction of the recent 'Classification and Diagnostic Criteria for Headache Disorders, Cranial Neuralgias and Facial Pain' (Headache Classification Committee 1988), one might think that there is little to be said on the subject, even about paediatric migraine. But many important questions remain unanswered.

The problem of the clinical meaning of the so-called equivalents of childhood migraine is not yet resolved, nor is that of the boundaries and relationships between migraine and tension-type headache. It is in fact very difficult to distinguish clinically between episodic tension-type headache and migraine: many workers have always maintained that they are both part of the same spectrum of benign headache and differ only in severity.

Appenzeller (1976), Lanzi (1980), Silberstein (1990) and Ziegler (1976) have emphasized that episodes of tension-type headache and attacks of migraine with or without aura can often be found in the history of the same subject. In his book, Lanzi (1980) stressed that in situations of particular stress and fatigue patients with migraine often face more frequent attacks which take on the clinical aspects of chronic tension-type headaches, and that a few months' anti-migraine treatment may bring the patient back to the previous condition with headache-free intervals of variable length between attacks. On the other hand, or in parallel, Silberstein (1990) indicates that both migraine and episodic tension-type headache may become chronic daily headache or chronic tension-type headache as a result of the abuse of analgesics or ergotamine. On interruption of the drug, the headache frequently returns to its previous form.

We therefore believe that recently most authors have insisted on the existence of a continuum, at least in childhood, between migraine and tension-type headache. It is thus difficult to discuss the semiology of migraine attacks, but we shall attempt to keep to the subject we have been given.

To come back to the main theme of this chapter, Condorelli's text may be our guide as it indicates that the semiology of a migraine attack is not limited to a list of symptoms and signs but must be characterized by a clinical approach to the patients and their parents, which begins with a meeting of the person-doctor with the person-patients and their parents following an open, free and sympathetic pattern, which has been described many times by us and by many other authors (Balottin et al., 1989).

The anamnestic investigation is the element that should be taken into consideration with the utmost accuracy for the semiological definition of the disorder and for the correct formulation of diagnosis and treatment.

The history of children with migraine should be investigated with special care. The approach should be of a particular type – aimed at establishing a relationship with the patients, getting alongside them and putting oneself in their shoes as much as is possible, and data should be gathered from both the children and their parents. Furthermore, the data we need cover a range that is greater than in adult patients; it is necessary to inquire about the family relations with particular attention, about certain aspects of the physiological anamnesis (pregnancy, birth, neurological and psychological development, learning, social relations, and interfamilial relations), about any previous neurological or behavioural problems or psychosomatic conditions, and about all the consequences that the disorder has on the social and the family life of the child.

Naturally it will be necessary to test for the presence of infections of the paranasal sinuses, recurrent abdominal pain, epilepsy, diabetes, cranial traumas, vertigo, the use and abuse of drugs, ataxia, impairment of consciousness, fever, systemic diseases, and exposure to toxic substances or smoke. A complete neurological examination will also be necessary, with the assessment of the arterial pressure, weight, height, the investigation of the skin for the presence of petechiae, stripes, coffee coloured blotches, hypopigmented lesions, sebaceous adenomas or traumas indicating maltreatment; examination of the fundus oculi, cranial circumference and careful listening to the head for the presence of cranial bruit are also necessary.

As Lance (1982) has stressed, the first semiological element to be considered concerning the headache attack is its timescale. Four patterns are usually described: first, *acute headache* which may suggest a migraine attack but also meningitis, a subarachnoid haemorrhage or possibly an encephalitis, a post-traumatic syndrome, a glaucoma or an optic neuritis.

The second pattern is *recurrent headache attacks*: these suggest migraine unless there are significant modifications or deteriorations in the characteristics of the headache.

The third possibility is *progressive chronic headache* attacks: these often indicate the presence of a primary neurological disorder which is caused by a tumour, a subdural haematoma, or a brain abscess.

The fourth possibility is *non-progressive chronic headache*. This pattern is found in chronic tension-type headache (chronic daily headache), in which all the literature indicates the presence of a significant psychological component.

Paediatric migraine has a variety of clinical expressions; the most common symptom is headache. Hockaday (1988) defines all recurrent paroxysmal headaches in childhood as migraine if there is a return to normal mental and physical health in the interval between attacks.

This type of diagnostic and semiological approach to the problem seems acceptable and simple even though it is clear that it does not resolve the problem of the boundary between migraine and episodic tension-type headache mentioned above.

We shall thus follow the 1988 international classification of headache disorders as a guide to the semiology of migraine attacks.

Migraine without aura may already occur, as has been emphasized in the literature, at an age of less than 2–3 years. In such circumstances it has been written that the headache is less intense but that the gastrointestinal symptoms should be more noticeable. There are generally very few characteristics in juvenile migraine which have been demonstrated to be really different from adults. Indeed the most frequent location is the frontal area, the pain is pulsating, but often also pressing or tightening, and tends to be bilateral rather than monolateral. It is associated with nausea and/or vomiting, and phonophobia and/or photophobia. The pain worsens with physical activity. Furthermore, in the majority of cases (60 per cent according to Manzoni *et al.*, 1989) the attack lasts less than an hour.

Some character features which make the migrainous child in some way 'different' from other children have been reported. Such children (Bille, 1989) are sadder, more vulnerable to frustration and anxiety, with less basic confidence and optimism. These features are not universally accepted; personally we believe, in line with numerous studies, that they are valid (Lanzi *et al.*, 1989).

Migraine with aura is an idiopathic chronic disorder with attacks of neurological symptoms which may be located in the cerebral cortex or brain stem, and headache. These disorders usually develop slowly, over 5–20 min, and last less than 60 min. Headache, nausea and photophobia generally follow the symptoms of the neurological aura after a short symptom-free interval or directly. The headache lasts between 4 and 72 h and may sometimes be absent (migraine aura without headache). In the form with a typical aura the main symptom is visual disturbance sometimes followed by unilateral sensorial disturbance, hemiparesis or dysphasia or a combination.

It has been amply demonstrated in the literature that migraine with aura is much less frequent than the form without aura, even though some workers, for example Zammarano *et al.* (1989) maintain the opposite view.

Hockaday (1988) writes that the attacks are shorter than is the case in adults, generally lasting less than an hour. There is agreement on this point.

Among the numerous forms of migraine with aura listed in the classification, as well as the form with a typical aura (1.2.1. in the International Headache Society classification) the following should be noted:

(1) Familial hemiplegic migraine (IHS: 1.2.3) and *sporadic hemiplegic migraine*. Both begin in childhood and cease in adulthood. The attacks may be precipitated by cranial traumas. In these cases the visual aura is followed by unilateral sensory, and rarely motorial symptoms which develop gradually. Dysarthria, aphasia and impairment of consciousness are frequently associated. These symptoms however rarely last more than an hour and in this case are included in the form of migraine with prolonged aura (IHS: 1.2.2.).

Differential diagnoses of this form include focal convulsions, vascular malformations and mitochondrial encephalomyopathy with lactic acidosis and stroke-like episode (MELAS).

(2) Alternating hemiplegia of childhood (IHS: 1.5.2). There is still much doubt concerning the nature of this form, a very rare disease which begins in infancy and is characterized by sudden,

rapid (and repeated) attacks of hemiplegia which affect the two sides of the body in alternation; they may last from some hours to some days, and are associated with dystonic disturbances. It is progressive, with onset before 18 months ending with permanent motorial defects, mental retardation and dyskinesia. 50 per cent of patients have a positive family history for migraine.

(3) Basilar migraine (IHS: 1.2.4) is more commonly observed. In the past it was called basilar artery migraine and is typical of adolescent or preadolescent girls. Barlow (1984) considers it a rare form, but it should be said that in a series of 27 patients described by Jacobi (1989) 13 had onset of this disorder at less than 10 years of age. Attacks usually last less than an hour and are followed by headache. Generally there is a bilateral visual disturbance, dysarthria, ataxia, bilateral vertigo, tinnitus, bilateral paresthesias, bilateral pareses, nausea, vomiting and a decreased level of consciousness. More rarely nystagmus, diplopia and hypoacusis may be found. Differential diagnoses include cerebrovascular disorders, Chiari's malformation, posterior fossa tumours and metabolic disorders such as homocystinuria and Leigh's disease.

(4) Ophthalmoplegic migraine (IHS: 1.3). Presents with acute attacks of paralysis of cranial nerves III (external or internal) which appear during a migraine attack; nerves IV and VI are rarely involved. The pain is located in the orbital region, is bilateral and pulsating or pressing. The duration of the ophthalmoplegia varies from months to years and often continues after the headache ceases. It presents in subjects who already suffered from migraine, characterized by orbital or post-orbital pain, which is often very intense. The onset, despite previous opinions in the literature, even occurs at less than 10 years of age: Jacobi (1989) indicates that two out of four subjects had onset between 6 and 10 years. Often there is a positive family history for migraine. Aneurysms and above all Tolosa–Hunt syndrome are differential diagnoses that should be mentioned. Tolosa–Hunt syndrome is characterized by orbital pain, involvement of the nerves of the cavernous sinus (III and/or IV and V), a tendency for spontaneous remission with recurrent attacks at intervals of months or years, a neuroradiological diagnosis of cavernous sinus disorder and finally a clear sensitivity to corticosteroids. It is attributed to an idiopathic granulomatosis of the cavernous sinus or the superior orbital fissure.

(5) Retinal migraine (IHS: 1.4). This form is very rare in children and presents with repeated attacks of scotoma or blindness of one eye, lasting less than an hour. It sometimes may be associated with headache which follows the visual disturbance after an interval of less than 60 min but on rare occasions may precede it.

(6) Confusional migraine. This occurs in children with an incidence of about 5 per cent. It is characterized by a typical aura and by a headache which may be mild, accompanied by mental confusion which may precede or follow the headache. There is inattention, distractibility, difficulties in speech and alterations of motor activity. Agitation, disturbances in memory, obscene phrases and violent behaviour are however not frequent. This migraine disturbance may last 2–5 days. Differential diagnosis naturally includes metabolic and viral encephalitis, postictal states and acute psychosis.

(7) The Alice in Wonderland syndrome. This is characterized by attacks, which are the prodrome of the headache, consisting of complex visual perceptive disturbances (Lilliputian, Brobdingnagian, mosaic vision and zoom effects), in which the child usually has the impression that his body, or parts of it, are changing size or shape.

Lastly we must describe some disorders which are very characteristic of paediatric migraine and have been much discussed in recent years. These are periodic syndromes of infancy, which are possible precursors of migraine or may be associated with it. Alternating hemiplegia of childhood, which we have already discussed, and benign paroxysmal vertigo of childhood have been placed in this group, while other aspects such as abdominal migraine, recurrent abdominal pain, periodic attacks of fever, growing pains and benign torticollis in infancy, etc., have been deliberately excluded from the classification. The reason for this exclusion is the opinion that such disturbances cannot by rights be considered to be precursors or equivalents of migraine.

(8) Benign paroxysmal vertigo of childhood (IHS: 1.5.1) consists of multiple episodic attacks of vertigo which occur in healthy children. They momentarily stop all activity and grab hold of something to steady themselves; they are frightened and pale, and often are nauseous and suffer from vomiting and headache. Naturally neurological examination, electroencephalogram and oto-vestibular examination should be negative.

We should also like to draw attention to one of the relatively frequent complications of paediatric migraine. This is *status migrainosus* (IHS: 1.7.1) which even presents in relatively young children, in whom the attack will last more than 72 h even if it is treated. It satisfies the diagnostic criteria for migraine without aura or migraine with aura. The headache is continuous or is interrupted by headache-free intervals lasting less than 4 h. The interruption during sleep is not considered. This form is important because many patients are urgently admitted to hospital in a state of serious physical and mental suffering. Accurate diagnosis to exclude other pathologies and fast and efficient treatment are necessary.

References

Appenzeller, O. (1976): *Pathogenesis and treatment of headache*. New York: SP.

Balottin, U., Borgatti, R. & Lanzi, G. (1989): The therapeutic approach to the migraine patient. In: *Headache in children and adolescents*, International Congress Series 1989, eds. G. Lanzi, U. Balottin & A. Cernibori, pp. 317–324. Amsterdam: Excerpta Medica.

Barlow, C.F. (1984): *Headache and migraine in childhood*. Oxford: Spastics International Medical Publications.

Bille, B. (1989): Migraine in children: prevalence, clinical features and a 30-year follow-up. In: *Migraine and other headaches*, eds. M.D. Ferrari & X. Lataste, pp. 29–38. New Jersey: Parthenon Publishing Group.

Headache Classification Committee of the International Headache Society (1988): Classification and diagnostic criteria for headache disorders, cranial neuralgias and facial pain. *Cephalalgia* **8** (suppl. 7).

Hockaday, J.M. (1988): Definitions, clinical features, and diagnosis of childhood migraine. In: *Migraine in childhood*, pp. 5–24, ed. J.M. Hockaday. London: Butterworths.

Jacobi, G. (1989): Complicated migraine in children and adolescents. In: *Headache in children and adolescents*, International Congress Series, eds. G. Lanzi, U. Balottin & A. Cernibori, pp. 101–108. Amsterdam: Excerpta Medica.

Lance, J.W. (1982): *Mechanism and management of headache*. 4th edn. London: Butterworths.

Lanzi, G. (1980): *La cefalea essenziale nell'età evolutiva*. Rome: Il Pensiero Scientifico.

Lanzi, G., Balottin, U., Borgatti, R., Guderzo, M. & Scarabello, E. (1989): Different forms of migraine in childhood and adolescence; notes on personality traits. *Headache* **28**, 618–622.

Manzoni, G.C., Granella, F., Malferrari, G., Cavalieri, R., Bissi, P. & Ferraru, A.M. (1989): An epidemiological study of headache in children aged between 6 and 13. In: *Headache in children and adolescents*, eds. G. Lanzi, U. Balottin & A. Cernibori, pp. 185–188. Amsterdam: Elsevier.

Rasario, G.M. (1972): *Manuale di semeiotica medica*. Naples: Idelson.

Silberstein, S.D. (1990): Twenty questions about headaches in children and adolescents. *Headache* **30**, 716–724.

Zammarano, C.B., Quaranti, E., Miceli, M.C. & Poli, D. (1989): A statistical analysis of the distribution of the clinical patterns of migraine. In: *Headache in children and adolescents*, eds. G. Lanzi, U. Balottin & A. Cernibori, pp. 67–74. Amsterdam: Elsevier.

Ziegler, D.K., Hassanein, R.S. & Ward, D.F. (1976): Migraine, tyramine and blood serotonin (L2). *Headache* **16**, 53–57.

Chapter 11

Migraine–epilepsy syndrome: intercalated seizures in benign occipital epilepsy

Mario Giovanni Terzano, Liborio Parrino, Vladimiro Pietrini and Laura Galli

Institute of Neurology, University of Parma, via del Quartiere, Parma, Italy

Summary

Migraine and epilepsy share several genetic, clinical, evolutive and neurophysiological features. Epileptic seizures and migraine attacks may also coexist independently within the same subject and occasionally they may mutually interact in succession. In the intercalated attacks of benign epilepsy with occipital EEG paroxysms during episodes of classic migraine, the epileptic manifestations are framed between the prodromal and the painful phases of the migraine attack. This time-locked association between migraine and epilepsy is highly suggestive of a direct interference between the pathophysiological mechanisms of the two clinical symptoms. Intracranial vascular disregulation can activate a massive neuronal phenomenon, described as spreading depression, in the occipital cerebral cortex of one or both hemispheres. If an epileptic focus coexists in the same area in which these reactions take place, the phase of intense neuronal activation that supports the migrainous prodrome may trigger the epileptic manifestations. This migraine–epilepsy syndrome represents a peculiar clinical entity included within the benign epilepsy of childhood with occipital paroxysms.

Common features in epilepsy and migraine

Among ictal disorders, migraine and epilepsy present some common clinical features, although aetiopathogenetic mechanisms and treatment may be extremely different. Both syndromes are characterized by stereotyped, reversible, recurrent and intrinsically modulated clinical manifestations. However, epileptic seizures correlate with neuronal dysfunction that produces abnormal activation of anatomo-functional cerebral systems, whereas migraine attacks derive from a transient imbalance of cranial vasomotricity with a secondary encephalic involvement only in the episodes with aura (Headache Classification Committee of the International Headache Society, 1988). The various clinical forms are defined on the basis of specific symptomatology, individual genetic factors and evolution. The risk of attacks throughout the years may induce severe limitations on the patient's lifestyle and in many cases a drug treatment – intermittent for migraine, chronic for epilepsy – is mandatory and may last for years or decades.

The identification of benign clinical entities is quite frequent in the headache field, while until a short time ago it concerned only a restricted set of epileptic syndromes. In the latter, the benign notion is based on a lack of detectable lesions, absence of neurological signs, regular psychomotor development, adequate therapeutical control and complete remission of attacks. These diagnostic criteria, once confined to some forms of generalized epilepsy, nowadays embrace a broad group of focal syndromes generally considered in the past to be of lesional origin.

Among these sydromes, the longest known is certainly benign epilepsy with centrotemporal spikes to which more recently further clinical entities have been added: benign epilepsy with affective symptoms (Dalla Bernardina et al., 1980), childhood epilepsy with occipital paroxysms (Gastaut, 1982), benign frontal epilepsy (Beaumanoir & Nahory, 1983) and benign epilepsy with extreme somatosensory evoked potentials (Tassinari & De Marco, 1985).

A possible connection between migraine and epilepsy has been repeatedly suggested in the past on the basis of the following issues: high incidence within the same family of subjects presenting with epileptic seizures and subjects suffering from migraine; clinical behaviour of specific epileptic seizures resembling migraine-like episodes; possible loss of consciousness during a migraine attack; emergence of cerebral symptoms in the prodromal phase of classical migraine; and chiefly, the presence of EEG paroxysmal patterns in migraine patients (Barolin, 1966).

Interictal EEG abnormalities are considered a quite specific pattern for epilepsy, whereas their occurrence in migraine patients is rarely associated with clinical epileptic manifestations. However, epileptic seizures and migraine attacks may coexist independently within the same subject. In centrotemporal epilepsy and, to a lesser degree, in absence epilepsy, the association with migraine is a non-fortuitous finding (Septien et al., 1991). Occasionally, migrainous and epileptic attacks, although separated, may mutually interact if arising in succession and in such a way that the one acts as a trigger mechanism for the other. In more limited cases the same individual may show a real migraine–epilepsy syndrome, in which the overlapping clinical symptoms and the connections among pathophysiological processes are entangled in such a way that a clear-cut separation between the two phenomena is questionable (Terzano et al., 1981).

Childhood epilepsy with occipital paroxysms

In the past years, two clinical syndromes that associate migraine and epilepsy within the same attack have been described separately: (1) basilar migraine, seizures and severe epileptiform EEG abnormalities (Camfield et al., 1978); (2) intercalated attacks of benign epilepsy with occipital paroxysms during episodes of classical migraine (Manzoni et al., 1979; Terzano et al., 1980).

In the international classification of epileptic syndromes these two clinical disorders have been merged into benign epilepsy of childhood with occipital paroxysms (Gastaut, 1985). This electroclinical entity, that Gastaut first described in 1982 (Gastaut, 1982), is characterized by specific occipital EEG discharges and visual symptoms that may be associated with convulsive manifestations. The prognosis is favourable and, despite some extreme cases, the disease is limited to the age range of 7–20 years.

These three syndromes share common EEG patterns of spikes or spike-and-wave complexes in the posterior regions of one or both hemispheres. The EEG abnormalities may differ among the different subjects or show morphological variations within the same individual (Fig. 1). They are blocked upon eye opening, while they are insensitive to hyperventilation and intermittent light stimulation. However, seizures may be provoked when strong environmental illumination alternates with sudden visual suppression (Panayiotopoulos, 1989).

Opposite to what occurs in benign epilepsy with centrotemporal spikes, slow wave sleep activates the occipital paroxysms only in 1/3 of the cases, while in most patients it exerts an inhibitory influence compared to the discharge rate when awake with closed eyes (Fig. 2). While the centrotemporal spikes are poorly modulated by the pseudoperiodic fluctuations of vigilance (Terzano et al., 1991) that compose the microstructure of sleep, i.e. the cyclic alternating pattern or CAP, the latter activates the occipital spike and waves, likewise the generalized EEG discharges (Terzano et al., 1989). In particular, the greater arousal swings of CAP exert a triggering influence upon the

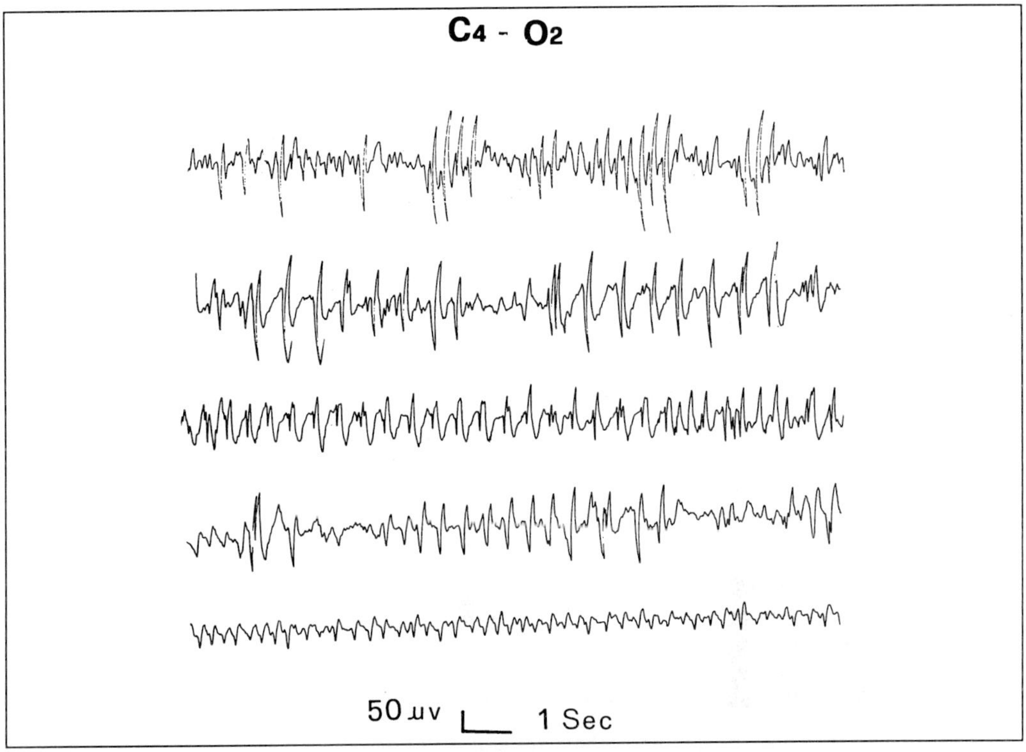

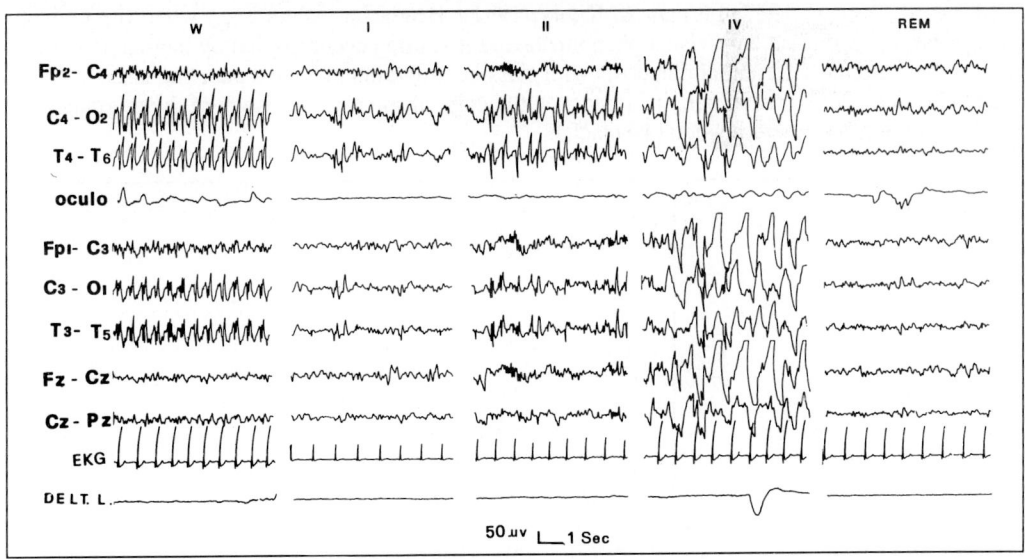

Fig. 1. Continuous morphological and voltage variation of EEG paroxysmal discharges in occipital foci during noctural sleep recordings (from Terzano et al., 1986).

Fig. 2. Patient with intercalated attacks of benign epilepsy with occipital paroxysms during episodes of classic migraine. Compared to wakefulness (W), the EEG activity of the right occipital focus is reduced in rapid eye movements (REM) sleep, and in stages 1 (I), 2 (II) and 4 (IV). EKG: electrocardiogram. Delt. L: left deltoid muscle activity (from Terzano et al., 1986).

occipital paroxysms which thus increase in frequency during transient activation phases and nocturnal awakenings (Fig. 3).

Clinical features of occipital lobe epilepsies

Although infrequent, the epileptic seizures are characterized by visual symptoms, and convulsive and non-convulsive manifestations.

(a) Visual disturbances are reported in almost all cases, as the seizures always originate from an occipital focus. They are subdivided into negative and positive symptoms: both may occur during the same attack. The negative symptoms consist of modifications in the visual field ranging from hemianopsia to amaurosis. The positive symptoms may include either scotomata or complex visual hallucinations (micropsia, macropsia, metamorphopsia). Patients often report visual experiences based on coloured spots, flashes, circles and other geometric figures or butterflies, dragonflies and moving flakes, intensely coloured with red prevalent.

(b) Panayiotopoulos (1989) reports that convulsive symptoms generally appear as hemiclonic attacks with initial turning of the head and eyes. At times, the attacks may rapidly generalize with tonic–clonic manifestations. The non-convulsive symptoms that emerge as perceptive hallucinations or illusions are usually associated with complex partial seizures (Commission on Classification and Terminology of the International League Against Epilepsy, 1989). The evolution is favourable since both seizures and EEG abnormalities classically disappear in adulthood. However, in about 5 per cent of the cases an active form of epilepsy may persist after the age of 20 (Gastaut, 1985).

Migrainous or postictal headache?

Postictal phenomena are an important characteristic of these syndromes. Headache is extremely frequent, constantly reported in the first two syndromes but described in about 1/3 of the patients with occipital epilepsy – between 11 per cent and 60 per cent according to the various investigations – (Roger & Bureau, 1987; Lerman & Kivity, 1991). Headache occurs even when the epileptic manifestations comprise only visual phenomena and it is often accompanied by nausea and vomiting. In this case the differential diagnosis with classical migraine may be a puzzling issue. According to Gastaut (1985), cranial pain in epilepsy with occipital spike-waves is not of the migraine-type but corresponds to a mere postictal headache.

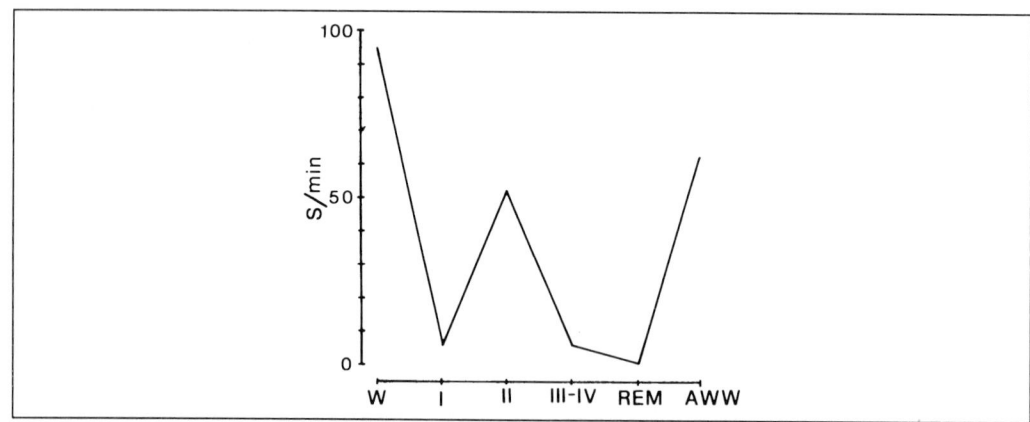

Fig. 3. Diagram of the different frequencies of paroxysmal discharges per minute (S/min) in sleep stages. W: wakefulness; I: stage 1; II: stage 2; III–IV: stages 3 and 4; REM: rapid eye movement sleep; AWW: arousal without wakefulness that corresponds to the A phase of cyclic alternating pattern. (from Terzano et al.,

The associated vegetative symptoms could be explained by the postictal propagation of the occipital discharge to the brainstem structures involved in the regulation of cerebral and gastrointestinal vasomotor activity (Gastaut, 1985).

Camfield *et al.* (1978) assign a different relevance to visual symptoms, headache and neurovegetative symptoms in the syndrome associating basilar migraine, seizures and severe epileptiform EEG abnormalities. A significant role in supporting these symptoms as well as convulsive manifestations is attributed to the vasomotor mechanisms typical of migraine in the vertebrobasilar territory.

In basilar migraine, described by Bickerstaff (1961), the arterial dysfunction induces brainstem impairment characterized by ataxia, dysarthria, diplopia and sensitive alterations followed by headache. It cannot be excluded that the recurrent migraine attacks, in relatively young subjects with high epileptic susceptibility, may produce, through ischaemic mechanisms, an epileptogenic focus with spikes and waves in the occipital regions. Afterwards, the same migraine attacks would act, once again through an ischaemic process, as triggering factors of the epileptic seizures. Thus, the interference between migraine and epilepsy involves both pathophysiological mechanisms and clinical symptoms.

Possible interference between occipital foci and migraine

In the intercalated attacks of benign epilepsy with occipital paroxysms during episodes of classic migraine, seizures are almost always merged with the visual aura of the headache process. The ictal event derives from the sudden change of the migraine prodrome, generally represented by total or partial visual impairment or by a scintillating scotoma in the optic field opposite to the epileptic focus. The scotoma is replaced by multiple, frequently spinning spots or by stylized figures that rapidly spread throughout the entire visual field. The conversion of optic perception from a negative to a positive symptom generally corresponds with the beginning of the epileptic seizure. Owing to its faster accomplishment in the succession of events, the seizure 'intercalates' between the prodromal and the painful phase of the migraine attack (Manzoni *et al.*, 1979).

Several genetic, clinical, evolutive and neurophysiological considerations indicate these clinical forms as a well-defined subgroup of epileptic syndromes with occipital spike-waves.

(1) Familial cases of this syndrome have been reported (Terzano *et al.*, 1986). In particular, we described a family with a high incidence of periodic migraine attacks and occipital EEG abnormalities. From this peculiar genetic combination it emerged that in the cases assessed epileptic seizures occurred only in the members affected by both occipital EEG paroxysms and classic migraine attacks with visual prodromes. The single detection of either EEG abnormalities or classical migraine could not activate the epileptic event.

(2) Clinically, these patients may suffer from migraine attacks independent of epileptic seizures. There may be a therapeutic dissociation between the two types of episodes if only antimigraine drugs (persistence of epileptic seizures) or only antiepileptic drugs (persistence of migraine attacks) are administered (Terzano *et al.*, 1987). In some cases, compounds effectively used for headache prophylaxis, i.e. flunarizine, may control both manifestations (Terzano *et al.*, 1986), although the combination of both kinds of drugs represents the most adequate approach.

(3) In these subjects the course of the syndrome is generally characterized by complete remission of epilepsy but by unchanged recurrence of migraine attacks that may persist in adulthood according to their typical evolution.

(4) The coexistence of an occipital epileptic focus and recurrent attacks of classic migraine is highly suggestive of a direct interference between the pathophysiological mechanisms of the two clinical symptoms. A preliminary involvement of the cranial arterial branches is likely to trigger a classic migraine attack. In the prodromal phase the vasoconstriction of the posterior intracranial arteries activates a series of cortical extrasynaptic events in the occipital cerebral cortex of one or both hemispheres. This neuronal phenomenon – described by the term spreading depression (Leao, 1944)

– could be the neurophysiological basis of the visual symptoms (Milner, 1958). The hypothesis has been confirmed by clinical and experimental evidence (Olesen *et al.*, 1981; Lauritzen *et al.*, 1983; Snow *et al.*, 1983). In the animal, spreading depression consists of a transient inhibition of the cortical electric activity preceded by a phase of intense neuronal excitation (Grafstein, 1956; Snow, 1983). The latter induces a massive activation of experimental epileptogenic foci with increased intracellular spiking, while discharges are suppressed during the inhibitory phase (Goldensohn, 1975). If an epileptic focus coexists in the same area in which these reactions take place (as occurs in epilepsy with occipital spike-waves), the phase of intense neuronal excitation that supports the migrainous scotoma may become the factor that changes the interictal activity into an ictal outcome. The modification of visual perception generally indicates the conversion of migrainous optic symptoms into the epileptic event that afterwards proceeds autonomously. However, for the rapidity of its development the ictal phenomenon is framed between the prodromal and the painful phases of the migraine attack.

In certain conditions in which epilepsy and migraine coexist within the same individual, postictal headaches and migrainous headaches may be hardly distinguished owing to common clinical features. The question of overlapping boundaries should not be overlooked since the pathophysiological mechanisms of both occipital epilepsy and migraine operate upon the same cortical target. Although limited in frequency, the 'intercalated' seizures should be taken into consideration especially when epileptic and migrainous manifestations appear as time-locked phenomena.

References

Barolin, G.S. (1966): Migraines and epilepsies: a relationship? *Epilepsia* **7**, 53–66.

Beaumanoir, A. & Nahory, A. (1983): Les épilepsies benignes partielles: 11 cas d'épilepsie partielle frontale à évolution favorable. *Rev. EEG. Neurophysiol* **13**, 207–211.

Bickerstaff, E.R. (1961): Basilar artery migraine. *Lancet* i, 389–396.

Camfield, P., Metrakos, K. & Andermann, F. (1978): Basilar migraine, seizures and severe epileptiform EEG abnormalities. *Neurology* **28**, 584–588.

Commission on Classification and Terminology of the International League Against Epilepsy (1989): Proposal for classification of epilepsies and epileptic syndromes. *Epilepsia* **26**, 268–278.

Dalla Bernardina, B., Bureau, M., Dravet, C., Dulac, O., Tassinari, C.A. & Roger, J. (1980): Epilepsie bénigne de l'enfant avec crises à séméiologie affective. *Rev. EEG Neurophysiol.* **10**, 8–18.

Gastaut, H. (1982): A new type of epilepsy: benign partial epilepsy of childhood with occipital spike-waves. *Clin. Electroencephalogr.* **12**, 13–22.

Gastaut, H. (1985): Benign epilepsy of childhood with occipital paroxysms. In: *Epileptic syndromes in infancy, childhood and adolescence*, eds. J. Roger, C. Dravet, M. Bureau, F.E. Dreifuss & P. Wolf, pp. 159–170. London: John Libbey.

Goldensohn, E.S. (1985): Initiation and propagation of epileptogenic foci. In: *Advances in neurology*, eds. J.K. Penry & D.D. Daly, pp. 141–162. New York: Raven Press.

Grafstein, B. (1956): Mechanism of spreading cortical depression. *J. Neurophysiol.* **19**, 154–171.

Headache Classification Committee of the International Headache Society (1988): Classification and diagnostic criteria for headache disorders, cranial neuralgias and facial pain. *Cephalalgia* **8** (suppl. 7), 1–96.

Lauritzen, M., Olesen, J., Lassen, N.A. & Paulson, O.B. (1983): Regulation of regional cerebral blood flow during and between migraine attacks. *Ann. Neurol.* **14**, 569–572.

Leao, A.A.P. (1944): Spreading depression of activity in cerebral cortex. *J. Neurophysiol.* **7**, 359–390.

Lerman, P. & Kivity, S. (1991): The benign partial nonrolandic epilepsies. *J. Clin. Neurophysiol.* **8**, 275–287.

Manzoni, G.C., Terzano, M.G. & Mancia, D. (1979): Possible interference between migrainous and epileptic mechanisms in intercalated attacks. *Eur. Neurol.* **18**, 124–128.

Milner, P.M. (1958): Note on a possible correspondence between the scotoma of migraine and spreading depression of Leao. *Electroencephalogr. Clin. Neurophysiol.* **10**, 705.

Olesen, J., Larsen, B. & Lauritzen, M. (1981): Focal hyperemia followed by spreading oligemia and impaired activation of rCBF in classic migraine. *Ann. Neurol.* **9**, 344–352.

Panayiotopoulos, C.P. (1989): Benign nocturnal childhood occipital epilepsy: a new syndrome with nocturnal seizures, tonic deviation of the eyes and vomiting. *J. Child. Neurol.* **4**, 43–48.

Roger, J. & Bureau, M. (1987): Les épilepsies partielles idiopathiques de l'enfant. *Rev. Neurol.* **143**, 381–391.

Septien, L., Pelletier, J.L., Brunotte, F., Giroud, M. & Dumas, R. (1991): Migraine in patients with history of centro-temporal epilepsy in childhood: a Hm-PAO SPECT study. *Cephalalgia* **11**, 281–284.

Snow, R.W., Taylor, C.P. & Dudek, F.E. (1983): Electrophysiological and optical changes in slices of rat hippocampus during spreading depression. *J. Neurophysiol.* **50**, 561–572.

Tassinari, C.A. & De Marco P. (1985): Benign partial epilepsy with extreme somato-sensory evoked potentials. In: *Epileptic syndromes in infancy, childhood and adolescence*, eds. J. Roger, C. Dravet, M. Bureau, F.E. Dreifuss & P. Wolf, pp. 176–180. London: John Libbey.

Terzano, M.G., Manzoni, G.C., Maione, R. & Mancia, D. (1980): Epilessia benigna con parossismi occipitali ed emicrania: problema delle crisi intercalate. In: *Atti del IX Congresso Nazionale della Società Italiana di Neuropsichiatria Infantile*, pp. 827–832. Repubblica di San Marino, San Giovanni in Persiceto: FARAP.

Terzano, M.G., Manzoni, G.C., Maione, R., Moretti, G. & Mancia, D. (1981): Association patterns between epileptic and migraine attacks. *Acta. Neurol.* **36**, 587–598.

Terzano M.G., Pietrini, V., Parrino, L. & Ferro-Milone, F. (1986): Migraine and intercalated seizures with occipital EEG paroxysms: observations on a family. *Headache* **26**, 509–512.

Terzano, M.G., Manzoni, G.C. & Parrino, L. (1987): Benign epilepsy with occipital paroxysms and migraine: the question of intercalated attacks. In: *Migraine and epilepsy*, eds. F. Andermann & E. Lugaresi, pp. 83–96. London, Boston: Butterworths.

Terzano, M.G., Parrino, L., Anelli, S. & Halasz, P. (1989): Modulation of generalized spike-and-wave discharges during sleep by cyclic alternating pattern. *Epilepsia* **30**, 772–781.

Terzano, M.G., Parrino, L., Spaggiari, M.C., Barusi, R. & Simeoni, S. (1991): Discriminatory effect of cyclic alternating pattern in focal lesional and benign rolandic interictal spikes during sleep. *Epilepsia* **32**, 616–628.

Chapter 12

An EEG contribution to the study of migraine and of the association between migraine and epilepsy in childhood

Anne Beaumanoir

Fondazione Pierfranco e Luisa Mariani, Viale Bianca Maria 28, 20129 Milano, Italy

Summary

The occurrence in migrainous children of spikes (S) and spike-and-wave complexes (S–W) morphologically similar to those characteristic of idiopathic partial epilepsies (IPE), particularly occipital (IPEO), the possible association in the same child or adolescent of occipital seizures and migraine (M), the frequency of postcritical headaches in epileptic seizures with visual symptoms and, most of all, the semiological similarities between some migraine attacks and some epileptic seizures starting in the occipital lobes, have led several authors to wonder about the relationship between IPE and M. A review of the recent literature and of personal data points out that posterior S and S–W, 'fixation-off sensitive spikes' (FOSS), are quite frequent when the two syndromes are associated in the same subject. Their proportion, on the other hand, is not significant in a population of migraine-free subjects. These observations suggest a different nature of the physiological processes responsible for the occipital epileptic seizure and the visual symptoms in the first phase of some migraine attacks. On the other hand, longitudinal studies assess a different evolution between migraine attacks and epileptic seizures typical of IPEO. Even if the association IPE-M seems quite frequent, though epidemiological studies are lacking, the analysis of intercritical, critical and postcritical EEG clearly distinguishes the two syndromes. Only the epileptic seizures of IPEO are, like the S and S–W of FOSS type, age-dependent, and tied to the process of cerebral maturation.

Introduction

In a lecture published in 1907, Gowers, discussing the uncertain borders of epilepsy and the differential diagnosis of cerebral 'attacks' (fainting, vagal symptoms, vertigo, migraine, parasomnias) concluded that migraine and epilepsy are two distinct syndromes which can, however, coexist in the same patient. A consensus conference was held following the studies of Terzano *et al.* (1987) on the time relationship between epileptic seizures and migrainous attacks, which can occur in the same patient independently or can be intercalated (Terzano *et al.*, 1993). Epileptic seizures in the course of a migrainous attack can be generalized or partial. In this latter event they frequently are occipital.

While Kinast *et al.* (1982) describe rolandic spikes identical to those of idiopathic benign childhood epilepsy with centro-temporal spikes (IBCECTS) in nine out of 100 migrainous non-epileptic children, aged 4 to 15 years, other authors underline the high frequency of migraine in the child with partial benign epilepsy and especially IBCECTS. Percentages of 60 to 80 per cent reported in some papers (Bladin, 1987; Giroud et al., 1986) are disputed by other authors, especially Giovanardi Rossi et al. (1987). The description by Camfield et al. in 1978 of four patients who presented, in association, epileptic seizures, migraine and 'epileptiform abnormalities on the EEG' corresponding to the spike focus described by Panayiotopoulos (1981) as fixation off sensitivity spikes (FOSS) focused attention on the association of occipital epilepsy and migraine.

Discussing the existence of the syndrome epilepsy-migraine (SyEM) in children, Andermann & Lugaresi (1987) suggested subdividing it into four categories, among them 'patients with occipital epilepsy' (which will be discussed in this paper) and 'patients with mitochondrial diseases' (Andermann, 1993).

Firstly, we propose to identify the limits of the syndrome SyOEM (syndrome occipital epilepsy-migraine) in the child. Then, we will compare ictal and postictal EEG data of occipital seizures and of migrainous attacks, with visual and/or autonomic symptomatology, with the aim of clarifying the pathogenic relationship among epileptic seizures, migraine and postictal headache in the child suffering from occipital epilepsy.

Is there a syndrome occipital epilepsy-migraine of childhood?

The association of occipital epilepsy (OE), migraine (M) and FOSS clearly represents a syndrome typical of children and adolescents. All the authors who studied this syndrome demonstrated that FOSS is age-dependent like idiopathic childhood epilepsy with occipital paroxysms (ICEOP), and represents a feature of its diagnosis (Beaumanoir, 1993; Panayiotopoulos, 1993: see Chapters 9 and 18 in this volume).

FOSS is described in the child with congenital visual deficits as well as in the child with signs of sensorimotor immaturity (Beaumanoir et al. 1981; Beaumanoir & Grandjean, 1987; Herranz Tanarro et al., 1984; Lerman & Kivity, 1981). FOSS may precede or accompany photosensitivity in the same subject (Panayiotopoulos, 1989a). In this case, an ICEOP, an idiopathic generalized epilepsy and a migraine may coexist (as in Case 1, Fig. 6, see above). Analysis of the electroclinical correlations in 63 patients from 7 to 12 years of age with FOSS shows that 69.8 per cent of them suffer from ICEOP (Table 1). Nine (14.2 per cent) present ICEOP and migraine together. Seven times out of nine, migraine is independent of epileptic seizures.

In two cases, headaches of more than 1 h duration, accompanied by nausea and vomiting in one patient, and by confusion in the other, occurred after a free interval of 15 to 30 min after an occipital epileptic seizure. This is not, then, strictly a postictal migraine, as was the case in one observation where all occipital epileptic seizures were followed by a migraine which could last even for 10 h.

Four patients (i.e. 6.3 per cent) had migraine but not epileptic seizures. This percentage of 6.3 per cent is identical to the one of Herranz Tanarro et al. in 1984. The proportion of migrainous children with FOSS then is not significant, considering the prevalence of migraine in children.

On the other hand, the association ICEOP-M-FOSS is an important one, about 15 per cent (16 per cent for Gastaut, 1982). This proportion is very close to the one demonstrated in IBCECTS by Beaumanoir et al. in 1974 (15.4 per cent) or by Giovanardi Rossi et al. in 1987 (13.9 per cent). As in the cases of Camfield et al. (1978), most children and adolescents who are or have been affected by FOSS (11 of our 13 patients) suffer from of basilar migraine (Bickerstaff, 1961; Lanzi & Balottin 1993, see Chapter 10 in this volume).

Eight of 13 patients (61 per cent) suffering from migraine (basilar migraine in seven out of eight cases) are girls, while in the whole sample the number of girls almost equals that of boys (32). The proportion of 61 per cent corresponds at the same time to the percentage of girls in the series of Panayiotopoulos (1989b), concerning 18 children with ICEOP whose seizures were mainly noctur-

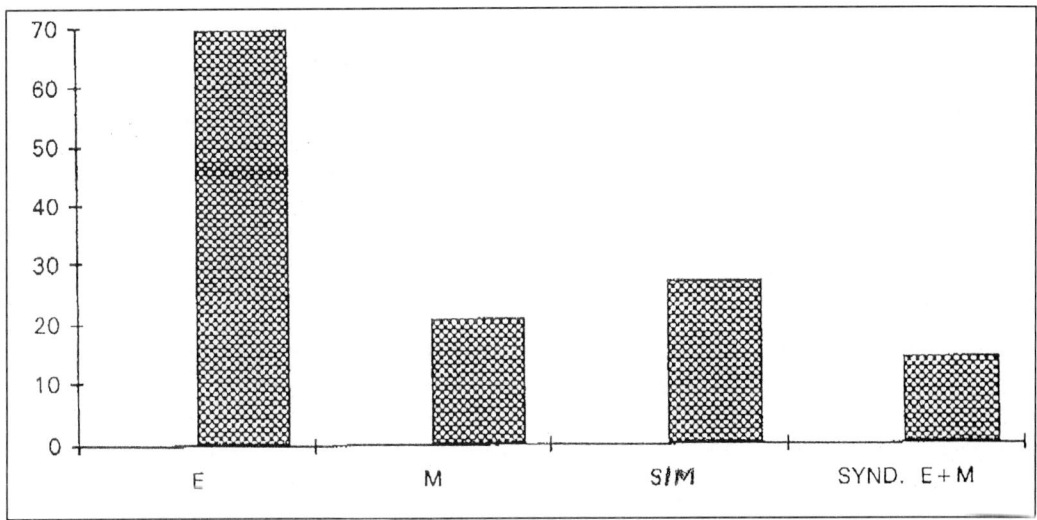

Table 1a. E = epilepsy; M = migraine
SMI = sensorimotor immaturity; Synd. E + M = association of epilepsy and migraine

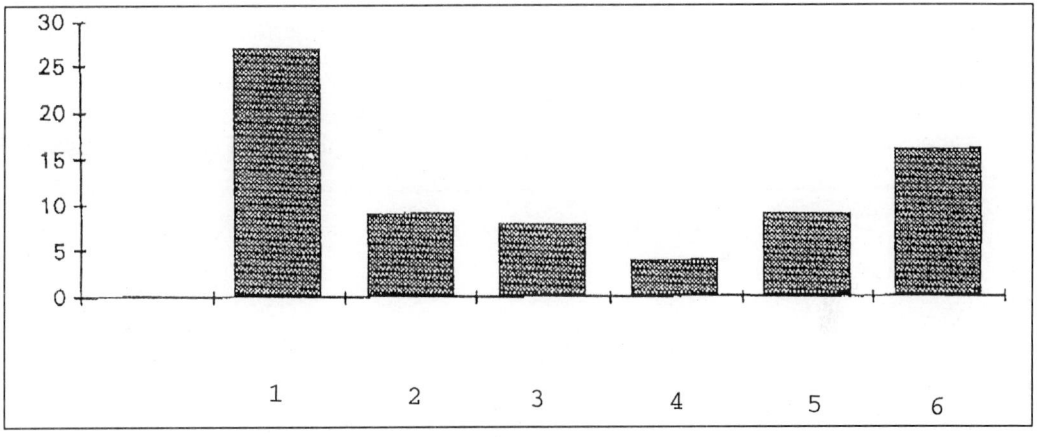

Table 1b.
1 = Idiopathic occipital epilepsy; 2 = epilepsy + migraine; 3 = epilepsy; 4 = migraine;
5 = sensorimotor immaturity; 6 = peripheral visual defect.

nal and whose symptomatology consisted of a sensation of malaise, vomiting and alteration of consciousness (Beaumanoir, 1993; Panayiotopoulos, 1993).

This kind of epileptic seizures is typical of the early onset variant of ICEOP (Panayiotopoulos, 1989b), while basilar migraine is more frequent in the adolescent (Bickerstaff, 1961). In eight out of 11 patients the first attack of basilar migraine occurred after age 9 years.

Epileptic seizures disappear as FOSS, while migrainous attacks may persist (Beaumanoir & Grandjean, 1987). SyME and particularly BM-OE-FOSS could then correspond to the combination of two syndromes occurring in the same age group, and more often in girls than in boys. However, the similarity of the semiology between migrainous attacks and occipital seizures increases the importance of EEG and cerebral metabolism investigation techniques in the differential diagnosis of these conditions.

EEG during migrainous attacks in children

EEG during migrainous 'aura' with negative and /or positive visual symptomatology

EEG records during the initial vasoconstrictor phase of migraine are rare and usually fortuituous as in two observations which we published in 1987 (Beaumanoir & Jekiel, 1987).

(a) EEG during deficitary signs

In these two cases as in the case of Huott *et al.* (1974), Swanson & Vick (1978), Gastaut & Zifkin (1987), and Sacquegna *et al.* (1987). EEG abnormalities are pseudoperiodic sharp waves in both occipital regions. The deficitary visual symptomatology can be precipitated by intermittent photic stimulation (IPS).

In a new observation (Fig. 1) an EEG taken only 30 min after the first symptoms and approximately 20 min after a total amaurosis shows monomorphic bioccipital slow waves. In the case of Sacquegna, however, EEG shows a paroxysmal theta rhythmic activity on the left occipital region.

(b) EEG during positive signs

In three of our patients (among them, Case No. 22, Beaumanoir & Jekiel, 1987) from 20 to 40 min after the beginning of the migraine, while sight is not completely recovered, the patients saw a brief positive visual phenomenon (Fig. 2). It consists of a coloured hallucination: in two cases a red colour, in the other a yellow ball shining like a sun. During these brief episodes, a low amplitude fast activity, similar to that recorded during epileptic visual seizures, is recorded (Beaumanoir, 1992).

(c) EEG during the prodromic phase of basilar migraine

During this phase, which may be short or prolonged, the EEG is rarely studied. In one of our observations the EEG was recorded while the patient was still complaining of vertigo or nausea and

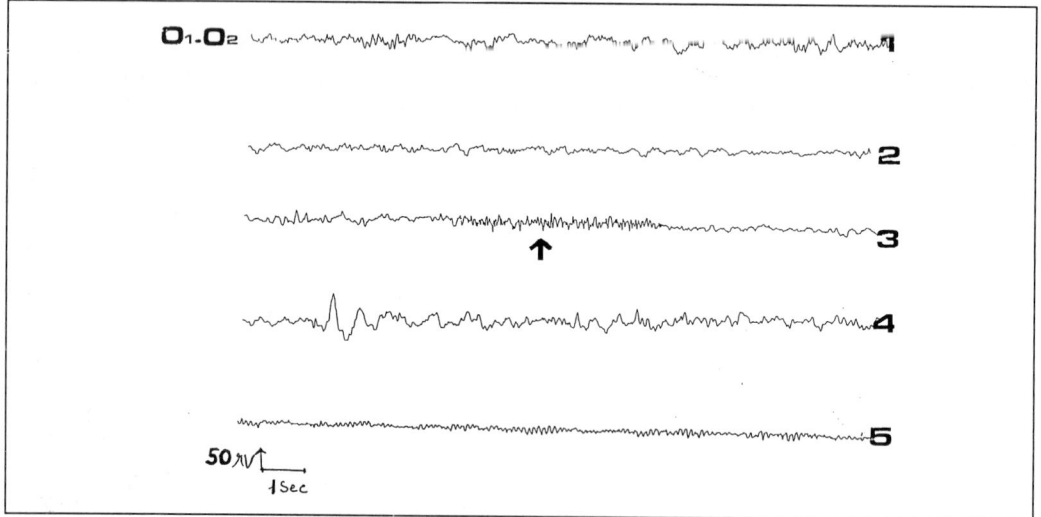

Fig. 1. Each recording corresponds to 15 s. 1, 2, 3, 4 are taken from the first 45 min of recording during a migraine attack in a 15-year-old girl with catamenial headaches since the age of 12 years. 5 is the normal intercritical reading. In 1 and 2 the patient complains of amaurosis; in 3, 10 min after 1, she sees non-coloured vague forms; at the moment of recording fast rhythms (arrow) she says 'The sun'. 4 corresponds to the recording 45 min after 1. Vision is normal after about 20 min. The patient has headache and photophobia. The migraine is going to last, as usual, about 12 h.

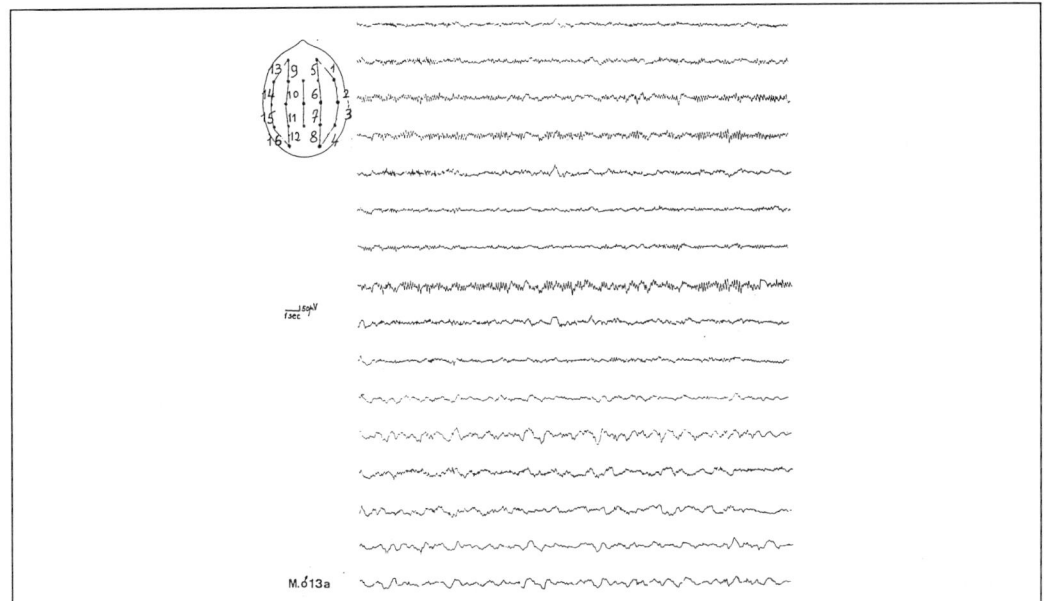

Fig. 2. Recording performed half an hour after the prodromic phase with hemianopia and aphasia during a left migraine in a boy whose father suffered from migraine too, most often on the left with an aphasic aura.

vomiting, and it showed diffuse monomorphic slow waves of higher amplitude in the occipital regions (Figs. 2 and 5). In a case of Amit *et al.* (1986) the EEG, during a state of acute confusional migraine in a 9-year-old child, showed diffuse slowing.

EEG of basilar migraine during the cephalalgic phase

(a) As long as autonomic symptoms, especially nausea, persist, the EEG is identical to the one recorded during the prodromic phase. However, very quickly the monomorphic activity becomes localized to the occipital poles, is increasingly fragmented, and disappears during visual stimuli resembling occipital intermittent rhythmic delta activity (OIRDA) (Fig. 7). This EEG pattern is described by Ziegler & Wong (1967), Matthis *et al.* (1976), Lapkin *et al.* (1977), and Beaumanoir & Jekiel (1987).

(b) EEG during the cephalalgic phase of simple migraine. According to many authors the EEG is always abnormal: the background activities are often of low amplitude and low frequency. Theta or delta monomorphic abnormalities are always present and diffuse but predominate in posterior areas. An asymmetry with reduction of amplitude on the side of migraine may be observed (Fig. 8). Slow abnormalities are progressively reduced, but persist after 6 to 48 h, or more, after the end of the attack.

The EEG mapping demonstrates slow abnormalities and shows that the reduction in amplitude is more marked in the posterior territories (Schoenen *et al.*, 1987).

Finally, during the cephalalgic phase of simple migraine and basilar migraine, predominating abnormalities are focalized monomorphic slow waves of higher amplitude in the occipital regions of the scalp. These abnormalities are progressively reduced after the end of the attack. Abnormalities described in migrainous attacks are not described in non-migrainous headaches following occipital epileptic seizures. Gastaut & Zifkin (1987) report postictal headaches accompanied by nausea and vomiting (migraine-like) in 17 per cent of their patients with ICEOP. Only one EEG was obtained during these manifestations, but the authors do not describe it, although they remark that no ictal discharge was observed during this phase.

Commentary on the role of EEG in the differential diagnosis between migraine attacks and occipital seizures in childhood

Negative visual signs (scotoma, loss of vision) are more frequent than positive visual phenomena (illusions, phosphenes, hallucinations) during migrainous aura. During an ischaemic process entailing visual deficits, the EEG shows monomorphic slow waves and/or pseudo-periodic sharp waves, while positive signs related to an irritative process are characterized by fast rhythms, which are identical to ictal epileptic discharges. These epileptic discharges during a migrainous aura with visual deficit, although very brief, probably reflect a mechanism described by Terzano et al. (1992, see Chapter 11 in this volume).

During the epileptic deficitary visual seizure, the EEG may present a pseudo-periodic sharp wave discharge as described during transient ischaemia; or slow waves as seen in migrainous attacks or in the hemiplegic attack in the syndrome of alternating hemiplegia of the young child, considered by some authors as an equivalent of migraine at this very early age (Verret & Steele, 1971; Dalla Bernardina et al., 1987).

In basilar migraine, autonomic manifestations always follow visual signs, and are accompanied by diffuse monomorphic slow waves which seem to confirm a transient involvement of the brainstem structures (Beaumanoir & Jekiel, 1987). Nocturnal seizures characteristic of ICEOP, whose symptoms consist also of autonomic manifestations (vomiting) and disturbances of consciousness, may reveal on the EEG slow delta monomorphic activities which are more marked in one or both posterior regions. However, these epileptic seizures, even if prolonged, are not followed by clinical and EEG postictal signs. Moreover, sleep, which is a facilitating factor in epilepsy, acts more rarely as such in migraine.

EEG during migrainous postictal headaches is not well known: in the cases where an electroclinical description is available, the EEG does not show the monomorphic abnormalities of migraine, but focal polymorphic slow waves.

All these electroclinical data contributing to the differential diagnosis between a migrainous attack involving the occipital lobe and visual seizures in childhood are illustrated by the following case of association between these two syndromes.

Case 1. Female, age 12. She is followed in Turin by Prof. G. Capizzi. Her mother suffers from migraine. A paternal uncle had febrile convulsions.

The first night-time seizure occured at 6 years of age. The EEG then showed a unilateral right FOSS, and an EEG at rest shows rare generalized spike and waves. IPS has no effect. CT scan is normal. The diagnosis of ICEOP is maintained. The first migraine attacks started at the age of 9 years. At 9 years the EEG when awake is unchanged with respect to the first EEG, but the focus is bilateral (Fig. 3).

The epileptic seizures most often occur during the night. Only one seizure was witnessed. The child had an agitated sleep. As soon as the lights in her room were switched on, her eyes and head deviated to the left. When her mother tried to put her head back in her axial position, the child spoke, but in an incomprehensible way, then she had a few clonic movements of the left superior limb. The overall duration of the seizure was about 2 min, then the patient went back to sleep. The next morning she presented her third daytime attack, characterized, as were the previous ones, by phosphenes in her left hemifield, followed very shortly – so shortly that the patient insists on the concomitance of the two manifestations – by the impression of objects coming nearer with brighter colours. These sensory phenomena lasted about 15 s and in this attack they were followed by ocular clonic movements with eye deviation to the left. An EEG was performed 1½ h after this seizure (Fig. 4).

The patient suffers from migraine headache, on the right with a visual defect aura (Figs. 5 and 6) or on the left (Fig. 8). The visual aura may be absent, but there are considerable vegetative reactions accompanying a diffuse headache (Fig. 7).

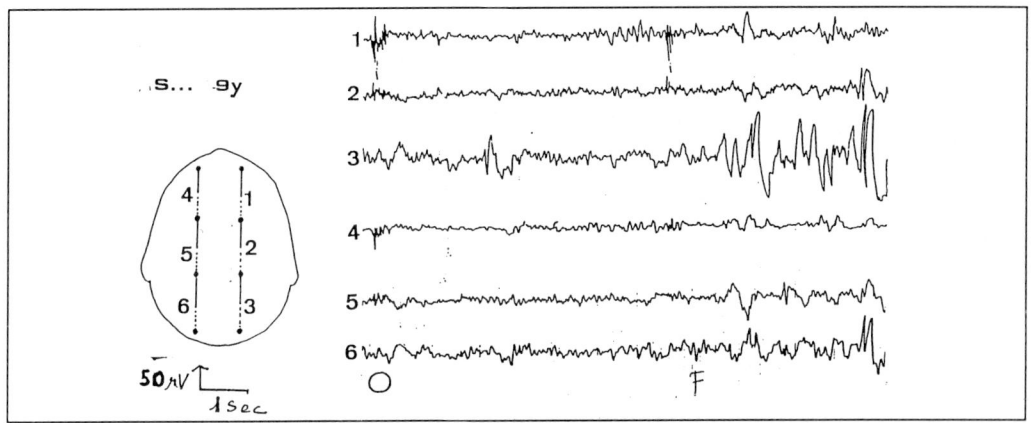

*Fig. 3. Intercritical recording. O = eyes open ; F = eyes closed
(1.5 cm = 1 s; 0.5 cm = 50 µV).*

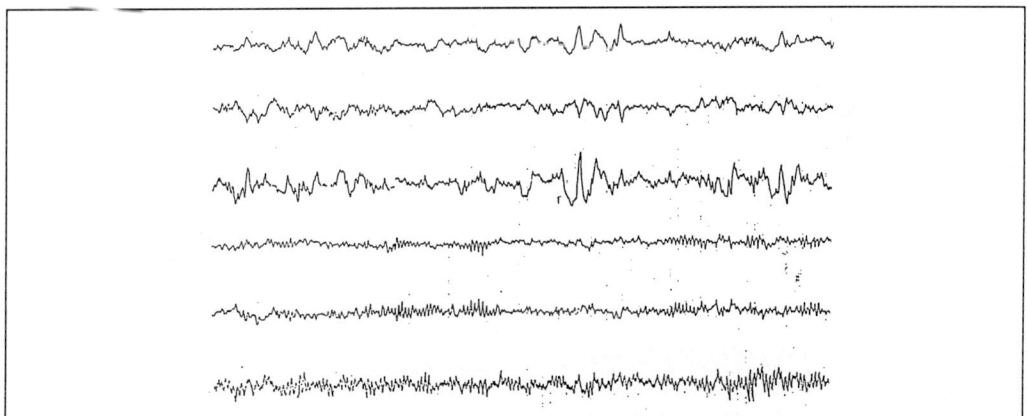

Fig. 4. Postcritical recording after two partial visual, oculomotor seizures and one right hemiclonic seizure occurring 8 h before (1.5 cm = 1 s; 0.5 cm = 50 µV).

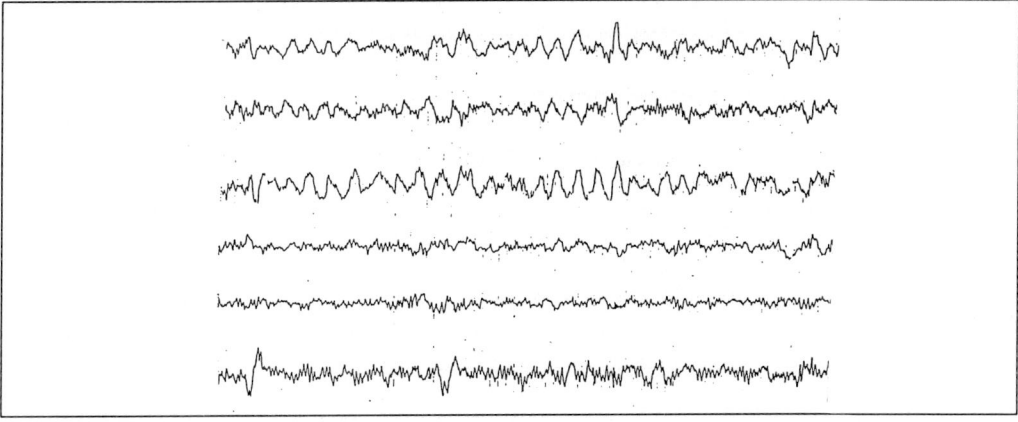

*Fig. 5. Recording after right migraine
(1.5 cm = 1 s; 0.5 cm = 50 µV).*

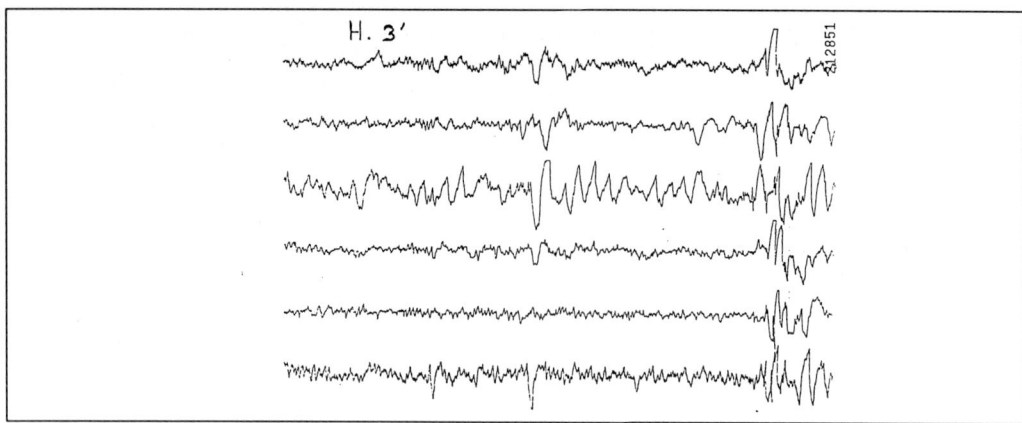

Fig. 6. Recording performed 4 h after Fig. 3 (1.5 cm = 1 s; 0.5 cm = 50 μV).

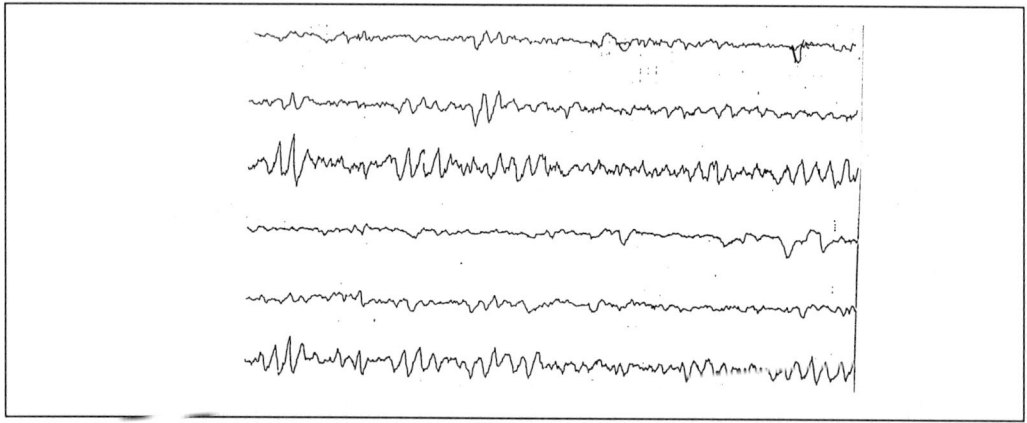

Fig. 7. Recording performed during a headache attack similar to basilar migraine; the patient still has nausea and is quite confused (1.5 cm = 1 s; 0.5 cm = 50 μV).

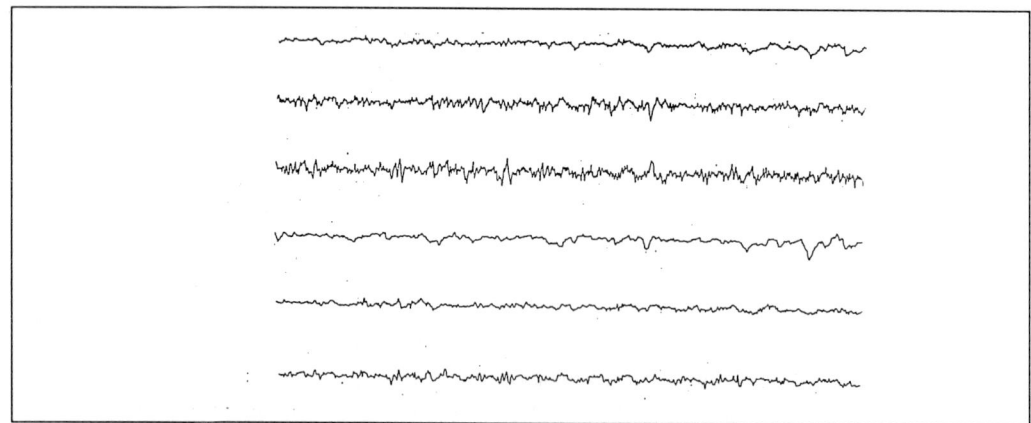

Fig. 8. Recording about 1 h after the onset of a left migraine of 5 h duration (1.5 cm = 1 s; 0.5 cm = 50 μV).

The postcritical EEG, performed less than 2 h after an epileptic seizure of right visual areas, shows slow polymorphic abnormalities (Fig. 4), morphologically different from those recorded less than 1 h after a right migraine attack (Fig. 5) and more than 3 h after this one (Fig. 6). After the migraine attack, IPS causes paroxysmal discharges, sometimes corresponding to a secondary hypersynchrony.

During a left migraine, 1 h after the onset of headache the recording shows a marked asymmetry, a disappearance of FOSS and monomorphic slow waves of low amplitude, more constant on the left (Fig. 8). In the hour following the onset of manifestations suggestive of basilar migraine, after the peak of autonomic disturbances, the EEG shows monomorphic slow waves, somewhat higher on the right (Fig. 7).

The six EEGs were performed between June 1990 and February 1992.

Conclusions

The study of EEG during paroxysmal visual manifestations (migrainous aura, epileptic seizure) shows different patterns according to the clinical symptoms (positive or deficient): firstly, fast rhythms probably represent epileptic phenomena accompanying positive semiology during the course of migraine as well as of epileptic seizure. Secondly, monomorphic slow waves or pseudoperiodic sharp waves in deficient ictal symptoms reflect the alterations due to ischaemia during the vasoconstrictor phase of migraine. These same EEG signs can be recorded during an ictal epileptic blindness, suggesting a non-epileptic (very likely ischaemic) origin of the deficit during an epileptic seizure in some, if not all, of these cases.

EEG reflects the pathogenic mechanism responsible for the clinical symptom, whatever the syndrome may be. The recording of the vasodilator phase of the migrainous attack is different from the postictal epileptic record. This observation confirms that a different pathogenesis originates the two events and gives a special value to the EEG, performed during and after the attack, in the not always easy differential diagnosis between migrainous attacks and epileptic seizures in children.

Acknowledgements: The author thanks Doctors Andrée Van Lierde and Laura Mira for their help in revising the English version of this paper.

References

Amit, R., Shapira, Y., Flusser, H. & Aker, M. (1986): Basilar migraine manifesting as transient global amnesia in a 9 year old child. *Headache* **26**, 17–18.

Andermann, F. (1993): Occipital epileptic abnormalities in mitochondrial disorders. In: *Occipital seizures and epilepsies in children*, eds. F. Andermann, A. Beaumanoir, L. Mira, J. Roger & C.A. Tassinari, pp. 111–120 London: John Libbey.

Andermann, F. & Lugaresi, E. (1987): *Migraine and epilepsy*. Boston, London: Butterworths.

Beaumanoir, A., Ballis, I., Varfis, G. & Ansari, K. (1974): Benign epilepsy of childhood with Rolandic spikes. A clinical, electroencephalographic and telencephalographic study. *Epilepsia* **15**, 301–315.

Beaumanoir, A., Inderwildi, B. & Zagury S. (1981): Paroxysmes EEG 'non-épileptiques'. *Médecine et Hygiène (Genève)*, **39**, 1911–1918.

Beaumanoir, A. & Grandjean, E. (1987): Occipital spikes, migraine, and epilepsy. In: *Migraine and epilepsy*, eds. F. Andermann & E. Lugaresi, pp. 97–110. Boston, London: Butterworths.

Beaumanoir, A. & Jekiel, M.E. (1987): Electrographic observations during attacks of classical migraine. In: *Migraine and epilepsy*, eds. F. Andermann & E. Lugaresi, pp. 163–180. Boston, London: Butterworths.

Beaumanoir, A. (1993): Semiology of occipital seizures in infants and children. In: *Occipital seizures and epilepsies in children*, eds. F. Andermann, A. Beaumanoir, L. Mira, J. Roger & C.A. Tassinari, pp. 71–86 London: John Libbey.

Bickerstaff, E.R. (1961): Basilar artery migraine. *Lancet* i, 15–17.

Bladin, P.F. (1987): The association of benign Rolandic epilepsy with migraine. In: *Migraine and epilepsy*, eds. F. Andermann & E. Lugaresi, pp. 145–152. Boston, London: Butterworths.

Camfield, P.R., Metrakos, K. & Andermann, F. (1978): Basilar migraine seizures and severe epileptiform EEG abnormalities. *Neurology* **28**, 584–588.

Dalla Bernardina, B., Capovilla, G., Trevisan, E., Colamaria, V., Andrighetto, G., Fontana, E. & Tassinari, C.A. (1987): Alternating hemiplegia in childhood. In: *Migraine and epilepsy*, eds. F. Andermann & E. Lugaresi, pp. 189–201. Boston, London: Butterworths.

Gastaut, H. (1982): L'épilepsie bénigne de l'enfant à pointe-ondes occipitales. *Rev. EEG Neurophysiol. Clin.* **12**, 179–201.

Gastaut, H. & Zifkin, B.G. (1987): Benign epilepsy of childhood with occipital spike and wave complexes. In: *Migraine and epilepsy*, eds. F. Andermann & E. Lugaresi, pp. 47–81. London: Butterworths.

Giovanardi Rossi, P., Santucci, M., Gobbi, G., D'Alessandro, R. & Sacquegna, T. (1987): Epidemiological study of migraine in epileptic patients. In: *Migraine and epilepsy*, eds. F. Andermann & E. Lugaresi, pp. 313–322. Boston, London: Butterworths.

Giroud, M., Soichot, P., Weyl, M., Dauvergne, M., Alison, M. & Dumas, R. (1986): L'épilepsie à pointe-ondes occipitales. *Ann. Pediatr.* **33**, 131–135.

Gowers, W.R. (1907): *The borderland of epilepsy*, pp. 6–87. London: J. & A. Churchill.

Herranz Tanarro, F.J., Lope, E.S. & Sassot, S.C. (1984): La pointe-onde occipitale avec et sans épilepsie bénigne chez l'enfant. *Rev. EEG Neurophysiol.* **14**, 1–7.

Huott, A.D., Madison, D.S. & Niedermeyer D. (1974): Occipital lobe epilepsy. A clinical and electroencephalographic study. *Eur. Neurol.* **11**, 325–339.

Kinast, M., Lueders, H., Rothner, D. & Erenberg G. (1982): Benign focal epileptiform discharges in childhood migraine (BFEDC). *Epilepsy* **32**, 1309–1311.

Lanzi, G. & Balottin, U. (1993): The semiology of migraine attacks in childhood. In: *Occipital seizures and epilepsies in children*, eds. F. Andermann, A. Beaumanoir, L. Mira, J. Roger & C.A. Tassinari, pp. 87–91 London: John Libbey.

Lapkin, M.L., French, J.H., Golden, G.S. *et al.* (1977): The electroencephalogram in childhood basilar artery migraine. *Neurology* **27**, 580–583.

Lerman, P. & Kivity, S. (1981): Focal epileptic EEG discharges in children not suffering from clinical epilepsy: etiology, clinical significance and management. *Epilepsia* **22**, 551–558.

Matthis, H., Pevriaud, P., Jekiel, M. E. & Beaumanoir, A. (1976): Serial EEG records during migrainous attacks, eds. H. Lenner & A. Ananbor, pp. 267–272. EEG and Clinical Neurophysiology International Congress Series.

Panayiotopoulos, C.P. (1981): Inhibitory effect of central vision on occipital lobe seizure. *Neurology* **31**, 1331–1333.

Panayiotopoulos, C.P. (1989a): Fixation-off-sensitive epilepsies. In: *Reflex seizures and reflex epilepsies*, eds. A. Beaumanoir, H. Gastaut & R. Naquet, pp. 203–217. Genève: Médecine et Hygiène.

Panayiotopoulos, C.P. (1989b): Benign childhood epilepsy with occipital paroxysms. A 15 year prospective study. *Ann. Neurol.* **26**, 51–56.

Panayiotopoulos, C.P. (1993): Benign childhood epilepsy with occipital paroxysms. In: *Occipital seizures and epilepsies in children*, eds. F. Andermann, A. Beaumanoir, L. Mira, J. Roger & C.A. Tassinari, pp. 151–164. London: John Libbey.

Sacquegna, T., Cortelli, P., Baldrati, A., De Carolis, P., Tinuper, P. & Lugaresi, E. (1987): Electrographic observations on migraine and transient global amnesia, confusional migraine, and migraine and epilepsy. In: *Migraine and epilepsy*, eds. F. Andermann & E. Lugaresi, pp. 153–161. Boston, London: Butterworths.

Schoenen, J., Jamart, B. & Delwaide, P.J. (1987): Cartographie électroencéphalographique dans les migraines en périodes critique et intercritique. *Rev. EEG Neurophysiol.* **17**, 289–299.

Swanson, J.W. & Vick, N.A. (1978): Basilar artery migraine. 12 patients, with an attack recorded electroencephalographically. *Neurology* **28**, 782–786.

Terzano, M.G., Manzoni, G.C. & Parrino, L. (1987): Benign epilepsy with occipital paroxysms and migraine: the question of intercalated attacks. In: *Migraine and epilepsy*, eds. F. Andermann & E. Lugaresi, pp. 83–96. Boston, London: Butterworths.

Terzano, M.G, Parrino, L., Pietrini, V. & Galli, L. (1993): Migraine–epilepsy syndrome: intercalated seizures in benign occipital epilepsy. In: *Occipital seizures and epilepsies in children*, eds. F. Andermann, A. Beaumanoir, L. Mira, J. Roger & C.A. Tassinari, pp. 93–99 London: John Libbey.

Verret, S. & Steele, J. C. (1971): Alternating hemiplegia in childhood: a report of 8 patients with complicated migraine beginning in infancy. *Pediatrics* **47**, 671–680.

Ziegler, D.R. & Wong, G.J (1967): Migraine in children: clinical and electroencephalographic study of families. The possible relations to epilepsy. *Epilepsia* **8**, 171–187.

Chapter 13

Occipital epileptic abnormalities in mitochondrial disorders – preferential involvement, illustrations of clinical patterns, current progress in neurobiology and a hypothesis

Frederick Andermann

Department of Neurology and Neurosurgery, McGill University; and the Montreal Neurological Hospital and Institute, 3801 University Street, Montreal, Quebec, Canada, H3A 2B4

Summary

The syndrome of malignant migraine, epilepsia partialis continua and predominantly occipital lesions has been shown to be characteristic of mitochondrial encephalopathy with lactic acidosis and stroke-like episodes (MELAS). The clinical spectrum of this disorder is rapidly growing but the reasons for the occipital predilection have not been clarified as yet. Patients often present with seemingly benign occipital seizures, sometimes several years before the typical catastrophic events. DNA point mutations have now been identified in MELAS but are found only in familial cases and not in the sporadic patients who seem to have a family history of common or classical migraine. Mitochondrial abnormalities can be demonstrated in small cerebral arteries.

In myoclonic epilepsy with ragged red fibres (MERRF) there is in addition to photic sensitivity a tendency for occipital spike discharges. Thus, in this syndrome also, occipital involvement is manifest. Migraine with aura, MELAS, MERRF, the other progressive myoclonus epilepsies and photosensitive epilepsy share a predisposition for involvement of the occipital structures. The pathophysiology of this preferential involvement may involve dopaminergic mechanisms but is at present not well understood.

Introduction

There appears to be a preferential involvement of the occipital lobe in patients with mitochondrial encephalomyopathy both in those with MELAS (mitochondrial encephalomyopathy with lactic acidosis and stroke like episodes) and in those with MERRF (myoclonus epilepsy with ragged red fibres). The recognition of this preferential involvement, illustrations of the clinical patterns, current progress in the neurobiology of mitochondrial disorders and a hypothesis attempting to explain this preferential involvement in sporadic patients with MELAS syndrome are the subject of this chapter.

Our interest in these disorders dates back to the late 1950s when a young man from Cuba was admitted for investigation of seizures to the service of Dr Wilder Penfield at the Montreal Neurological Hospital. The following are a verbatim quote from Dr Penfield's case notes: Patient J.R.: 'The outstanding features as I understand them, are as follows: Normal young man aged 18. He has had migraine, which is regularly left-sided, from childhood. Age 9: Operation for obstruction of the intestinal tract by Dr. Gross in Boston. In 1954, age 15: Fell from a motorcycle. He was riding on the back, and when he was picked up he was found to be having a seizure, and an old lady says that the movement was in the right hand. Attacks at intervals following this, usually associated with left-sided migraine headaches, and with stars of a scintillating variety. The side of the stars is not certain. This is followed by nausea and at times convulsive movements of the right hand.

20 October 1957: While watching a moving picture, his friend noticed that he was covering his eyes. He asked him what was the matter and he said he was seeing stars. A little later, he was having a severe left-sided headache and the friend noticed that the right hand was jerking. The friend became alarmed and insisted on his leaving the moving picture. They walked out together. On 23 October, he went into frequent attacks which were followed by hemiparesis or a hemiplegia, lasting about 3 weeks. On 13 November, there was vomiting due to intestinal obstruction.

On 1 December, the attacks became severe. On 9 December, he had an abdominal operation following which he was free of attacks for five days. At the end of the fifth day, the attacks returned and have been continuous up to the present in spite of medication which he was given in very large amounts; phenobarbital and dilantin and intravenous paraldehyde.

As seen this morning, he is having clonic movements of the right shoulder, right abdominal musculature and sometimes in the right leg at the hip. This may spread so that there is twitching of the eyelids and of the hands at times. On inquiry, he says that there is a tingling numbness of the right arm. He seems to have a right homonymous hemianopsia as judged by a very rough test. He showed no evidence of aphasia although he is right-handed.

X-rays slowed slight comparative smallness of the left cranial chamber. In the pneumogram carried out last October in Havana, there was very slight comparative enlargement of the anterior part of the left lateral ventricle. The inferior horns appear quite symmetrical. There was a superficial collection of air in the central region of Rolando near the midline; side not quite certain. There is an unusual bony vascular channel in the left occipital region. The electrogram shows spike activity in the left occipital and left central areas, sometimes appearing independently.

Family history: All members of the family including mother and father who are first cousins and the other three children have migraine. In the father's case, it is either right-sided or left-sided, interchangeably.

Investigation of J.R.: CSF protein 76 mg per cent with 2WBC, Lange curve 0012332100. Left carotid angiogram was normal. Left vertebral angiogram revealed, despite adequate injection of contrast, non-filling of the basilar system with the dye remaining in the vertebral artery, compatible with either partial or complete occlusion of the upper left vertebral artery. EEG demonstrated focal electrographic status from the posterior half of the left hemisphere involving the left occipital and left central region.'

The patient underwent a left craniotomy with removal of the left occipital lobe. Again we quote from Dr Penfield's operative note: 'There was true abnormality of the occipital lobe particularly in the vicinity of the calcarine fissure. There was a second area in the region of the precentral gyrus, where shoulder movement could be produced. The occipital lobe has been removed ... . Progress very guarded.' The pathology of the operative specimen revealed cortical neuronal degeneration and gliosis similar to the pathological process found at the patient's brother's autopsy.

Summary: Migraine started in childhood in a boy with strong family history of classical migraine.

Seizures developed at age 15 leading to left occipital and central status epilepticus. A left occipital lobectomy was carried out in an attempt to reduce the epileptogenic abnormality. He continued to deteriorate and died some years later. No autopsy could be obtained.

The pathological specimen obtained at surgery was studied by Dr Gordon Mathieson who concluded the presence of polioencephalopathy of undetermined type. This pathological finding explained poorly the very striking clinical picture which combined features of migraine and epilepsy and provided a stimulus for trying to understand patients with similar clinical problems who were studied later at the Montreal Neurological Hospital. Furthermore, this boy's brother had a similar problem and Dr Penfield obtained the following history: 'Patient R.R., the brother of J.R. was normal until, as a boy of 8 or 9, he had a seizure beginning in the right hand at the time of a very severe febrile illness. The illness was due to an intestinal parasite which produced dysentery. He spent from July 1945 to March 1946 in the Boston Children's Hospital. When he left the hospital, he was normal physically and mentally. On leaving however, the father pointed out to Dr Lennox and to Dr Bronson Crothers, that if they held the boy's right hand quietly they would feel a periodic contraction of the grip which came at regular intervals of some seconds. The patient was changed from Phenobarbital to Dilantin and that same day or the next day, he called to his mother and when she went to him he was having a seizure. Following this, he continued to have attacks which consisted in bilateral symmetrical simultaneous jerking of the arms and perhaps the legs but without loss of consciousness. When he was anaesthetized to try to stop them the attacks returned, first on the right.'

This boy died without cessation of the attacks and an autopsy of the brain was carried out at Boston Children's Hospital by Dr Betty Banker, in 1947. 'There was severe loss of nerve cells particularly in the lower layers of cortex. Large astrocytes infiltrated the cortex and replaced areas of neuronal loss. Many gemistocytic astrocytes were seen throughout the cortex. All areas of cortex were affected but the necrosis in the lower layers was most severe. There was no perivascular inflammatory reaction. Histiocytes occasionally surrounded the blood vessels and were also seen in the subarachnoid space. The white matter was normal. In the cerebellum, there was a striking loss of Purkinje cells with a replacement hyperplasia of Bergmann's astrocytes. The grey matter of pons and medulla also showed nerve cell loss and replacement gliosis.'

In summary, the brother of the previous patient developed seizures at age 8 or 9 progressing to status epilepticus and death at age 10. Neuronal degeneration and gliosis were found at autopsy. Dr Banker thought the changes were reminiscent of Alpers' disease.

In this family the consanguinity raised the possibility of autosomal recessive inheritance which did really nothing to clarify the unusual clinical picture. Dr Betty Banker's diagnosis of Alpers' disease in the younger boy was extraordinarily prescient considering recent progress in our understanding of this disease, now considered to be a mitochondrial disorder of the nervous system.

The relationship of this malignant disorder to migraine was further highlighted by several other patients referred over the years to the Montreal Neurological Hospital because of their intractable epilepsy. Three of these patients all with occipital involvement serve to illustrate this characteristic clinical presentation.

Patient A.K.: A 19-year-old right-handed male. His mother had common migraine. At age 13 he developed generalized tonic–clonic seizures associated with myoclonic jerks. An occipital spike focus was found on EEG. He was treated with phenytoin, valproic acid and clonazepam and had occasional seizures. At age 18, he experienced an episode of throbbing headaches associated with nausea and vomiting. Six months later, he developed bioccipital headache associated with scotomata in both visual fields followed by profuse vomiting. For 3 days, he was noted by the family to be somnolent and confused. Generalized convulsions followed and he was taken to hospital. Physical examination documented a confused and inattentive young man with a dense right homonymous hemianopia. He had almost continuous spike wave discharges from the left posterior quadrant on EEG. CT revealed a hypodense lesion suggesting an infarct in the left occipital lobe. Angiography demonstrated a complete block of the left calcarine artery. The headache resolved on the fourth hospital day and he was discharged 3 weeks later with a persistent right homonymous hemianopia.

Two months later, he again developed pounding occipital headache interrupting sleep. He became aware of being completely blind. On admission to hospital, he complained of nausea, vomited and had severe occipital headache. He was found to have cortical blindness. He was treated with i.v. decadron but remained lethargic, nauseated and complained of severe pounding headache for 3 days. Investigations revealed acellular CSF with protein of 59 mg per cent. CT scan showed a right occipital hypodense lesion suggesting infarction and an angiogram demonstrated attenuation of the right calcarine artery. His vision gradually improved although he remained unable to read.

Four months later, he was noted to have visual acuity of 20/200 bilaterally with inferior arcuate field defects. There was mild flattening of the left nasolabial fold and fine movements on the left were clumsily performed. His reflexes were slightly diminished on the left and plantar responses were flexor.

Laboratory examination revealed normal sedimentation rate, CBC, PT, PTT, fibrinogen clot-time, bleeding-time, platelet retention, platelet aggregation, antithrombin III, factor VIII, haemoglobin, electrophoresis, cholesterol; C3, C4, rheumatoid factor, ANA, and cryoglobulins. Triglycerides were 245 mg per cent and protein electrophoresis indicated a type IV hyperlipidaemic pattern. The electrocardiogram showed a Wolff–Parkinson–White pattern and the EEG revealed an intermittent generalized paroxysmal disturbance without epileptic activity. Visual evoked responses indicated bilateral latency delay: P100 OD–180 ms, P 100 OS–184 ms. A CT scan suggested the presence of bioccipital infarcts.

His vision improved somewhat but he continued to have episodes of migrainous headache followed by generalized seizures. A year and a half later, he had an episode of status epilepticus. He was intubated and treated with intravenous diazepam, phenytoin and phenobarbital, leading to cessation of the clinical manifestations, but continued to have electrical seizure activity. He could not be weaned from the respirator and developed repeated pulmonary infections and septicaemia. He did not respond to treatment and died at 20 years of age. Autopsy revealed multiple cortical infarcts of varying age.

Summary: Occipital seizures initially easily controlled started at 13 in a boy with family history of common migraine. Five years later he developed severe migraine leading to a left occipital and later to a right occipital infarct. He died at age 20 following status epilepticus. Multiple cortical infarcts were found at autopsy.

Patient D.S: An 18-year-old right-handed girl with a family history of common migraine developed seizures starting with visual changes going on to secondary generalization at age 9. An occipital EEG spike focus was found. She was treated with phenytoin and phenobarbital with good control. At age 17, she developed daily episodes of flashing lights in the right visual field. One month later, one of these episodes was followed by a generalized seizure. Her seizures became refractory to control and she began to have both generalized seizures and partial simple status with involvement of the right arm and leg. During her neurological examination she had episodes of occasional staring and right facial twitching. She had profound non-fluent dysphasia with good comprehension, right homonymous hemianopia, right central facial weakness and mild hemiparesis as well as hemisensory loss to all primary modalities. During hospitalization, she developed epilepsia partialis continua arising from the left posterior temporal and parietal areas. Seizures were temporarily controlled with large doses of carbamazepine, phenytoin and phenobarbitone. Investigations revealed leucocytosis, elevated sedimentation rate (52 mm) and raised liver enzymes all of which returned to normal spontaneously. CSF protein was 83 mg per cent, 135 mg per cent and 104 mg per cent on three different occasions. CSF IgG was 7.6 mg per cent. Platelet count was elevated at 561,000 (N:

140/440,00). PT, PTT, fibrinogen, factor VIII, serum protein electrophoresis and immunoelectrophoresis were normal. Rheumatoid factor and ANF were negative, C3 was 245 (slightly increased); CT scans revealed a hypodense non-enhancing lesion in the left occipital lobe. Four-vessel angiography showed delayed circulation in the distal branches of the left posterior cerebral artery. The middle inferior temporal branch of the posterior cerebral acted as collateral circulation supplying the posterior, inferior, and medial aspect of the occipital lobe. This suggested the presence of an infarct though no definite occlusion was seen.

She continued to have episodes of left-sided partial status with secondary generalization. A left temporal brain biopsy was carried out; this showed focal ischaemic changes.

She gradually improved but her right hemiparesis and hemianopia persisted. She continued to have occasional episodes of flashing lights followed by generalized seizures. Six months after discharge, she began having seizures from the opposite, right, occipital region, documented by EEG studies. These became uncontrollable and culminated in status epilepticus from which she died. No autopsy was obtained.

Summary: Occipital seizures initially easily controlled and appearing benign started at age 9 in a girl with family history of common migraine. Eight years later she developed frequent headaches, exacerbation of epilepsy and recurrent focal status epilepticus. First a left, then a right, occipital lesion developed and cerebral biopsy suggested ischaemic changes. She died at age 19 in status epilepticus.

Patient A.V.: A 41-year-old right-handed Indian male engineer with the beta thalassaemia trait had a long history of classical migraine with visual aura. One brother had a similar history. He began having generalized seizures at age 27. Initial EEG and brain scan were normal. He was treated with phenytoin and phenobarbital.

At age 30, he suffered an episode in which he saw 'stars and colours' throughout his visual field, his head turned to the right and this was followed by a generalized tonic–clonic seizure.

During the following 3 years, he had one seizure per year similar to the one described above. He was completely seizure free for 3 years, then again had one attack yearly.

At age 38, he experienced three of his typical seizures in one day. On examination he was in a postictal state without focal signs.

One month later, he experienced an episode of migraine status lasting 10 days. This consisted of visual phenomena, stars and colours associated with severe, generalized and pounding headache. There was no overt convulsive activity during this 10-day period. The family felt that his hearing was impaired and physical examination revealed receptive aphasia. An EEG showed delta activity throughout the left cerebral hemisphere. Five days later a record showed depression of cerebral activity over the left occipital lobe and the left temporal region. A CT scan revealed asymmetry of the lateral ventricles, the left being smaller than the right. A space-occupying lesion left of the midline was suspected.

Over the next few weeks, he gradually improved and his speech became normal. EEGs showed improvement of background activity but continued to show paroxysmal irregularities over the left temporal region with depression of cerebral activity over temporo-occipital areas. One month later, he again developed a confusional state, nausea and vomiting and this time a left hemiparesis and homonymous hemianopsia. The EEG now showed sharp and slow waves over the right temporal and parieto-occipital regions. A CT scan with and without contrast showed luxury perfusion in the territory of the right posterior cerebral artery and the posterior insular region. He was treated with steroids in high doses. A CT scan 1 month later showed a hypodense lesion in the right temporal and right capsular lenticular areas. He again improved gradually with resolution of the left hemiparesis although the hemianopia remained as a static deficit. Repeated EEGs during this time paralleled the clinical improvement. A ^{68}Ga PET scan revealed no focal abnormalities.

Four months later, he suffered a relapse with sudden loss of vision, hearing and aphasia. EEG revealed severe left frontal slow wave activity with epileptogenic bursts. A CT scan suggested breakdown of the blood–brain barrier in the left temporal, posterior parietal and occipital regions.

The patient underwent a left parietal brain biopsy which revealed ischaemic changes. Haemoglobin, platelets, PTT, cholesterol, triglycerides, C3, C4, IgG, IgA, rheumatoid factor, ANA, B12, echocardiogram and VDRL were normal. Serum IgG was elevated at 490 (N: 50–200). CSF was acellular with a protein of 86 mg per cent. CSF IgG was 13 mg per cent and oligoclonal banding was positive.

At 41, he was dysphasic, cortically blind, had cortical deafness and was psychotic with violent rage reactions. The psychosis was considered to be secondary to his deaf and disoriented state and chronic steriod therapy. The steroids were gradually decreased and he improved over the ensuing 3 weeks. Six months later resting lactic and pyruvic acid were 11 mg/dl (N: 9–16) and 0.7 mg/dl (N: 0.5–0.9) respectively. Post-exercise arterial lactic acid was 110 and 90 and 1 h later 2 mg/dl. Pyruvic acid was 5.2, 5.5 and 0.83 respectively. CSF lactate was 18 mg/dl (N: 9–16). A muscle biopsy showed mild denervation and no ragged red fibres. Visual, auditory and somatosensory evoked responses were abnormal but were difficult to evaluate in the presence of visual and auditory cortical deficit.

Summary: Seizures developed at age 27 in a man with classical migraine and family history of classical migraine. Eleven years later exacerbations of migraine led to a left temporo-occipital, then to a right-sided and later to a second left-sided lesion. Biopsy revealed ischaemic changes. At age 41 he had cortical deafness, blindness, dysphasia and profound mental changes. He had several recurrences and died at the age of 46.

Malignant migraine of MELAS syndrome

Thus, in these patients there was consistently a family history of classical or common migraine and they themselves had migrainous manifestations. They also had initially benign or easily controlled occipital epilepsies and then catastrophic deterioration with epilepsia partialis continua leading to stroke-like episodes with narrowing or amputation of branches of the posterior arteries. This was followed by partial recovery but then stepwise deterioration ensued. Characteristically the patients developed cortical blindness, cortical deafness and dementia and the disease was fatal in a few years.

At an international symposium on migraine epilepsy relationships in Bologna, Dr Elio Lugaresi presented a young patient with a similar history. This clinical pattern was not familiar to Dr Gastaut who was participating in the meeting but was remarkably similar to the patients just described. Unlike the preceding patients, this young man had an affected parent: his mother had a history of migraine and had had a few generalized epileptic seizures with atypical spike and wave discharges between the ages of 20 and 40. His father and paternal uncle had severe classical migraine. Obviously the disease was similar but the relationship to migraine and to the mother's clinical picture remained obscure. Shortly thereafter, Dr Louis Rowland in a presentation on progressive encephalopathies mentioned MELAS syndrome (Rowland, 1983), later described in extenso by Pavlakis *et al.* (1989), working with Di Mauro and Rowland at the Neurological Institute of New York. Dr Daune McGregor of the Hospital for Sick Children in Toronto was aware of Dr Rowland's presentation and followed a similar patient. When he had an acute recurrence she arranged for a muscle biopsy. This revealed ragged red fibres indicative of mitochondrial dysfunction (personal communication). When Dr Lugaresi was informed of this association he was incredulous but proceeded to carry out a muscle biopsy in his patient and this confirmed the diagnosis. The family was later reported in *Neurology* by Montagna *et al.* (1989) who have shown that the mother was affected by a mitochondrial disorder as well.

Mitochondrial disorders tend to present to epileptologists either with progressive myoclonus epilepsy with ragged red fibres (MERRF) associated with system degeneration or with occipital seizures followed by epilepsia partialis continua and with migrainous symptoms which have strong occipital localizing features. Reviewing a series of patients including the ones described above it appeared very likely that they suffered from MELAS syndrome. There was however no good evidence for lactic acidosis in some of these individuals and ragged red fibres were also not always found (Dvorkin et al., 1987). This led to considerable scepticism about the significance of the highly characteristic clinical pattern which these patients presented and which, by many, was not considered to be adequate for a diagnosis of mitochondrial disease. Over the years however it has become abundantly clear that ragged red fibres need not be present in all patients or in all biopsies: in a patient with MERRF we have seen a normal biopsy from one muscle and a great many ragged red fibres in a different muscle a few days later (Berkovic et al., 1989b). Lactic acidosis might be present in blood or in CSF but need not be present when the sample is obtained. Thus the clinical picture and especially the course of the illness in these patients is highly characteristic and can lead to a strong clinical suspicion of mitochondrial encephalopathy.

A variety of additional clinical features may be found in patients with MELAS syndrome. These include small stature, calcification of the basal ganglia, optic atrophy, peripheral nerve involvement, and clinical evidence for muscle involvement. In one patient we have recently studied, external ophthalmoplegia and severe peripheral neuropathy developed.

It soon became clear that patients with MELAS were either sporadic or that the disease was transmitted by maternal inheritance. The variation in the recognized phenotypes of MELAS constantly increased. Acute fatigue such as plane trips, long marches or extra hours at work are now known to precipitate attacks. A family history of migraine is quite striking in sporadic patients but is also found in the familial ones (Dvorkin et al., 1987; Berkovic et al., 1987, 1989b, 1991). Epilepsia partialis continua is a very prominent symptom in acute attacks, often associated with or following severe throbbing headaches with visual changes; these are highly suggestive or reminiscent of a migrainous aura. The lesions of MELAS are often visible by CT but at times can be found only by magnetic resonance imaging (Matthews et al., 1990). An abnormal MRI signal is highly characteristic. There are however patients with an otherwise strongly characteristic history and muscle abnormalities who do not have the characteristic MRI signals (personal observation).

Current progress in the neurobiology of MERRF and MELAS

Initial studies of various components of the respiratory chain yielded quite variable results and such studies are now not considered reliable indices of specific mitochondrial abnormality. A specific point mutation at tRNA$^{Leu\ UUR}$ has been identified by Goto et al. (1990) and subsequently two other point mutations have been described (Goto et al., 1991; Morton, et al., 1992). These mutations have been found only in patients with evidence for maternal inheritance and have not been encountered in patients with sporadic MELAS syndrome. The diagnosis now may be made by DNA analysis from peripheral tissues such as blood (Hammans et al., 1991). The ratio of the mutated to the wild type of DNA is constant in different portions of the brain in some patients with proven MELAS syndrome (Durcan et al., 1992). The ratio was found to be similar in different organs of affected sisters but was different in the organs of their affected mother (Macmillan et al., 1993). A variety of trials of treatment have been attempted with conflicting results. A recent careful trial of treatment of various forms of mitochondrial disease has shown no consistent improvement (Matthews et al., 1993) but only a single patient with MELAS syndrome was included in this trial.

Hypothesis

In a previous review of patients with malignant migraine indicative of MELAS syndrome (Dvorkin et al., 1987) we wondered about mitochondrial abnormality in smooth muscles of cerebral blood vessels to explain the stroke-like episodes. This has subsequently been demonstrated by Lach et al. in autopsies of patients of a family with the MELAS syndrome (Lach et al., 1986) who had the most frequently encountered DNA point mutation. This finding does however not explain the predilection for involvement of posterior structures which MELAS syndrome shares with classical migraine. It also does not explain the occurrence of catastrophic MELAS syndrome in sporadic patients who have a family history of migraine but not of any other mitochondrial abnormality. In that situation the possibility of secondary mitochondrial dysfunction may be postulated (Arnold, personal communication).

The possibility of mitochondrial abnormality in some patients who have migraine with aura has been studied by Barbiroli and Montagna from the University of Bologna (Montagna et al., 1988; Bresolin et al., 1991; Barbiroli et al., 1990, 1992). They have found a low phosphocreatine content in patients by measuring brain ^{31}P. MRS, accompanied by high adenosine diphosphate concentration, a high percentage of $V–V_{max}$ adenosine triphosphate, and low phosphorylation potential. These are features of an unstable state of metabolism. The same group has also demonstrated ragged red fibres and a five kilobase deletion without a point mutation at nucleotide pair 3243 in the mitochondrial RNA in a person with migraine. Their patient had defective energy metabolism in both muscle and brain, judging from phosphorus magnetic resonance spectroscopy. An increase in organic phosphate to phosphocreatine ratio due to decreased phosphocreatine content was found in the occipital lobes. Montagna and colleagues have postulated a defect of brain oxidative metabolism in patients with migraine predisposing to development of cerebral deficits when subjected to stressful events. Such trigger factors could provoke an increase in brain metabolic demands. This hypothesis is attractive and would explain the occurrence of MELAS syndrome in sporadic patients with migraine and who have a family history of migraine. Certainly further molecular genetic studies should provide better understanding of the mechanism of MELAS syndrome and of its relation to migraine.

A point mutation at tRNA^{Lys} in patients with MERRF has been described by Shoffner et al. (1991). In this disorder action myoclonus, epilepsy, ataxia and mental deterioration are the cardinal features. Hearing loss, optic atrophy, short stature, muscular or peripheral nerve involvement may also be found. Hearing loss may be the only symptom for many years and onset at different ages within one family may suggest the diagnosis in this second major mitochondrial disorder associated with epilepsy (Berkovic et al., 1989b; Rosing et al., 1985). A number of other familial disorders are most likely also due to mitochondrial dysfunction. These include multiple symmetric lipomatosis (Berkovic et al., 1991a), the May–White syndrome (May & White, 1968), Ekbom's syndrome (Ekbom, 1975) and perhaps biotin deficiency (Bressman et al., 1986). The overlap between MERRF and MELAS has been recognized by Fukuhara et al. (1980) and we have also encountered this in three patients.

The epilepsy in MERRF is often not very difficult to control and it is the action myoclonus which represents the major disability (So et al., 1989). This is then usually superseded by the progressive dementia although some patients show little deterioration over the years. Unlike what is seen in MELAS syndrome, classical migraine or migraine with aura is not a striking feature of MERRF. A positive family history of migraine is not as obviously present in patients with the familial or sporadic forms of this disorder.

Patients with MERRF are usually photosensitive, suggesting that occipital factors are involved or participate in the generalized epileptic process. Furthermore, focal epileptic abnormalities involving the occipital regions are common as well (So et al., 1989).

It has been recognized since Roger's original description (Roger et al., 1983) that patients with progressive myoclonus epilepsy of the Lafora type have in addition to the generalized and photosensitive epileptic abnormalities, occipital focal discharges. Such abnormalities have been encountered not only in MERRF and Lafora disease but also in other forms of progressive myclonus epilepsy, such as Unverricht–Lundborg disease, or in neuroaxonal dystrophy with myoclonus epilepsy. A common dopaminergic mechanism in myoclonus epilepsies due to a variety of causes has been demonstrated by Mervaala et al. (1990). This mechanism is similar to that seen in primary generalized photosensitive epilepsy as previously shown by Quesney (see Mervaala *et al.*, 1990 for review).

The progressive myoclonus epilepsies also share a tendency to the development of progressive ataxia. It is likely that a specific neuronal system is responsible for the action myoclonus, the generalized epilepsy, the occipital focal epileptogenic abnormalities and the progressive ataxia. Such a common denominator of the progressive myoclonus epilepsies has not yet been identified. Interestingly it seems to be shared by autosomal recessive or maternally inherited and even by an autosomal dominant disorder (some patients with Kufs disease).

One may conclude that migraine with aura, mitochondrial disorders such as MELAS and MERRF and also other progressive myoclonus epilepsies as well as primary generalized photosensitive epilepsy share a predisposition to involvement of occipital structures. Clarification of the basis for this preferential involvement must await progress in our understanding of the neurobiology of the occipital lobes.

References

Barbiroli, B., Montagna, P., Cortelli, P., Martinelli, P., Sacquegna, T., Zaniol, P. & Lugaresi, E. (1990): Complicated migraine studied by phosphorus magnetic resonance spectroscopy. *Cephalalgia* **10**, 263–72.

Barbiroli, B., Montagna, P., Cortelli, P., Funicello, R., Iotti, S., Monari, L., Pierangeli, G., Zaniol, P. & Lugaresi, E. (1992): Abnormal brain and muscle energy metabolism shown by ^{31}P magnetic resonance spectroscopy in patients affected by migraine with aura. *Neurology* **42**, 1209–1214.

Berkovic, S.F., Andermann, F., Karpati, G., Carpenter, S., Andermann, E. & Shoubridge, E. (1987): Mitochondrial encephalomyopathies: a solution to the enigma of the Ramsay Hunt syndrome. *Neurology* **37** (Suppl.), 125.

Berkovic, S.F., Carpenter, S., Evans, A. *et al.* (1989b): Myoclonus epilepsy and ragged-red fibres (MERRF). 1. A clinical, pathological, biochemical, magnetic resonance spectroscopic and positron emission tomographic study. *Brain* **112**, 1231–1260.

Berkovic, S.F., Shoubridge, E.A., Andermann, F., Andermann, E., Carpenter, S. & Karpati, G. (1991): Clinical spectrum of mitochondrial DNA mutation at base pair 8344. *Lancet* **338**, 457.

Berkovic, S.F., Andermann, F., Shoubridge, E.A. *et al.* (1991a): Mitochondrial dysfunction in multiple symmetrical lipomatosis. *Ann. Neurol.* **29**, 566–569.

Bresolin, N., Martinelli, P., Barbiroli, B., Zaniol, P., Ausenda, C., Montagna, P., Gallanti, A., Comi, G.P., Scarlato, G. & Lugaresi, E. (1991): Muscle mitochondrial DNA deletion and ^{31}P-NMR spectroscopy alterations in a migraine patient. *J. Neurol. Sc.* **104**, 182–189.

Bressman, S., Fahn, S., Eisenberg, M., Brin, M. Maltese, W. (1986): Biotin-responsive encephalopathy with myoclonus, ataxia, and seizures. In: *Myoclonus (Advances in Neurology,* Vol. 43*)*, pp. 199–225. New York: Raven Press.

Durcan, L., Carpenter, S. & Shoubridge, E. (1992): Distribution of the tRNA Leu MTDNA mutation in MELAS brain (abst). p. 282. *Neurology* **42** (Suppl. 3).

Dvorkin, G.S., Andermann, F., Carpenter, S., Melanson, D., Verret, S., Jacob, J.C., Sherwin, A., Bekhor, S., Lugaresi, E., Sackellares, C., Willoughby, J. & MacGregor, D. (1987): Classical migraine, intractable epilepsy and multiple strokes: a syndrome related to mitochondrial encephalomyopathy. In: *Migraine and epilepsy*, eds. F. Andermann & E. Lugaresi, pp. 203–232. London, Boston: Butterworths.

Ekbom, K. (1975): Hereditary ataxia, photomyoclonus, skeletal deformities and lipoma. *Acta Neurol. Scand.* **51**, 393–404.

Fukuhara, N., Tokiguchi, S., Shirakawa, K. & Tsubaki, T. (1980): Myoclonus epilepsy associated with ragged-red fibres (mitochondrial abnormalities): disease entity or a syndrome? *J. Neurol. Sci.* **47**, 117–133.

Goto, Y., Nonaka, I. & Horai, S. (1990): A mutation in the RNA (Leu UUR) gene associated with the MELAS subgroup of mitochondrial encephalomyopathies. *Nature* **348**, 651–653.

Goto, Y., Nonaka, I. & Horai, S. (1991): A new mitochondrial DNA mutation associated with the mitochondrial myopathy encephalopathy, encephalopathy, lactic acidosis and stroke-like episodes (MELAS). *Biochem. Biophys. Acta* **1097**, 238–240.

Hammans, S.R., Sweeney, M.G., Brockington, M., Morgan-Hughes, J.A. & Harding A.E. (1991): Mitochondrial encephalopathies: molecular genetic diagnosis from blood samples. *Lancet* **337**, 1311–1313.

Lach, B., Preston, D., Servidei, S., Embree, G., Di Mauro, S. & Swirenga, S. (1986): Maternally inherited mitochondrial encephalomyopathy. A vasculopathy. *Muscle Nerve* **9, 55,** 184. (Abst.)

Macmillan, C., Lach, B. & Shoubridge, E. (1993): Variable distribution of mutant mitochondrial DNA (tRNA Leu 324) in tissues of symptomatic relatives with MELAS: the role of mitotic segregation. *Neurology* (in press).

Matthews, P.M., Tampieri, D., Andermann, F., Carpenter, S. & Arnold, D.L. (1990): MRI shows specific features in patients with the MELAS syndrome. *Neurology* **40**, (Suppl.), 435.

Matthews, P.M., Ford, B., Dandurand, R.J., Eidelman, D.H., O'Connor, D., Sherwin, A., Karpati, G., Andermann, F. & Arnold, D.L. Coenzyme Q 10 with multiple vitamins is generally ineffective in the treatment of mitochondrial disease. (in press).

May, D.L. & White, H.H. (1968): Familial myoclonus, cerebellar ataxia, and deafness: specific genetically determined disease. *Arch. Neurol.* **19**, 331–338.

Mervaala, E., Andermann, F., Quesney, L.F. & Krelina, M. (1990): Common dopaminergic mechanism for epileptic photosensitivity in progressive myoclonus epilepsies. *Neurology* **40**, 53–56.

Montagna, P., Sacquegna, T., Martinelli, P., Cortelli, P., Bresolin, N., Moggio, M., Baldrati, A., Riva, R. & Lugaresi, E. (1988): Mitochondrial abnormalities in migraine. Preliminary findings. *Headache* **28**, (No. 7), 477–480.

Montagna, P., Sacquegna, T., Cortelli, P. & Lugaresi E. (1989): Migraine as a defect of brain oxidative metabolism: a hypothesis. *J. Neurol.* **236**, 123–125.

Morten, K., Brown, G., Lake, B., Wilson, J. & Poulton, J. (1992): EUROMIT, 2nd International Congress on Mitochondrial Pathology, Rome, 21–23 September 1992, abstr., p. 39.

Pavlakis, S.G., Philips, P.C., Di Mauro, S., De Vivo, D.C. & Rowland, L.P. (1989): Mitochondrial myopathy, encephalopathy, lactic acidosis and stroke-like episodes. A distinctive clinical syndrome. *Ann. Neurol.* **16**, 481–488.

Roger, J., Pellissier, J.F., Bureau, M., Dravet, C., Revol, M. & Tinuper, P. (1983): Le diagnostic précoce de la maladie de Lafora: importance des manifestations paroxystiques visuelles et interêt de la biopsie cutanée. *Rev. Neurol.* **139**, 115–124.

Rosing, H.S., Hopkins, L.C., Wallace, D.C., Epstein, C.M. & Weidenheim, K. (1985): Maternally inherited mitochondrial myopathy and myoclonic epilepsy. *Ann. Neurol.* **17**, 228–237.

Rowland, L.P. (1983): Molecular genetics, pseudogenetics and clinical neurology. The Robert Wartenberg lecture. *Neurology* **33**, 1189–1195.

Shoffner, J.M., Lott, M.T., Lezza, A.M.S., Seibel, P., Ballinger, S.W. & Wallace, D.C. (1991): Myoclonic epilepsy and ragged-red fiber disease (MERRF) is associated with a mitochondrial DNA tRNA Lys mutation. *Cell* **61**, 931–937.

So, N., Berkovic, S.F., Andermann, F., Kuzniecky, R., Gendron, D. & Quesney, L.F. (1989): Myoclonus epilepsy and ragged fibers (MERRF) 2. Electrophysiological studies and comparison with the other progressive myoclonus epilepsies. *Brain* **112**, 1261–1276.

Chapter 14

Occipital epilepsy in neonates and infants

Anne Lortie*, Perrine Plouin[†§], Jean Marc Pinard* and Olivier Dulac*[§]

Neuropediatric Department (Prof. G. Ponsot); †EEG Department; §INSERM U.29; Hôpital Saint Vincent de Paul, 82 av. Denfert Rochereau, 75674 Paris Cedex, France

Summary

We report 12 neonates and infants who had occipital epilepsy. The diagnosis was based on the association of seizures with an occipital lesion and/or persistence of an occipital focus on serial EEGs. Seizures were often generalized, including spasms in seven cases, and visual and behavioural development was severely disturbed even in patients who experienced seizure control months of treatment. Results are preliminary, all children will be re-evaluated.

Introduction

Seizures originating in the occipital lobe have been well described in adults by Penfield & Kristiansen (1951), and by Penfield & Jasper (1954). Since then, many authors have reported the clinical signs and symptoms that suggest an occipital lobe origin for seizure (Gastaut, 1960; Takeda *et al.*, 1969; White, 1971; Ludwig & Ajmone-Marsan, 1975; Holtzman & Goldensohn, 1977; Beun *et al.*, 1984; Williamson *et al.*, 1981, 1986, 1988, 1992; Kaplan & Lesser, 1989; Tusa *et al.*, 1990). The semiology of occipital lobe seizures includes subjective symptoms (elementary visual hallucinations, ictal amaurosis, sensations of eye pulling or moving); and clinical signs (rapid bilateral eye blinking also called eyelid flutter, eye and/or head deviation, nystagmoid movements).

However, occipital lobe seizures remain difficult to recognize. Because of the very frequent propagation of the ictal discharge from the occipital lobes to more anterior regions, the symptomatology is often associated with sensory, motor or visceral symptoms (Takeda *et al.*, 1969: Williamson *et al.*, 1986, 1988, 1992; Huott *et al.*, 1974.) Even in patients with a proven occipital origin for seizures, ictal and interictal scalp findings may be misleading (with temporal, bifrontal or large posterior foci) and they seldom suggest an occipital origin (Williamson *et al.*, 1981, 1986, 1988, 1992; Takeda *et al.*, 1969).

Aso (1978) studied 21 children with occipital paroxysmal discharges. The age of the children at the onset of the seizures was between 4 months and 14 years (one case younger than 12 months), and the characteristics, in regard of semiology and EEG data, were similar to findings in adults. However, there is no description of occipital lobe seizures in newborns and infants and an occipital epileptic syndrome has not yet been defined in this age group.

In order to determine clinical and electroencephalographic particularities which could help in recognizing such a condition in this age group, we report 12 patients with occipital epilepsy starting in the first year of life.

Patients and methods

All patients were referred to the paediatric neurology department of the Hopital St. Vincent de Paul from 1983 to 1991 and met the following criteria: onset before 1 year, at least two unprovoked seizures, occipital origin of seizures based on evidence of an occipital lesion on magnetic resonance imaging (MRI) or cerebral computed tomography (CT scan), and/or persistent interictal focus on repeat EEG recordings, and follow-up of over 1 year. There were 12 cases, seven girls and five boys. Eight had an occipital lesion, and four had a persistent occipital focus on serial EEGs without occipital abnormalities on radiological studies. Follow-up ranged from 1 to 10 years with a mean of 5.25 years. All were evaluated in regard of their clinical outcome (neurological, behavioural and neurodevelopmental).

Results

1. Groups: Patients were divided into two groups, according to neuroradiological data (Table 1). The eight patients of group A had neuroradiological and/or neuropathological abnormalities. Three infants had occipital dysplasia, two had hemimegaloencephaly predominating in the parieto-occipital region, and three had structural abnormalities of the white and/or grey matters in the occipital areas. Four patients from group A underwent surgery (three with dysplasia, one with hemimegaloencephaly). The surgical tissue showed neuronal dysplasia in all cases. The four patients of group B had no radiological evidence of brain malformation.

2. Age (Table 1): all patients experienced first seizures before the age of 2 months.

3. Neurological status at the onset of the first seizures (Table 1): Two children had strabismus, one of whom had poor visual contact and was thought to have hemianopsia. The other 10 children had no other evident neurological defect.

4. Seizure types (Table 1 and Fig. 1): The seizures were of three types: partial, partial with secondary generalization, and generalized including spasms. Partial seizures were oculoclonic, versive, with eye and/or head deviation or hemiclonic, with flutter, and eye and/or head deviation. When they were complex, they were always associated with flutter or abnormal eye movements. The seizures were sometimes secondarily generalized.

Spasms were symmetrical or asymmetrical. They were called asymmetrical if preceded by eye and/or head deviation, or if limb flexion or extension was more severe on one side. Generalized seizures were tonic, atonic, tonico-clonic or myoclonic. Abnormal ocular movements were frequent features.

5. Clinical signs suggesting occipital lobe involvement included strabismus and/or poor visual contact that were seen before the first seizures or initial ictal signs, as described previously. Seven children in group A and three in group B had such clinical signs. The other two children developed strabismus in the month following their first seizures (Table 1).

6. EEGs at the onset of the seizures showed two patterns:

    (a) Good electroclinical correlation between the seizures, which were partial, and the EEGs which showed a focus of spikes. This was observed in four patients (all in group A) and is illustrated by the case of a 1-month-old boy who had partial seizures with eyelid flutter and eye deviation (Case No. 2). His first EEGs showed a right occipital focus, recorded ictally and interictally. At 4 years, he had the same focus (Figs. 2a, b, c).

    (b) Poor electroclinical correlation, noticed in six patients (four of group A and two of group B), illustrated by the case of a 1-month-old boy with epileptic spasms (Case No. 11). His

Groups	Patients (No.)	Neuroradiology (MRI)	Age at seizure onset	Neurological findings at onset	1st seizure types and signs	Age at last visit	Neurological outcome	Behavioural outcome	Neurodevelopmental outcome
Group A	1	4 m: hemimega	D1	None	P, flutter, eye and head deviation to the left	18 m	Strabismus disappeared after surgery, hemiplegia, hemianopsia	Pseudo-autism disappeared after surgery	Sits, isolated words, slow global acquisitions
	2	4 y: dysplasia	D9	None	P, flutter, eye and head deviation to the right	6 y 3 m	Strabismus, hemianopsia etc.	Hyperkinesia, disappeared 10 m after surgery	Walks, speaks, almost normal acquisitions
	3	7½ y: dysplasia	D3	Strabismus	P, nystagmus, eye and head deviation to the right, flutter	10 y 7 m	Strabismus	Aggressiveness, pseudo-autism	Walks, speaks, no acquisitions
	4	*	1 month	None	P, eye deviation to the left, flutter	9 y 9 m	Strabismus, hemianopsia	Hyperkinesia, pseudo-autism improved after surgery	Autonomous, delayed visuo-spatial acquisitions
	5	9 m: hemimega	D21	Strabismus, hemianopsia	AS	5 y 2 m	Hemianopsia, strabismus, hemiplegia	Hyperkinesia, disappeared at 3 y 2 m	Walks, speaks, slow verbal and fine motor acquisitions
	6	5 y 5 m: posterior abnormalities	1 month	None	P, flutter	6 y 7 m	None	Hyperkinesia, disappeared at 6 y 6 m	Walks, speaks, slow verbal and fine motor acquisitions
	7	3 y: posterior abnormalities	1½ months	None	SS, preceded by nystagmus	8 y 5 m	Nystagmus, PVC	Pseudo-autism	Walks, speaks, slow global acquisitions
	8	1 y: posterior abnormalities	3 weeks	None	P, secondarily generalized	6 y 6 m	Strabismus, nystagmus, PVC	Pseudo-autism, hyperkinesia	Walks, speaks, slow global acquisitions
Group B	9		D1	None	GT	3 y 6 m	Strabismus	Hyperkinesia disappeared at 6 m	Walks, monosyllables, slow fine motor and no verbal acquisitions
	10		2 months	None	GT, flutter	19 m	Strabismus, PVC	Sleep problems, pseudo-autism, hyperkinesia disappeared at 14 m	Sits, monosyllables, slow global acquisitions
	11		2 months	None	P, AS, eye and head deviation to the left	4 y 4 m	Hypotonia	Pseudo-autism, hyperkinesia	Sits, isolated words, slow global acquisitions
	12		2 months	None	P, AS, flutter, eye and head deviation to the left	2 y 10 m	Hypotonia	Pseudo-autism	Sits, monosyllables, slow global acquisitions

AS = asymmetrical spasms; SS = symmetrical spasms; GT = generalized tonic; P = partial; PVC = poor visual contact; *CT scan and MRI normal; neuropathological results: dysplasia.

interictal EEG showed bioccipital spikes. At 4 years, he still had spasms, associated with partial seizures. On his interictal EEG, there were left occipital spikes with contralateral diffusion (Fig. 3a, b). The first EEGs were not available for two patients.

Table 2. Evolution of EEGs

Groups	Patients	Age of appearance of foci	Generalized or multifocal EEGs
Group A	1	Left occipital: 3 m (subclinical discharges) Left rolandic: 4 m (ictal) Left temporal: 12 m (subclinical discharges)	*Left multifocal: 4 m
	2	Right occipital: 7 m (interictal) Right temporo-occipital: 9 m (ictal)	*Right multifocal: 18 days Generalized: 3 y 11 m
	3**	Left occipital: 7 y 6 m (interictal) Left fronto-temporal: 7 y 6 m (ictal) Left rolando-temporo-occipital: 7 y 7 m (interictal)	Generalized: 7 y 6 m
	4	*Right occipital: 4 m (interictal) Left frontal: 18 m (interictal) Right temporal: 18 m (interictal)	
	5**	Right temporo-occipital: 5 y 3 m (interictal) Left temporal: 5 y 5 m (interictal)	Generalized: 5 y 3 m
	6	Left posterior: 6 m (interictal)	*Generalized, suppression–bursts: 1 m Generalized: 3 m 13 m 23 m
	7	Left occipital: 6 m (ictal) Right temporo-occipital: 2 y (interictal)	*Generalized, hypsarrhythmia: 3 m
	8	Left occipital: 7 m (interictal) Left temporo-occipital: 10 m (interictal) Left frontal: 10 m (interictal)	*Generalized, hypsarrhythmia: 6 m
Group B	9	*Right rolandic: D4 (interictal) Bifrontal: D22 (ictal) Bioccipital: 2 m (subclinical discharges) Right temporo-occipital: 5 m (interictal) Left temporo-occipital: 13 m (interictal)	Generalized: D29, 1 m, 4 m
	10	Right rolandic: 3 m (interictal) Right temporo-occipital: 4 m (interictal) Right occipital: 7 m (interictal) Left fronto-rolandic: 7 m (interictal)	*Generalized: 2 m Generalized: 6 m
	11	*Left temporo-occipital: 3 m (interictal) Right frontal: 4 m (interictal) Left temporal: 5 m (interictal) Left frontal: 9 m (interictal) Left occipital: 4 y 6 m (interictal)	Generalized: 4 m Multifocal: 12 m
	12	*Bioccipital: 3 m (interictal) Bifrontal and left fronto-temporal: 6 m (interictal) Left occipital: 6 m (interictal) Birolandic: 16 m (interictal)	Generalized: 4 m, 6 m

*First EEG at Hôpital St-Vincent de Paul; **First EEG not available.

7. Outcome:

(a) Evolution of seizures (Fig. 1.) During follow-up, all children from group A, i.e. with a neuroradiological occipital lesion, developed partial seizures. Four had partial seizures (Cases No. 1–4) as their first seizure type (with secondary generalization in three cases). Case No. 2 also had spasms for a short period of time (1 month). They underwent surgery, after the demonstration of an occipital lesion. Two patients became free of seizures, and one was still treated with medication 1 year after surgery. The other two patients still had seizures, 11 and 33 months after surgery, but one had less than one seizure per month.

Cases No. 5–7 had a more complex seizure evolution. Two started with spasms that were noticed very early (D 21 and 1½ months) and lasted less than 5 months. All also had generalized seizures. At the last visit, two children had partial seizures treated with antiepileptic drugs, one having both partial and generalized seizures. Case No. 5 was not treated, as she stopped having seizures. The last patient, Case No. 8, had only partial seizures, except for spasms during 1 month. His seizure history during follow-up was unclear.

The four patients without evidence of brain malformation (Cases No. 9–12) were the only ones to present generalized tonic seizures as their first seizure type (Cases No. 9–10)). Two of these four patients initially had both partial seizures and asymmetrical spasms (Cases No. 11–12). During follow-up, all four patients had partial seizures, but in three cases they lasted for less than 3 months. Three patients had spasms (at 2 months, Cases No. 11 and 12 and 5 months, Case No. 10) which lasted less than 5 months in Cases No. 10 and 12 and almost 2 years in Case No. 11. Generalized seizures (tonic) were noticed in three cases. At last visit, two were controlled with antiepileptic drugs.

(b) Evolution of EEGs (Table 2). During follow-up, all children developed a focus of spikes in the posterior regions. It was restricted to the occipital region in 10 cases, and more diffuse in the two others (temporo-occipito-parietal or temporo-occipital). In one patient (Case No. 6), it was always associated with generalized abnormalities. All children had spikes recorded at least once in the temporal regions. Seven also had discharges in the frontal regions, and five in the rolandic regions. In three cases, a multifocal activity was noticed on one EEG. Finally, all except Case No. 4 had abnormal generalized abnormalities at least once during the evolution, usually early in the follow-up.

(c) Neurological outcome (Table 1): nine patients developed ocular symptoms. They appeared very early in the evolution and persisted. Strabismus was the most frequent.

(d) Behaviour (Table 1): all patients had abnormal behaviour during the evolution noticed soon after the beginning of the disease. Eight children developed pseudo-autistic behaviour consisting of poor contact with the examiner, as if patients were in their own world without any interpersonal communication. In addition there was sleep disturbance and/or hyperkinesia or aggressiveness. These behaviours improved in three of the four children who underwent surgery, and spontaneously disappeared in Cases No. 5, 6, 9, 10.

(e) Neurodevelopment (Table 1): all 12 patients had poor developmental progression, and even some regression of developmental abilities (language, gross and fine motor skills) during severe bouts of seizures. Three of the four patients who underwent surgery showed better developmental progression after surgery (Cases No. 1, 2, 4). At the last visit, the other nine patients still had delay in verbal, motor and cognitive development, although they continue to make slow progress.

Discussion

This work provides the first attempt to describe occipital epilepsy in infants and newborns. Some clinical characteristics are isolated, including ictal oculomotor signs, very early onset of seizures,

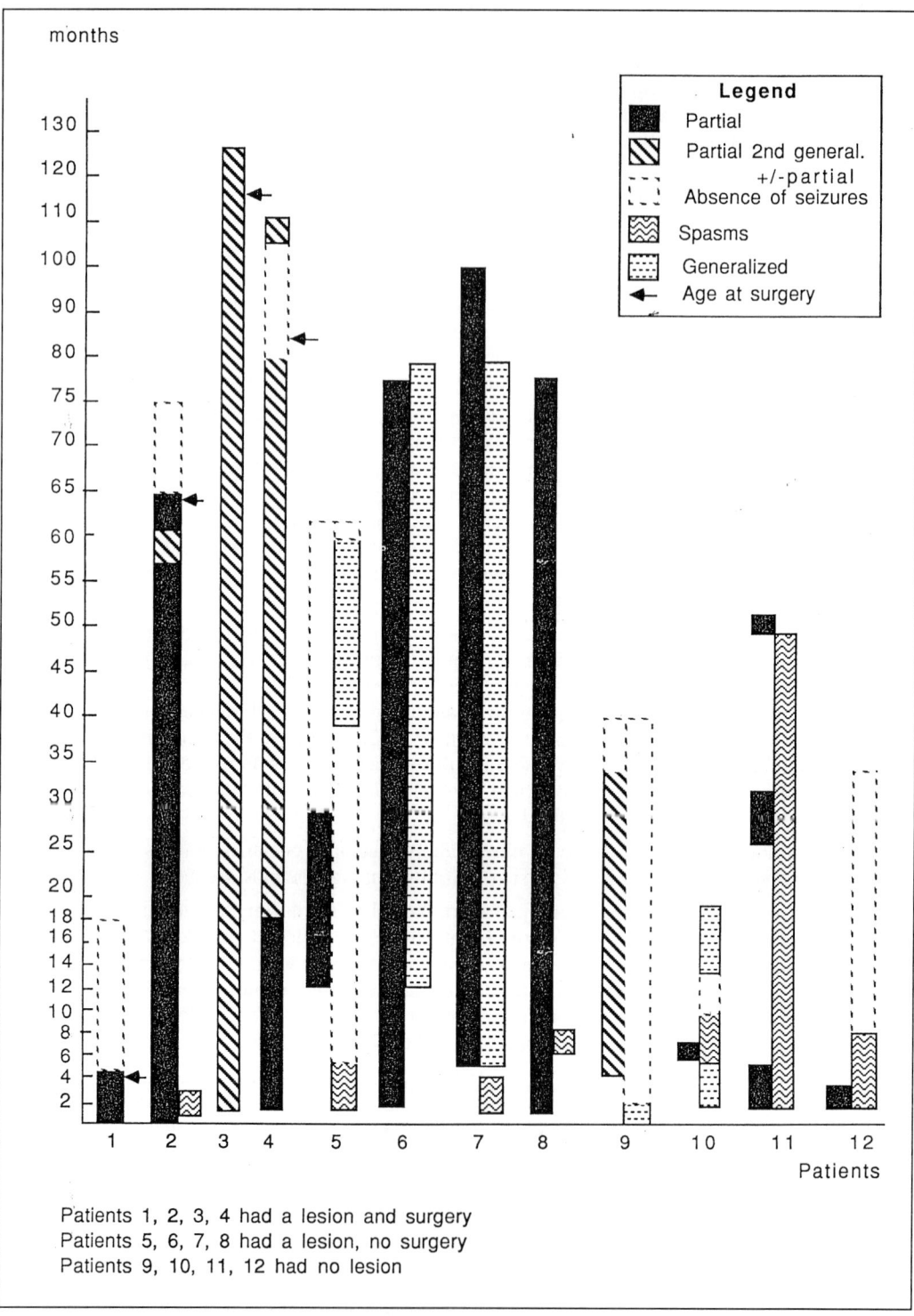

Fig. 1. Evolution of seizures.

Chapter 14 Occipital epilepsy in neonates and infants

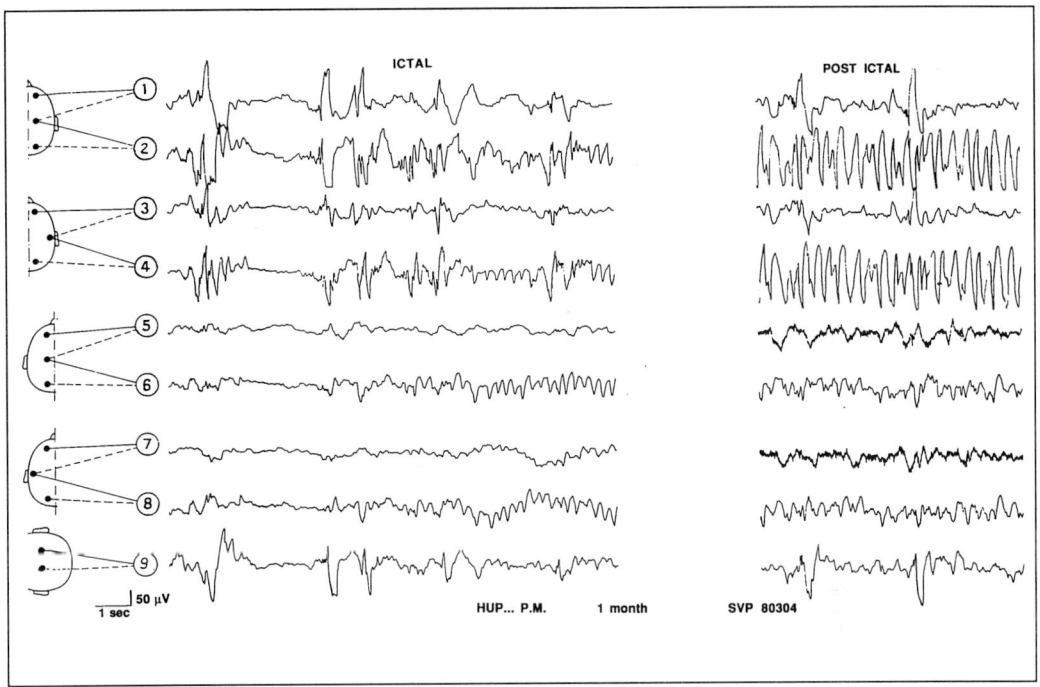

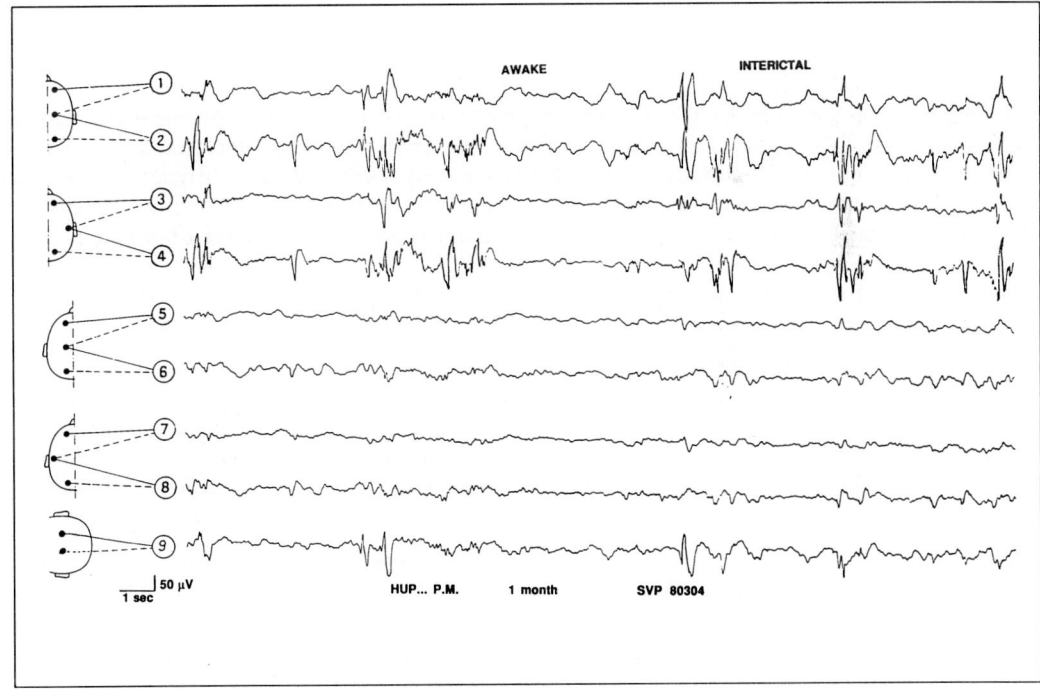

Fig. 2 (a,b). Good electroclinical correlation. First EEGs of a 1-month-old boy who had partial seizures (eyelid flutter and eye deviation) recorded ictally (a, top) and interictally (b, bottom).

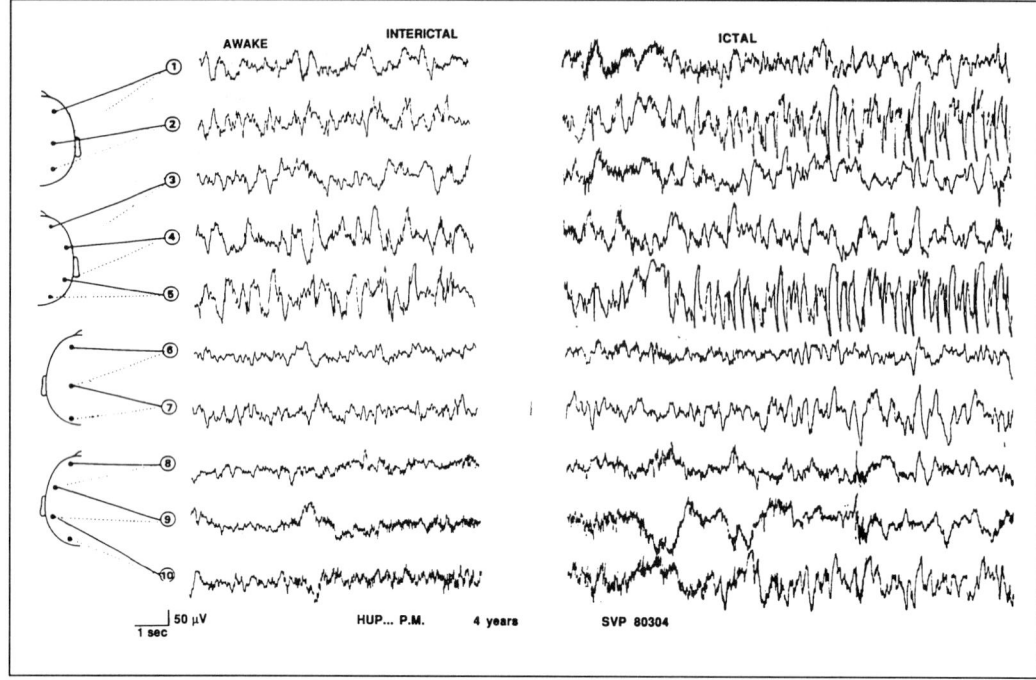

Fig. 2(c). EEG of the same boy, who still had partial seizures at 4 years.

early spasms, no tendency to spontaneous remission, and severe mental and behavioural disorders. Such features may be useful in recognizing occipital epilepsy at this age.

It is clear from the literature that the occipital origin of seizures is not always obvious. Both clinical and electrophysiological data are very often imprecise, or so varied that the exact diagnosis is delayed or even ignored. In our population, occipital epilepsy was particularly difficult to diagnose. It is impossible, in a newborn or an infant, to obtain the description of subjective symptoms. Discrete ictal signs such as flutter or oculoclonic movements require careful observation from parents and physician to be recognized. Therefore our patients were selected according to neuro-radiological evidence of an occipital lesion, or a persistent occipital focus on serial scalp EEGs. But this method is imprecise for two reasons.

First, the occipital lesion was defined according to cerebral MRI. And we know that the visualization of abnormalities partly depends on the myelination of the white matter, which is insufficient for the grey–white matter border to be well visualized before 2 years of age (Valk & van der Knaap, 1989). Therefore it is possible that infants included in group B because of a normal MRI obtained before 2 years, may be later classified into group A after repeat MRI. For the same reason, even if MRI reveals a focal occipital dysplasia, the brain malformation may be in fact more diffuse.

Secondly, the occipital focus was recorded on scalp EEGs, which is very imprecise according to Williamson (1992) and Takeda (1969). This is particularly true with interictal EEGs which almost never demonstrate spikes in the occipital regions. And if spikes are recorded in posterior areas, it is impossible to be certain that they originate in the occipital lobe, and not in the association cortex. When possible, depth electrodes should be used, as illustrated by Williamson (1992). Nevertheless, for the four children who exhibited no MRI abnormalities, the diagnosis was based on the persistence of an occipital focus on interictal scalp EEGs, together with clinical descriptions of seizures consistent with an occipital origin and abnormal neurodevelopment and behaviour.

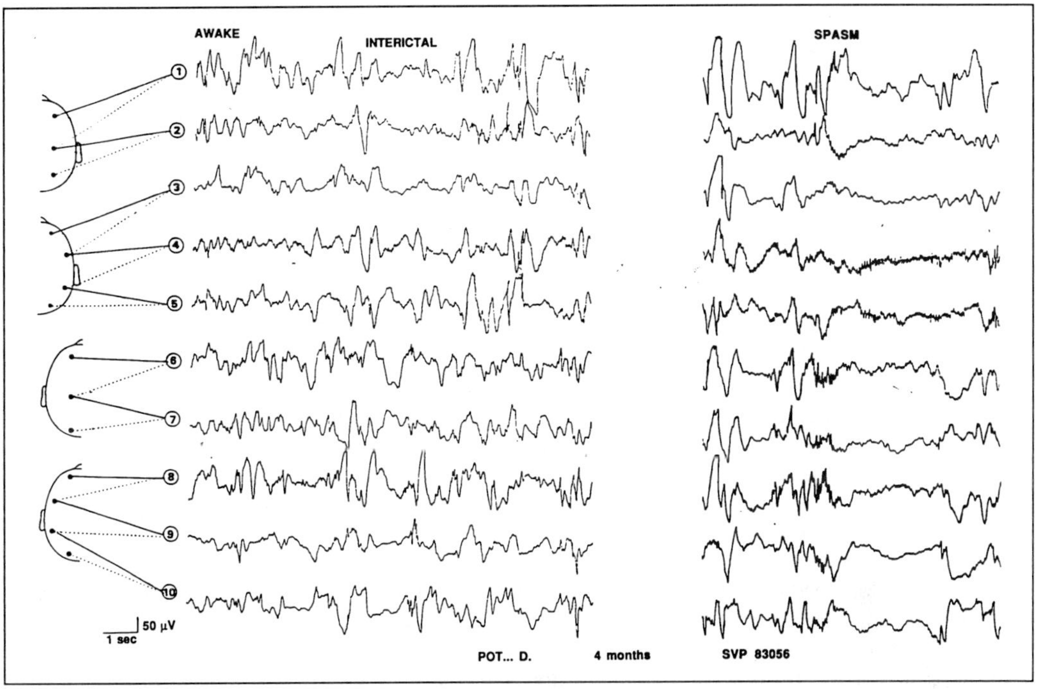

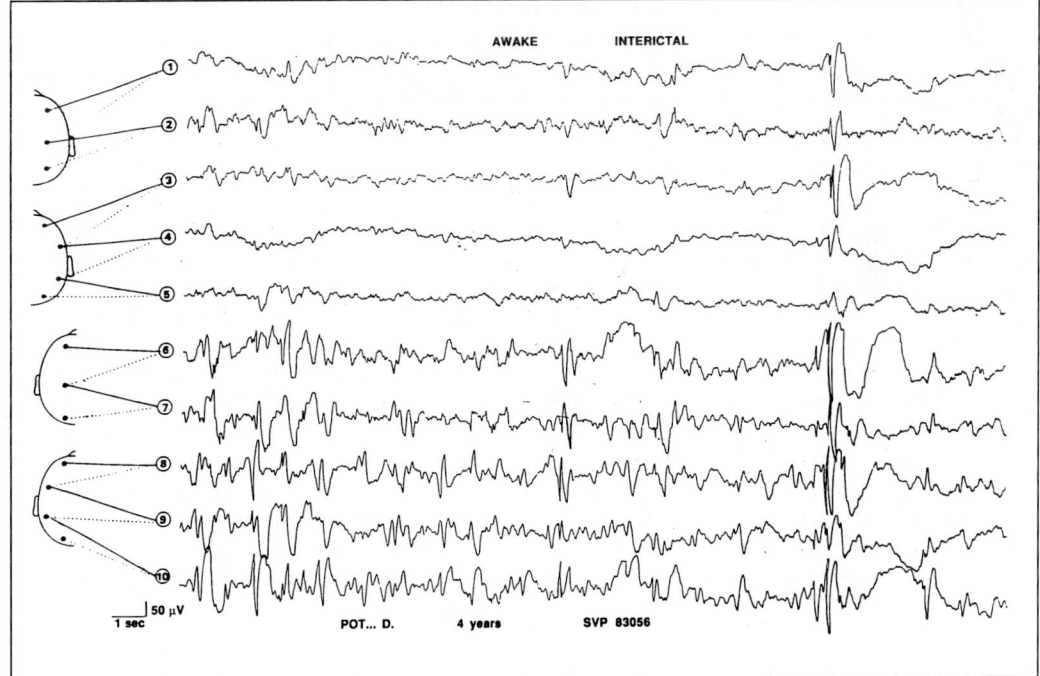

Fig. 3 (a,b). Poor electroclinical correlation. First EEGs of a 1-month-old boy who had asymmetrical spasms. His EEGs showed bioccipital spikes, recorded interictally, and spasms (a, top). At 4 years he still had spasms, associated with partial seizures. On his interictal EEGs there were left occipital spikes with contralateral diffusion (b, bottom).

It is important to note that the diagnosis of occipital epilepsy cannot be made only according to the type of seizures. Indeed, even if all children finally exhibited focal features during seizures, they were often lacking early in the evolution, a finding previously reported in infants with focal epilepsy (Luna et al., 1989). In some of our cases, partial seizures were noticed only after a period of generalized seizures including spasms. Indeed, spasms have already been shown to result from focal brain lesions (Alvares et al., 1987; Cusmai et al., 1988; Chugani et al., 1990), and West syndrome has been reported to be associated with occipital lesions (Dulac et al., 1987; Chugani et al., 1990). It may pose a difficult diagnostic problem, only solved by the precise observation of the ictal event (eye deviation, nystagmus) and by the existence of an interictal occipital focus modifying hypsarrhythmia, combined with neuroradiological and functional imaging investigations. Spasms were noticed in seven of the 12 children of our series, occurring before the age of 4 months in five of them. This is in agreement with the observation that symptomatic spasms begin earlier in life than cryptogenic.

The age of occurrence of epilepsy produced by an occipital lesion is interesting to consider. All children had their first seizures during the first 2 months of life, a period at which occipital lobes undergo rapid functional development. Functional neuroimaging, i.e. positron emission tomography (PET) and single photon emission computed tomography (SPECT), clearly shows that glucose metabolism and cerebral blood flow increase during the first 6 months of life in occipital cortex (Chugani et al., 1987; Chiron et al., 1992). Both investigations are markers of neuronal and synaptic activity. It has also been demonstrated that glutamate, which may be the primary neurotransmitter in the developing visuals pathways, has an overexpression of its receptors in the occipital regions early in postnatal life (McDonald & Johnson, 1990). As a consequence, any stimulation of the visual cortex during the process of maturation is likely to induce an enhanced response of the synaptic circuitry. In our patients, including those without evidence of brain malformation, some occipital neurons may be abnormal and particularly prone to become epileptogenic. It is possible that their overstimulation by excitatory amino acids (EAA) facilitates the creation of an epileptogenic focus during this period of rapid development (McDonald & Johnson, 1990).

Phenomena of generalized expression of epilepsy in this age group could also be considered according to functional development. Postnatal synaptic plasticity is characterized by an initial period of synaptic overactivity followed by a synaptic regression or stabilization (Changeux & Danchin, 1976). The existence of redundant cortico-cortical fibers in the first 6 months of life is likely to facilitate the spread of epileptic discharges. This could be the cause for the generalized symptomatology of West syndrome. In cases of lesional epilepsy, especially when it is dysplasia with imprecise limits, the lesion can always be incriminated for delays in development and cognitive problems. But delayed neurodevelopment and abnormal behaviour might also result from paroxysmal discharges occurring early during postnatal synaptic maturation. If an epileptic focus appears during the process of brain development, the excessive release of EAA in association with the overexpression of EAA receptors could induce neuronal injuries, and alter synaptic connections which could compromise the development of later maturing association cortex (McDonald & Johnson, 1990). This process might well be the result of an occipital focus, because the occipital cortex is the first cortical area to mature. Its connections with contralateral and more anterior regions may result in widespread abnormal reorganization. Visual unresponsiveness and autistic features are indeed frequent in patients with occipital epileptogenic foci, even if unilateral, including patients with West syndrome (Jambaqué et al., in press).

Early control of occipital seizures is therefore a prerequisite for the improvement of long-term prognosis, particularly for cognitive and behavioural outcome. No children had spontaneous remission. Only three patients were controlled with antiepileptic drug treatment alone. Seizure control was obtained after several months of very high seizure frequency and patients were left with major cognitive troubles, suggesting that seizures had stopped after much of the brain had lost plasticity and therefore the ability to recover sensorial integration. Early detection, with radiological and/or functional imaging of localized structural abnormalities and eventual removal of focal dysplasia may prevent the occurrence of such a severe outcome.

Conclusions

The recognition of the occipital origin of seizures in infancy is a difficult challenge. The seizure types are varied. When partial seizures are present, they are not always typical of seizures originating in the occipital lobe. Clinically, they can be more compatible with temporal or frontal seizures. Scalp EEGs are not always helpful: spikes are often recorded over a diffuse posterior area, or they are only noticed in frontal or temporal lobes. However, occipital epilepsy should be suspected in certain conditions: (1) when the visual development of the infant is abnormal, (2) when ictal signs, characteristic of an occipital origin of the discharge, are noticed, (3) when seizures begin before the age of 12 months, or when spasms are present before 3 months.

If an occipital epilepsy is suspected, an ictal scalp EEG recording becomes mandatory and an occipital lesion should be looked for by conventional radiology and, if needed, by functional imaging. In patients resistant to antiepileptic medication, surgery should be considered.

References

Alvarez, L.A., Shinnar, S. & Moshé, S.L. (1987): Infantile spasms due to unilateral cerebral infarcts. *Paediatrics* **79**, 1024–1026.

Aso, K., Watanabe, K., Negoro, T., Takaesu, E., Furune, A., Takahashi, I., Yamamoto, N. & Nomura, K. (1987): Visual seizures in children *Epilepsy Res.* **1**, 246–253.

Beun, A.M., Beintema, D.J., Binnie, C.D., Debets, R.M.Chr., Overweg, J. & Van Heycop ten Ham, M.W. (1984): Epileptic nystagmus. *Epilepsia* **25**, 609–614.

Changeux, J.P. & Danchin, A. (1976): Selective stabilization of developing synapses as a mechanism for the specification of neuronal network. *Nature* **264**, 705–712.

Chiron, C., Raynaud, C., Mazière, B., Zilbovicius, M., Laflamme, L., Masure, M.C., Dulac, O., Bourguignon, M. & Syrota, A. (1992): Changes in regional cerebral blood flow during brain maturation in children and adolescents. *J. Nucl. Med.* **33**, 696–703.

Chugani H.T., Phelps M.E. & Mazziotta J.C. (1987): Positron emission tomography study of human brain functional development. *Ann. Neurol.* **22**, 487–497.

Chugani H.T., Shields W.D., Shewmon D.A., Olson D.M., Phelps M.E. & Peacock W.J. (1990): Infantile spasms: I. PET identifies focal cortical dysgenesis in cryptogenic cases for surgical treatment. *Ann. Neurol.* **27**, 406–413.

Cusmai R., Dulac O. & Diebler C. (1988): Lésions focales dans les spasmes infantiles. *Neurophysiol. Clin.* **17**, 169–182.

Dulac, O., Raynaud, C., Chiron, C., Plouin, P., Syrota, A. & Arthuis, M. (1987): Etude du débit sanguin cérébral dans le syndrome de West idiopathique: corrélations avec les données électroencéphalographiques. *Rev. EEG Neurophysiol. Clin.* **17**, 169–182.

Gastaut H. (1960): Un aspect méconnu des décharges neuroniques occipitales: la crise oculoclonique ou 'nystagmus occipital'. In: *Les grandes activités du lobe occipital*, ed. T. Alajouanine, pp. 169–185. Paris: Masson.

Holtzman R.N.N. & Goldensohn E.S. (1977): Sensations of ocular movements in seizures originating in occipital lobe. *Neurology* **27**, 554–556.

Huott A.D., Madison D.S. & Niedermeyer E. (1974): Occipital lobe epilepsy: a clinical and electroencephalographic study. *Eur. Neurol.* **11**, 325–339.

Jambaqué I., Chiron C., Dulac O., Raynaud C. & Syrota A. (in press): Autistic features in West syndrome: a neurophysiological and functional cerebral imaging study by SPECT. *Epilepsia*.

Kaplan P.W. & Lesser R.P. (1989): Vertical and horizontal epileptic gaze deviation and nystagmus. *Neurology* **39**, 1391–1393.

Ludwig B.I. & Ajmone-Marsan C. (1975): Clinical ictal patterns in epileptic patients with occipital electroencephalographic foci. *Neurology* **25**, 463–471.

Luna D., Dulac, O. & Plouin P. (1989): Ictal characteristics of cryptogenic partial seizures in infancy. *Epilepsia* **30**, 827–832.

McDonald J.W. & Johnson M.V. (1990): Physiological and pathophysiological roles of excitatory amino acids during central nervous system development. *Brain Res. Rev.* **15**, 41–70.

Penfield W. & Kristiansen K. (1951): *Epileptic seizure patterns.* pp. 116–126. Springfield Il: Charles C. Thomas.

Penfield W. & Jasper H. (1954): *Epilepsy and the functional anatomy of the human brain.* pp. 116–126. Boston: Little, Brown and Company.

Takeda A., Bancaud J., Talairach J., Bonis A. & Bordas-Ferrer M. (1969): A propos des accès épileptiques d'origine occipitale. *Rev. Neurol.* **12**, 306–315.

Tusa R.J., Kaplan P.W., Hain T.V.C. & Naidu S. (1990): Ipsiversive eye deviation and epileptic nystagmus. *Neurology* **40**, 662–665.

Valk J. & van de Knaap M.S. (1989): *Magnetic resonance of myelin, myelination, and myelin disorders.* Heidelberg: Springer-Verlag.

White J.C. (1971): Epileptic nystagmus. *Epilepsia* **12**, 157–164.

Williamson P.D., Spencer S.S., Spencer D.D. & Mattson R.H. (1981): Complex partial seizures with occipital lobe onset. *Epilepsia* **22**, 247–248.

Williamson P.D. & Spencer S.S. (1986): Clinical and EEG features of complex partial seizures of extratemporal origin. *Epilepsia* **27** (suppl 2), s46–s63.

Williamson P.D., Boon P.A., Spencer, D.D., Spencer S.S. & Mattson R.H. (1988): Occipital and partial epilepsy. *Epilepsia* **29**, 682.

Williamson P.D., Thadani V.M., Darcey T.M., Spencer D.D., Spencer S.S. & Mattson R.H. (1992): Occipital lobe epilepsy: clinical characteristics, seizure spread patterns, and results of surgery. *Ann. Neurol.* **31**, 3–13.

Chapter 15

Benign occipital epilepsy of childhood with prolonged seizures and autonomic symptoms

Federico Vigevano and Stefano Ricci

Section of Neurophysiology, Bambino Gesù Children Hospital, IRCCS, Piazza S. Onofrio 4, 00165 Rome, Italy

Summary

Fourteen children presented with prolonged epileptic seizures that started in sleep and were characterized in sequence by nausea, vomiting, lateral deviation of the eyes, impaired consciousness and hemiconvulsions. The seizures lasted from 15 to 120 min. All the children were neurologically normal and no aetiological factors were identified. Seven patients had a family history of epilepsy or febrile convulsions. The onset of seizures occurred between 2 and 5 years of age. Seizures were sporadic: four patients had only one. EEGs in 11 patients showed occipital spikes; three patients had normal recordings. Three patients also had rolandic spikes. During the follow-up the occipital spikes sometimes migrated to one side then disappeared, whereas the rolandic spikes persisted longer. The follow-up period ranges from 1 year 4 months to 9 years. The seizures respond well to therapy. In our opinion, these children have a distinct form of idiopathic epilepsy with occipital spikes. This should be included with the known occipital and rolandic forms, already listed in the classification.

Introduction

In 1982 Gastaut described a type of epilepsy that he called 'benign partial epilepsy of childhood with occipital spikes' (Gastaut, 1982). Universally recognized, this entity now has its place in the latest Classification of Epilepsies and Epileptic Syndromes among the idiopathic focal, age-related epilepsies (Commission, 1989).

Various other authors have contributed further to delineating this epilepsy (Beaumanoir, 1983; Deonna *et al.*, 1984; Niedermeyer *et al.*, 1988), which is characterized mainly by visual seizures with simple or complex symptomatology. Most authors agree, however, that non-symptomatic epilepsies with occipital EEG anomalies can also manifest with seizures that are not visual. In particular, Panayiotopoulos (1988, 1989) has reported, as we have (Vigevano *et al.*, 1989; Ricci *et al.*, 1991), the occurrence in childhood of prolonged occipital seizures with autonomic nervous system symptoms, including nausea and vomiting, accompanied by motor symptoms such as eye deviation and clonic jerks. This type of epilepsy manifests with sporadic seizures in otherwise healthy children and has an excellent prognosis. Because of its consistent clinical and constant EEG characteristics, we agree with Panayiotopoulos that this is a new benign occipital epileptic syn-

Table 1: Clinical and EEG data of 14 patients

Patient	Sex	Family history	Age at onset (yr.month)	Febrile convulsions	Maximal duration of seizures (min)	Total number of seizures	Body side	EEG Beginning of FU	EEG End of FU	Therapy	Follow-up yr.month
1	M	–	3.6	–	60	4	L	R Occ. + B Rol	N	PB	8.4
2	M	–	2.0	–	90	2	R	L Occ + B Rol	N	PB	9.0
3	M	FC	4.8	–	15	2	L	R Occ	R Occ + L Rol	–	4.10
4	M	E	5.0	2	30	3	R	L Occ	B Rol	VPA	3.0
5	F	E + FC	3.11	–	120	3	L	R Occ	R Occ	PB	3.9
6	F	E	3.5	–	40	6	R	L Occ	R Occ	PB	3.4
7	M	E	5.10	–	25	1	R	L Occ + R Rol	B Rol	–	2.10
8	F	–	4.1	–	120	2	L	R Occ	N	CBZ	2.11
9	F	–	2.2	–	120	1	L	R Occ	N	–	4.6
10	M	FC	3.2	3	60	1	R	N	L Rol	PB	4.3
11	F	–	2.2	–	30	2	R	N	N	PB	2.2
12	M	–	3.10	–	20	3	L	R Occ	B Occ	VPA	2.0
13	M	–	4.8	2	15	2	R	L Occ	R Occ	PB	4.6
14	F	FC	3.8	2	60	1	L	N	R Occ	VPA	1.4

Abbreviations:
M: Male; F: Female; FC: Febrile convulsions; E: Epilepsy; L: Left; R: Right; B: Bilateral; Rol: Rolandic; Occ: Occipital; N: Normal; PB: Phenobarbital; VPA: Valproic acid; CBZ: Carbamazepine.

drome of childhood, that should be included in the classification along with the form described by Gastaut.

Patients and methods

Our study concerns 14 patients, observed at the Epilepsy Center at the Bambino Gesù Children's Hospital during the period 1983 to 1992, whose seizures were characterized by nausea, vomiting, lateral deviation of the eyes, and lateralized or bilateral clonic jerks. Autonomic symptoms, especially vomiting, occurred in every seizure and began early in the sequence of ictal events. Patients who vomited after a seizure or experienced a symptom-free interval between vomiting and a subsequent seizure were excluded, as were those with a clinical picture of hemiplegic migraine.

Clinical, neurological, and serial EEG data were obtained in all patients at the onset of the disease and during follow-up. All patients had CT scans.

The follow-up period in the 14 patients ranged from 1 year 4 months to 9 years (mean, 3 years 7 months).

Results

Clinical data

Table 1 summarizes the data from the 14 patients, eight boys and six girls. Three patients had a family history of epilepsy, one of epilepsy and febrile convulsions, three of febrile convulsions alone.

The ages at onset of seizures ranged from 2 years 2 months to 5 years 10 months (mean age 3 years 7 months).

In all cases pregnancy, birth, and psychomotor development were normal. Patients 4, 10, 13 and 14 had a history of simple febrile convulsions occurring between 10 and 36 months of life. In all cases, neurological findings were normal, as were those from CT scan.

Ictal features

Seizures showed an unusual pattern, with a constant sequence of symptoms, shown in Table 2. The initial symptom was always a feeling of malaise and nausea. This was followed by vomiting and lateral deviation of the eyes. Impairment of consciousness was hard to assess at this phase of the seizure. The seizure stopped 5 to 10 min after the onset (brief seizure) or persisted even for 1 or 2

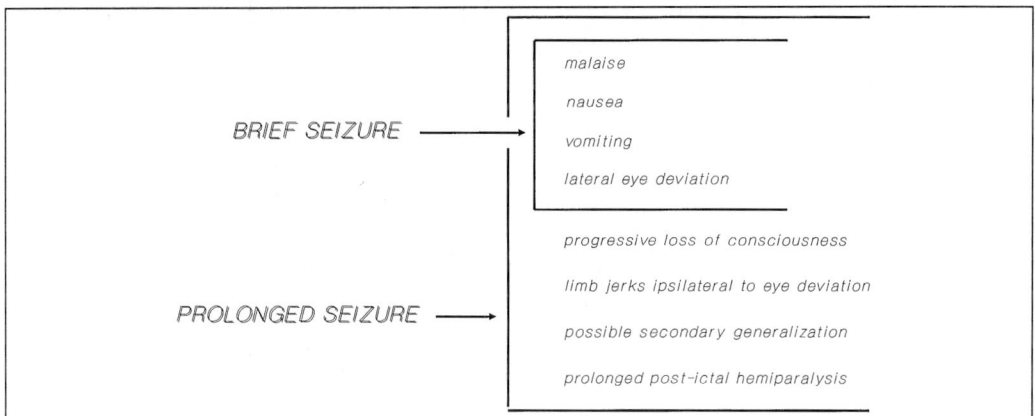

Table 2. Sequence of ictal symptoms

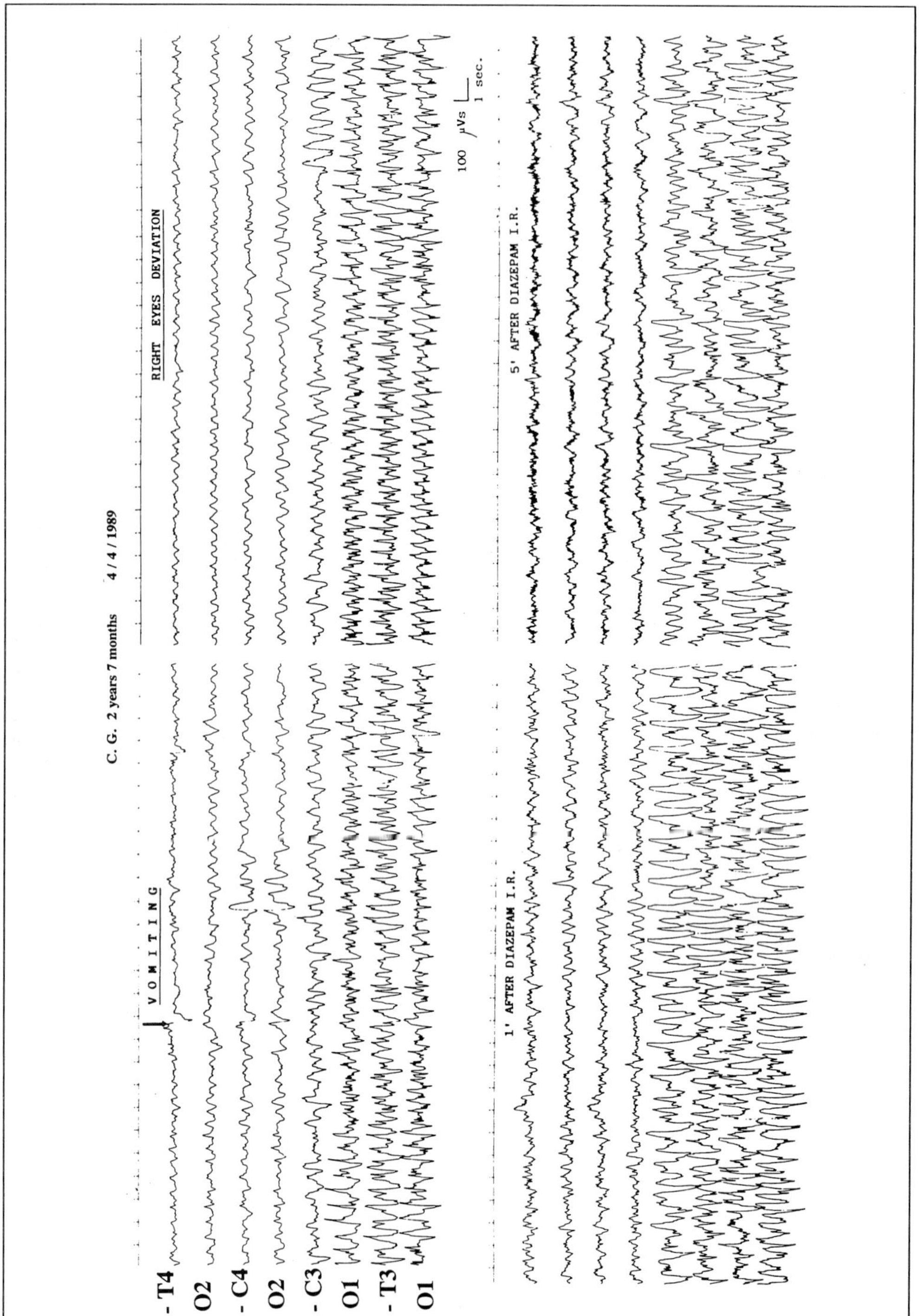

Fig. 1. Ictal EEG in Patient 11 (see text).

Chapter 15 Benign occipital epilepsy of childhood with prolonged seizures and autonomic symptoms

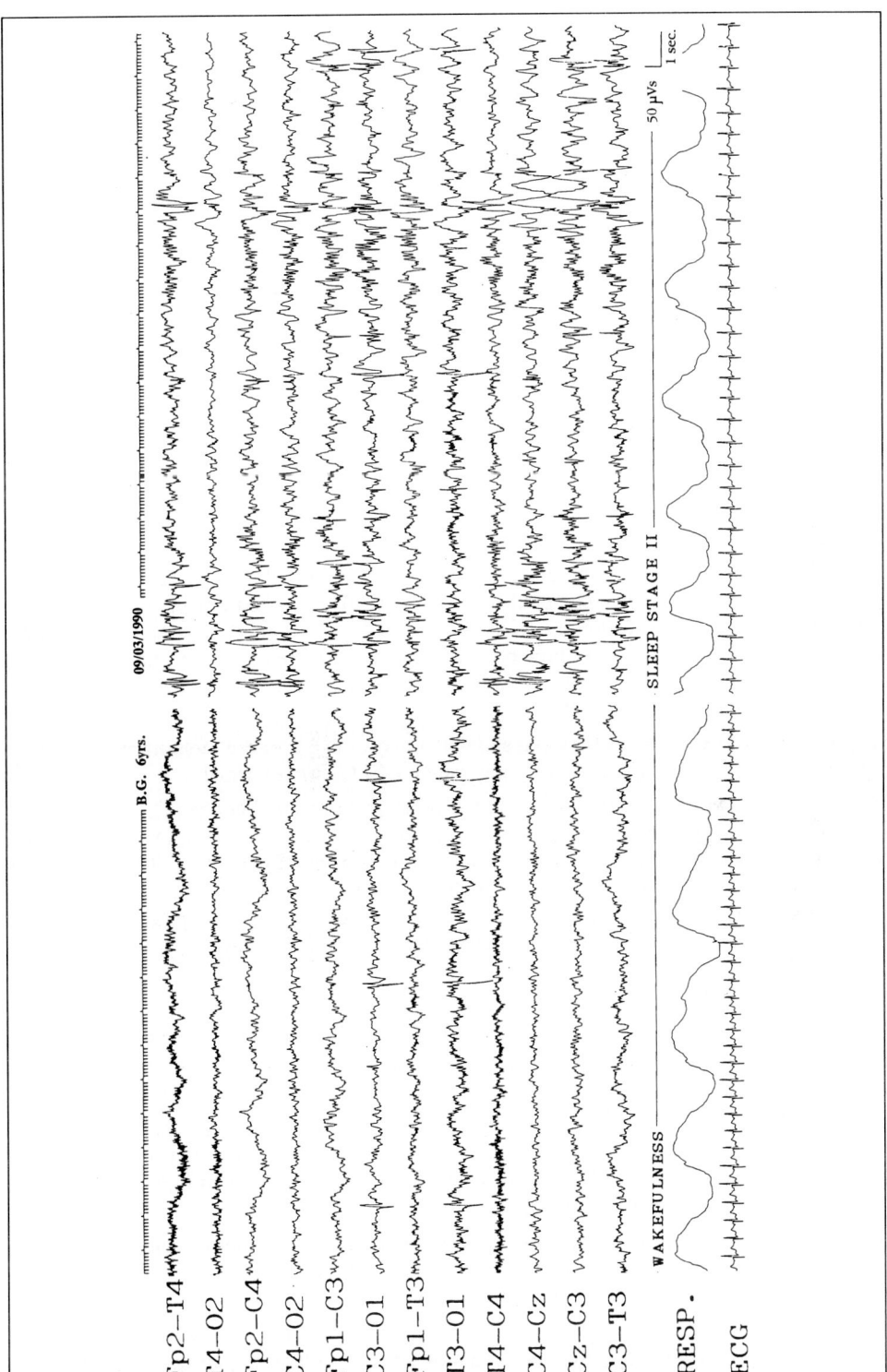

Fig. 2. Interictal EEG in Patient 4. Left: left occipital spikes during wakefulness. Right, left occipital and independent bilateral rolandic spikes during sleep.

h (prolonged seizure). In this case, eye deviation and vomiting continued, consciousness became progressively impaired, and clonic jerks appeared in the side of the body ipsilateral to the eye deviation. A secondary tonic-clonic generalization sometimes ensued. Prolonged seizures were always followed by postictal hemiparesis.

In all patients seizures were precipitated by sleep; only four patients also had sporadic seizures during wakefulness. Every patient had at least one prolonged episode, lasting from 15 to 120 min. Because these seizures responded promptly to intravenous or intrarectal administration of diazepam, their duration depended upon the timeliness of therapy.

Seven patients also had short seizures, which ceased spontaneously a few minutes after the onset. In some children these brief events, consisting only of night-time vomiting, were not considered epileptic.

In nine patients, at least one prolonged seizure was precipitated by fever.

EEG findings

In one patient (Case 11) we were able to record a seizure that had just started (Fig.1). Seizure activity was characterized by widespread 1 to 2 Hz temporo-occipital waves intermingled with spikes. The patient had nausea, vomiting and deviation of the eyes to the right. Intrarectal administration of diazepam stopped the seizure. The postictal EEG showed high amplitude delta waves throughout the left hemisphere and pharmacological fast activity in the right hemisphere.

The interictal EEGs recorded in wakefulness and sleep exhibited normal background activity. In 11 patients spikes were evident in the occipital areas. Spikes always occurred in the hemisphere contralateral to the clinical manifestations. Spikes were of high amplitude and were sometimes followed by a slow wave. The EEGs in three patients also disclosed unilateral or bilateral rolandic spikes occurring mainly during sleep (Fig. 2). In Patient 4, tactile stimulation of the fingers evoked spikes in the contralateral rolandic regions.

Occipital spikes appeared with the eyes closed and with the eyes open. Intermittent light stimulation failed to provoke a pathological response. In three patients EEGs were normal.

During the follow-up period the EEG exhibited diverse patterns. In Patients 1, 2, 8 and 9 it normalized; in Patient 3 in addition to occipital spikes rolandic spikes appeared; in Patients 4 and 7, occipital spikes were replaced by bilateral rolandic spikes; in Patients 5, 6, 12 and 13, the occipital spikes remained unchanged, became bilateral or changed side; in Patients 10 and 14, normal at the beginning of follow-up, spikes appeared in the rolandic and occipital areas respectively; and in Patient 11 the EEG remained normal throughout the follow-up.

Treatment and course of epilepsy

The follow-up period ranged from 1 year 4 months to 9 years (mean, 3 years 7 months).

The seizures occurred sporadically in all cases; the total number was always low. All the patients treated responded promptly to anticonvulsant therapy.

Patients 7, 9, 10 and 14 had one seizure only; the first two patients were never treated. The other two patients were treated because a prolonged seizure supervened, in one case after three and in the other after two febrile convulsions. Patient 3 was not treated because she had only two seizures, separated by a seizure-free interval of 18 months.

Eleven of our patients were treated: seven with phenobarbital, three with valproic acid and one with carbamazepine. All of them responded to treatment, with disappearance of the seizures, except Patient 3, who had an isolated seizure during therapy, followed by 2 years without seizures.

Patient 2, at the age of 9, 5 years after the occipital seizures, had several seizures during sleep clinically characterized by right facial twitching, loss of speech, without impairment of consciousness and lasting about 1 min.

Discussion

The 14 patients we have described had a uniform clinical picture. They were all neurologically normal children, without aetiological factors, apart from a high family incidence of family history of epilepsy or of febrile convulsions.

Between the age of 2 and 5 years these children began to have prolonged seizures, occurring during sleep and characterized in sequence by nausea, vomiting, lateral deviation of the eyes and hemiconvulsion. The epilepsy had a benign course. EEGs disclosed occipital spikes subsequently migrating to the other side or towards the rolandic areas. Some children had short seizures, of the same type, consisting only of the initial phase, that is up to the eye deviation. Because eye deviation was difficult for the parents to recognize these seizures were mistaken for harmless episodes of nocturnal vomiting.

Our patients never had visual seizures; nor did they have photic-induced seizures. The EEGs never showed occipital spike-wave complexes in response to eye closure or to intermittent light stimulation. These cardinal elements sharply distinguish the epilepsy described here from the known occipital forms (Gastaut, 1982, 1985; Beaumanoir, 1983; Deonna et al., 1984).

Our patients' seizures also differed markedly from the so-called 'intercalated seizures' (Terzano et al., 1987), a visual type of focal epileptic seizures between migrainous aura and headache.

In addition, our EEG documentation demonstrates that the autonomic nervous system symptoms are epileptic, thus excluding other nonepileptic phenomena such as migraine (Ricci et al., 1991).

The EEG anomalies consist principally of spikes with only rare spike-wave complexes. They closely resemble those of benign epilepsy with centro-temporal spikes and more generally resemble those of benign partial epilepsies (Dalla Bernardina, 1985). An interesting point is the evolution of the EEG. In some patients we found either a migration of the spikes to the rolandic areas, or the coexistence of rolandic and occipital spikes. In cases with a longer follow-up, the EEG tends to normalize. And finally, the similarity with benign epilepsy with rolandic spikes becomes even clearer if we consider Patient 2, who between 2 and 4 years of age had two prolonged occipital seizures starting with vomiting, and at 9 years had typical rolandic seizures.

In 1985 Dravet drew attention to an epileptic syndrome that was characterized exclusively by unilateral seizures of long duration (Dravet, 1985). Some of these patients had hemiparesis; others were neurologically normal. In the latter, seizures appeared between 1 and 5 years, were sporadic and had a benign course. Even though the authors attributed little importance to the autonomic symptoms in these seizures, some of these patients might have overlapped with ours.

Our cases closely resemble those described by Panayiotopoulos (1989), who first proposed this entity as a new form of occipital epilepsy. Some differences are, however, noteworthy. Our patients have a high family incidence of epilepsy and febrile convulsions. The occipital EEG anomalies in our cases are not strictly linked to eye opening and fixation. And last, our cases exhibit a high percentage of rolandic spikes.

All these elements provide further evidence that we are indeed describing a new benign partial epilepsy of idiopathic origin.

References

Beaumanoir, A. (1983): Infantile epilepsy with occipital focus and good prognosis. *Eur. Neurol.* **22**, 43–52.

Commission on Classification of Epilepsies and Epileptic Syndromes (1989): Proposal for revised classification of epilepsies and epileptic syndromes. *Epilepsia* **30**, 389–399.

Dalla Bernardina, B. (1985): Benign partial epilepsies In: *Epileptic syndromes in infancy, childhood and adolescence*, eds. J. Roger, C. Dravet, M. Bureau, F. E. Dreifuss & P. Wolf, p. 322. London: John Libbey.

Deonna, T., Ziegler, A. L. & Despland, P. A. (1984): Paroxysmal visual disturbance of epileptic origin and occipital epilepsy in children. *Neuropediatrics* **15**, 131–135.

Dravet C. (1985): Comment on an epileptic syndrome with unilateral seizures. In: *Epileptic syndromes in infancy, childhood and adolescence*, eds. J. Roger, C. Dravet, M. Bureau, F.E. Dreifuss & P. Wolf, pp. 222–227. London: John Libbey.

Gastaut H. (1982): A new type of epilepsy: benign partial epilepsy of childhood with occipital spike-waves. *Clin. Electroencephalogr.* **12**, 13–22.

Gastaut H. (1985): Benign epilepsy of childhood with occipital paroxysms. In: *Epileptic syndromes in infancy, childhood and adolescence*, eds. J. Roger, C. Dravet, M. Bureau, F.E., Dreifuss & P. Wolf, pp. 159–170. London: John Libbey.

Niedermeyer E., Riggio S. & Santiago M. (1988): Benign occipital lobe epilepsy. *J. Epilepsy* **1**, 3–11.

Panayiotopoulos C.P. (1988): Vomiting as an ictal manifestation of epileptic seizures and syndromes. *J. Neurol. Neurosurg. Psychiatr.* **51**, 1448–1451.

Panayiotopoulos C.P. (1989): Benign nocturnal childhood epilepsy: a new syndrome with nocturnal seizures, tonic deviation of the eyes and vomiting. *J. Child Neurol.* **4**, 43–48.

Ricci S., Cusmai R., Di Capua M., Fusco L. & Vigevano F. (1991): Seizures with vomiting, eye deviation and hemiconvulsion: epilepsy or migraine? In: *Juvenile headache*, eds. V. Gallai & V. Guidetti, pp. 193–196. Amsterdam: Elsevier.

Terzano M. G., Manzoni G. C. & Parrino L. (1987): Benign epilepsy with occipital paroxysms and migraine: the question of intercalated attacks. In: *Migraine and epilepsy*, eds. F. Andermann & E. Lugaresi, pp. 83–96. Boston, London: Butterworths.

Vigevano F., Ricci S., Di Capua M., Claps D. & Fusco L. (1989): Vomito, deviazione oculare, emiconvulsione: una particolare forma di stato epilettico nel bambino. *Boll. Lega. It. Epil.* **66–67**, 315–316.

Chapter 16

Television-induced occipital seizures

Roberto Michelucci and Carlo Alberto Tassinari

Department of Neurology, University of Bologna, Bellaria Hospital, Bologna, Italy

Summary

Photosensitive epilepsy is usually considered to belong to the generalized epilepsies and the most common EEG pattern associated with it is diffuse and bilateral spike and wave (SW) activity. We describe a group of 12 patients with television (TV)-induced tonic–clonic seizures, who proved to suffer from true occipital focal seizures with secondary generalization. The occipital origin of such seizures could be suspected on the basis of EEG and clinical findings. From the clinical point of view, these patients usually reported, at the seizure onset, elementary visual hallucinations, metamorphopsia, blurring of vision or blindness. A deviation of the eyes and head was sometimes observed. From the EEG point of view, TV or intermittent photic stimulation (IPS) could provoke both generalized SW discharges or recruiting rhythms in the occipital regions. Polygraphic recording of several seizures induced by TV (one patient) or IPS (two patients) confirmed the clinical suspicion that the ictal discharges initially involved one occipital region before a secondary generalization into a tonic–clonic seizure occurred. All the patients had normal neurological examination and CT scan. The evolution was usually benign, with rare seizures easily controlled by antiepileptic treatment. Although it is usually held that TV-induced seizures belong to idiopathic generalized epilepsies, our study demonstrates the existence of visually-induced seizures of occipital origin in a context of idiopathic focal epilepsy.

Introduction

Photosensitive epilepsy is by far the commonest form of stimulus-sensitive epilepsy (Jeavons & Harding, 1975; Newmark & Penry, 1979). Visual triggering factors include environmental flicker stimulation (usually television), patterns or eye closure. Photosensitive epilepsy may be classified into three major groups (Jeavons, 1982; Tassinari *et al.*, 1990):

1. Pure photosensitive epilepsy;
2. Photosensitive epilepsy associated with spontaneous seizures;
3. Non-flicker visually evoked seizures, which may be divided into two subgroups: (a) Pattern-induced seizures; (b) Seizures induced by eye closure.

The seizure types associated with these different forms of epilepsy are shown in Table 1. Tonic–clonic seizures are usually seen in pure photosensitive epilepsy whereas absences predominate in patients with pattern-induced or eye closure-induced attacks. The resting EEG may show generalized paroxysmal abnormalities and photosensitivity is common (Jeavons & Harding, 1975). Therefore, electro-clinical evidence suggests a generalized nature of the seizures, and a close link related abnormalities Figs. 2, 3. Panayiotopoulos, 1976, 1977, 1978; 1989c). The clinical manifestations of these children were as interesting as their EEG features and made me initiate this study. It was already apparent in our early reports that motor partial seizures were more common than visual partial seizures in children with occipital paroxysms:

> 'The attacks of long lasting tonic deviation of the eyes, sometimes followed by tonic–clonic seizures, occurred in seven of our patients during sleep. The remaining three patients experienced elementary visual hallucinations during daytime. Elementary visual hallucinations were also experienced by two of the patients with sleep seizures.'
>
> Panayiotopoulos & Siafacas (1980).

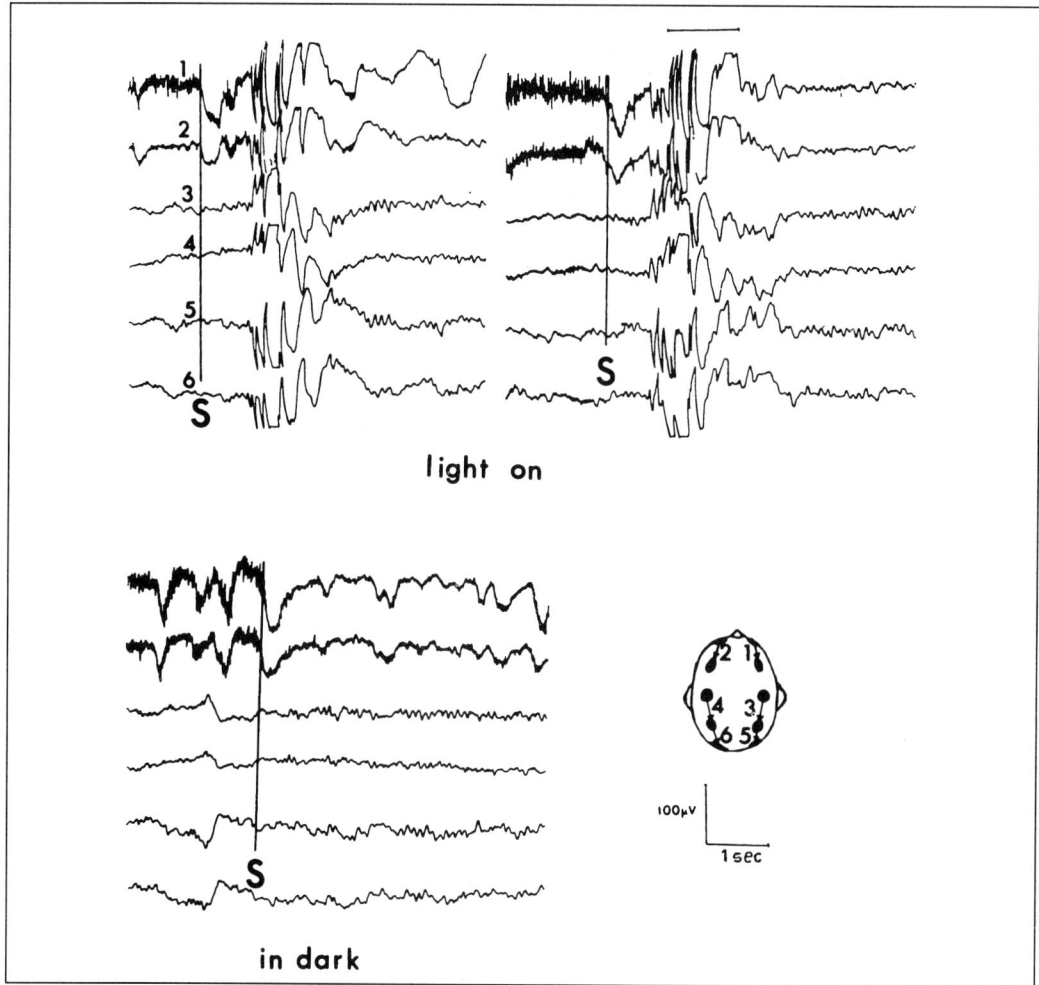

Fig. 1. 'Eye-closure' abnormalities in a photosensitive patient. These are generalized discharges which occur immediately (within 1–2 s) after closing of the eyes (eye-closure). They last for a few seconds and are not maintained during the phase of eyes closed (upper part of figure). Darkness has an inhibitory effect i.e. 'eye-closure' abnormalities are eliminated if eye-closure is performed in total darkness (lower part of figure) (from Panayiotopoulos (1974) with permission of Journal of Neurological Sciences).

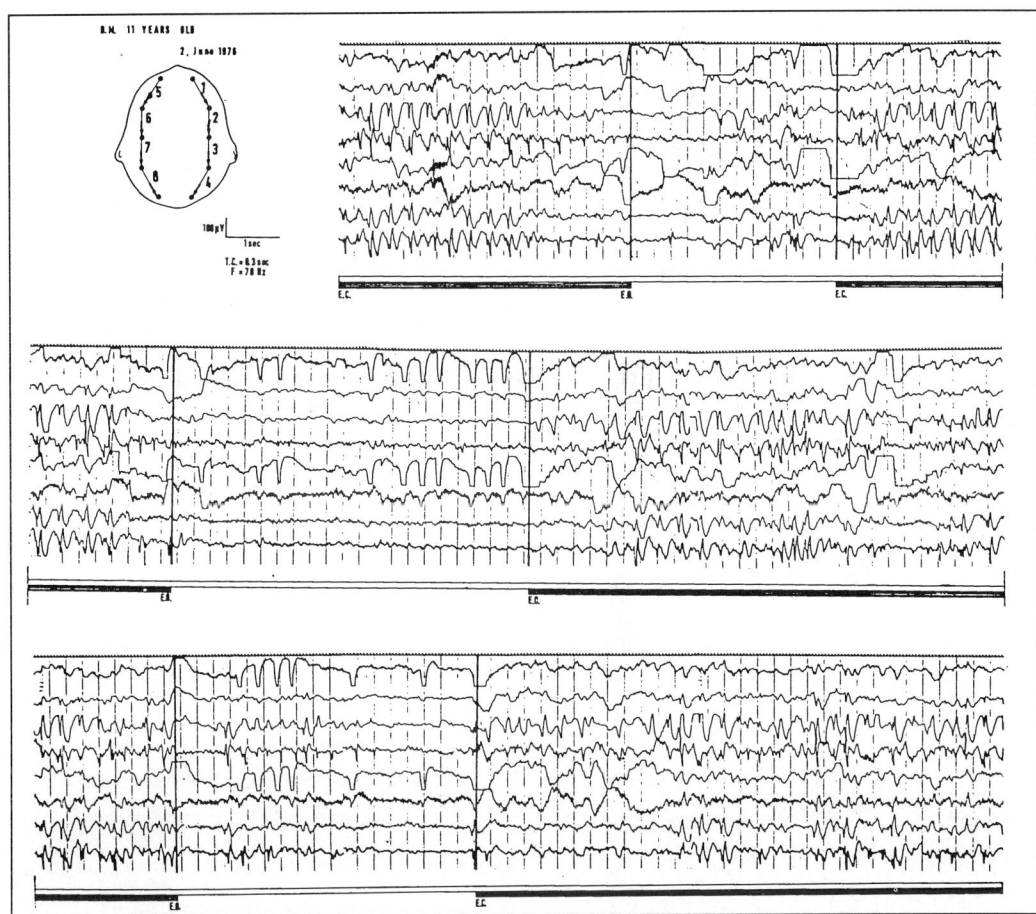

Fig. 2. EEG of Case 6, in 1976. Occipital paroxysms are continuously recorded as long as the eyes are closed (black bars). They are totally inhibited when the eyes are opened (from Panayiotopoulos (1978) by permission of Materia Medica Greca).

However, it was children with visual symptoms that attracted international interest (Camfield et al., 1978; Panayiotopoulos, 1980; Gastaut, 1982) and dominated BCEOP as defined by the ILAE (1989). The other group, with motor partial seizures, has been neglected despite well-presented evidence (Panayiotopoulos & Siafacas, 1980; Panayiotopoulos, 1981, 1987, 1989a, b; Beaumanoir, 1983). Therefore, it is rewarding that our observations have been confirmed by other authors in this book (see Vigevano et al., Chapter 15; Guerrini et al., Chapter 19). It is surprising to me that fixation-off sensitivity of occipital paroxysms, which was described in association with BCEOP before any other report of the syndrome, had not been studied or cited in the original and subsequent reports and reviews.

The age at onset appeared to be earlier for those with motor than with visual partial seizures (Fig. 4). Furthermore, children with motor partial seizures predominate, have different clinical manifestations and a better prognosis.

This I called 'the early onset variant of BCEOP' (Panayiotopoulos, 1989b). I had originally proposed that it is a different syndrome (Panayiotopoulos, 1987, 1989a). I still maintain that view (clinical features and evolution are different, despite identical EEG abnormalities) but I felt that its

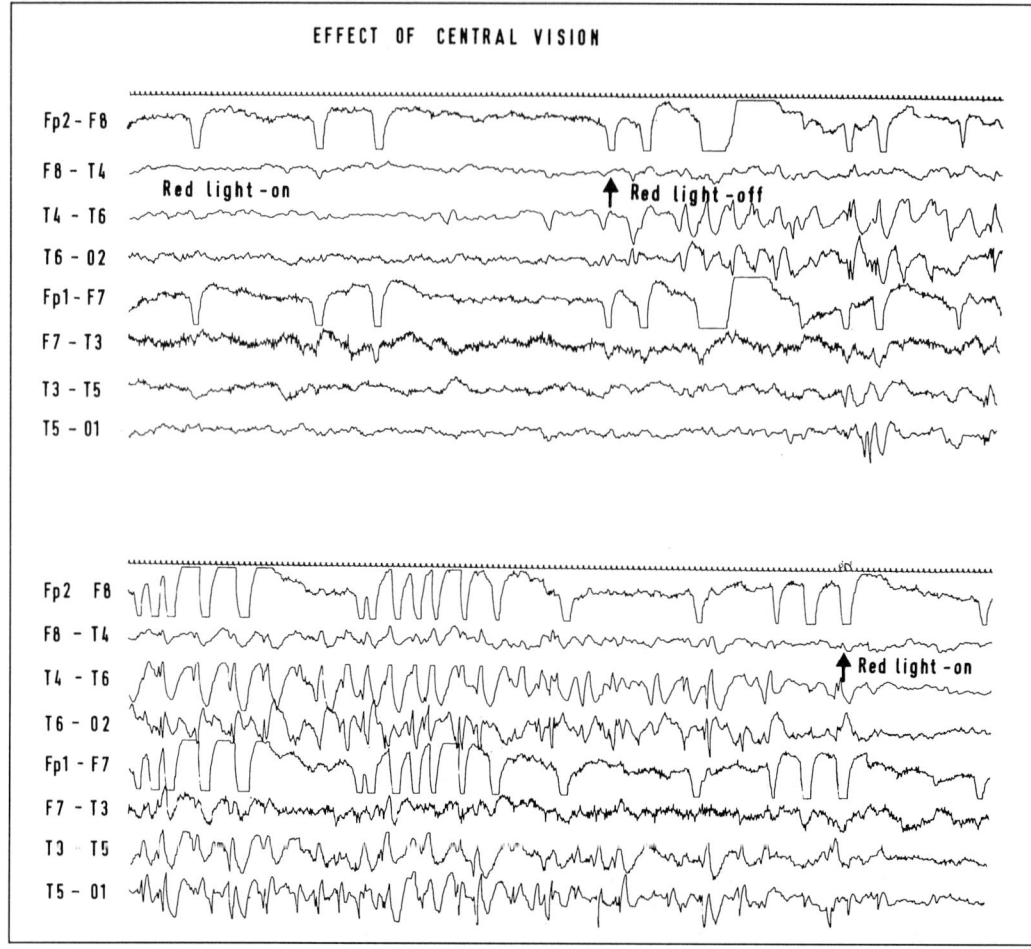

Fig. 3. EEG of the same patient as in Fig 2. Fixation-off sensitivity is demonstrated. Recording with eyes open either in total darkness or with patient fixating on a small red spot in an otherwise totally dark room. Occipital paroxysms are induced by darkness and eliminated by fixating on the red spot (from Panayiotopoulos (1980) by permission of Neurology).

classification as a variant of an entity already recognized by the ILAE would make it easier for others to accept (see for example Panayiotopoulos, 1989a, and associated reservations in the commentary by Aicardi, 1989).

Cumulative results

Cumulative results from the prospective study of 18 children with BCEOP (seen 1973–1983) and a review of the literature have been published elsewhere (Panayiotopoulos, 1989b) and need not be repeated. Briefly, in 16 patients, 10 girls and six boys, the cardinal features consisted of nocturnal seizures (all patients, additional diurnal seizures can be experienced) with tonic deviation of the eyes (13 children) and vomiting (12 children). Eye opening, retching, aphemia and oropharyngeal movements were seen infrequently (one to two patients each). Consciousness was preserved throughout the ictus in four patients. In all the other children consciousness was impaired or lost,

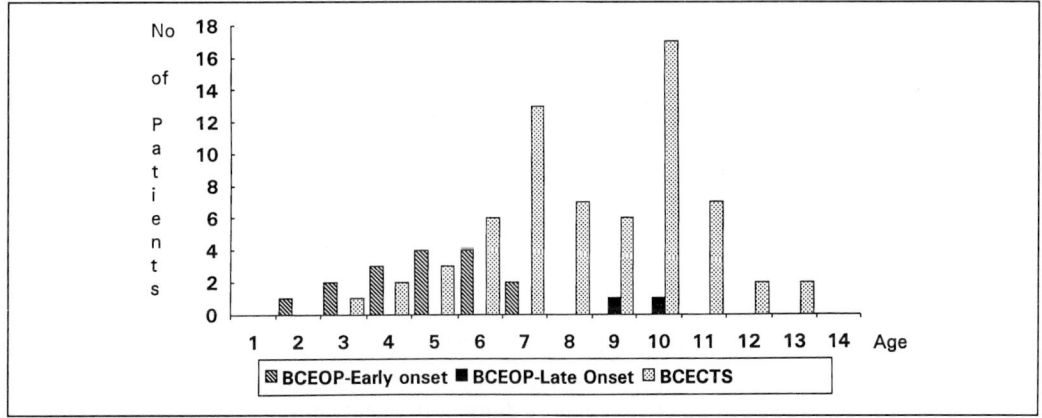

Fig. 4. Histogram of the age at onset of benign childhood epilepsy (years) with centrotemporal spikes (BCECTS) and the early and late onset variants of benign childhood epilepsy with occipital paroxysms (BCEOP).

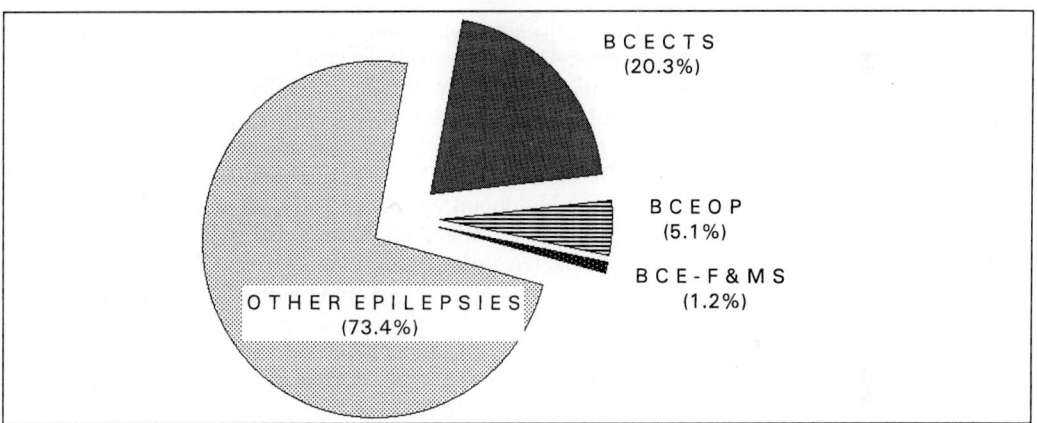

Fig. 5. Prevalence of benign childhood epilepsies (94 patients) amongst 354 children with onset of seizures at 2–13 years of age.

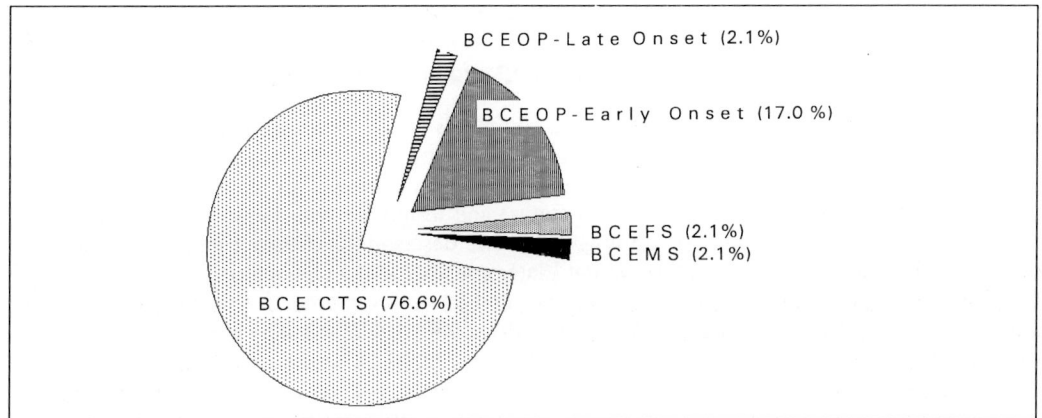

Fig. 6. Prevalence of age- and localization-related benign childhood epilepsies amongst 94 children with these syndromes.

either from the onset or during the course of the fits. Seizures lasted for only a few minutes (eight patients) or were prolonged for several hours (more than half an hour in eight children) eventually evolving into unilateral or generalized convulsions (12 patients).

The frequency of the seizures was remarkably low (range 1–12, mode 1 and 3 seizures), five children having only single fits. Five children developed diurnal seizures. These were either similar to the nocturnal fits, simple partial seizures, unclassifiable non-specific fainting episodes or infrequent episodes of perceptual abnormalities and automatisms occurring mainly in darkness or when the eyes were closed. Peak onset was at 5 years (early onset variant of BCEOP) and remission consistently occurred within 1–2 years from onset of seizures and never after the age of 12 years. None of the children experienced postictal headache, migraine or ictal visual symptoms in the long follow-up period. Two children revealed on questioning that, when they were concentrating with closed eyes, they saw a diffuse coloured light. One child had episodes of distorted visual perception (see Case 3, below).

The remaining two of the 18 children had mainly diurnal, frequent partial visual seizures, postictal headache and occasional nocturnal hemi-convulsions. Onset was at late childhood (late onset variant of BCEOP) and prognosis was less favourable than those with the early onset variant of BCEOP.

Prevalence is shown in Figs. 5 and 6. The results are from a study (Panayiotopoulos, 1989b) of 900 patients (of all ages) with epileptic disorders; 418 had onset of disease before age 13 years and 354 of them between 2 and 13 years (which is the age of onset of benign childhood epilepsies). Ninety-four of the 900 patients had benign childhood epilepsies: 72 benign childhood epilepsy with centrotemporal spikes (BCECTS), 16 early onset BCEOP, two late onset BCEOP, two benign childhood epilepsy with frontal spikes (BCEFS) and two benign childhood epilepsy with midline spikes (BCEMS). The prevalence of benign childhood epilepsies (94 patients) amongst the 354 children with onset of seizures at 2–13 years of age was 20.3 per cent for BCECTS, 4.5 per cent for the early onset BCEOP, 0.6 per cent for the late onset BCEOP, 0.6 per cent for BCEFS and 0.6 per cent for BCEMS. The remaining 73.4 per cent had other symptomatic or idiopathic epilepsies. The prevalence of the various syndromes amongst the 94 children with benign childhood epilepsies was 76.6 per cent BCECTS, 19.2 per cent BCEOP, 2.1 per cent BCEFS and 2.1 per cent BCEMS. The early onset variant of BCEOP was found in 16 (17.1 per cent) and the late onset variant of BCEOP in two (2.1 per cent). In BCEOP (18 children), 16 (88.9 per cent) had the early onset variant of BCEOP and two only (11.1 per cent) had the late onset BCEOP.

Sex: In the early onset BCEOP there was a preponderance of girls (10 out of 16) with a female/male ratio of 1.7.

Early onset variant BCEOP and illustrative cases

The typical clinical picture is of a child, more commonly a girl, who wakes up from sleep with vomiting and tonic deviation of the eyes to one side. Although usually impaired (complex partial seizures), consciousness may be preserved (simple partial seizures). This state may last for a few minutes to hours (simple or complex partial status) and terminate with hemi- and/or generalized convulsions. I had initially omitted vomiting from case descriptions (Cases 1 and 4 in Panayiotopoulos, 1981) as irrelevant or coincidental but I later considered it a characteristic manifestation of BCEOP as it became apparent that vomiting was consistently reported in children with the syndrome (12 out of 16 patients; Panayiotopoulos, 1987, 1988, 1989a, b). The early onset variant of BCEOP has infrequent seizures (sometimes solitary) which, although dramatic and prolonged (partial motor status) at their initial presentation, remit within 1–2 years and no later than age 12. In this respect it is at least as benign as BCECTS. This variant is illustrated below:

Case 1. K. H., born 26.3.71 (see Case 4, Panayiotopoulos, 1981). Her first seizure occurred at age 5½ (29.7.76) with the following sequence of events:

She went to sleep at 9 pm. At 11 pm she was found by her parents vomiting vigorously, eyes turned to one side, pale and unresponsive. She was taken to hospital and her condition remained unchanged, but at 2 pm developed 'generalized tonic clonic seizures for 5–7 min'. She gradually improved and was normal next morning.

A second nocturnal episode occurred 4 months later. She awoke, told her mother that she wanted to vomit and vomited. She was able to speak and reply. Within minutes her eyes turned to the right but she was still responsive. Her mother who was on her left asked 'Where am I?'. 'There, there,' K replied, showing to the right. Ten minutes later she closed her eyes and became unresponsive. Generalized convulsions occurred 1 h from the onset. She recovered quickly. There was no family history of epilepsy or migraine. K and her sister had infrequent classical vasovagal syncopal episodes.

She is reviewed annually from 1976. She remains well and successfully finished a business administration course in an American college in Athens.

Prolonged simple and complex partial motor status epilepticus imitating cerebral insult is common. Such episodes are usually nocturnal (see Case 1), rarely diurnal or both. They may be solitary (i.e. the only clinically detected epileptic event in the life of a child; Panayiotopoulos, 1981, 1987, 1989a, b). Single diurnal partial status epilepticus is illustrated below:

Case 2. Kath. C., a British girl of Chinese origin, born 8.5.84 (Panayiotopoulos & Igoe, 1992). No family history of migraine or epilepsy.

21.2.90. One single, prolonged (7–8 h) episode of vomiting, impairment and loss of consciousness, deviation of the eyes and generalized convulsions. The events are described as follows:

13.30. She became suddenly unwell after running a race at school. She had just finished running. She vomited and complained that she wanted to be sick again. All of a sudden she stood still, urinated and became confused. She was helped to walk to the school bus. Unable to climb the steps, but on arrival at the school she was able to walk up the stairs. Lay on the floor.

14.30. Unconscious. Eyes wide open and deviated to one side (left?). She became limp and pale and did not respond to commands. In the ambulance she was noted to froth at the mouth and dribble saliva.

16.15. Taken to St. Thomas' Hospital, London; twitching (all four limbs) and unresponsive. Diazepam 2 mg i.v. was administered and she was admitted. Unconscious over the next 4–5 h, gradually her level of conscious improved.

22.00. She was conscious and well. No medication was prescribed.

On review on 17.12.91 she was well with normal EEG on no medication.

In children with the early onset BCEOP, visual perceptions or other partial seizures in addition to the motor seizures are extremely rare. This is illustrated by the case E.K. who has been followed-up from 1973 to a few days before completing this report (Case 1, Panayiotopoulos, 1981):

Case 3. E. K., was born in 1967. There is no family history of migraine and epilepsy. At age 5 years she had a nocturnal episode of vomiting and tonic deviation of the eyes. She was limp and unable to speak. Recovered in 15 min without convulsions. Similar nocturnal episodes occurred 9 months and 1 year later. The last episode was not associated with vomiting. She was woken by a strong feeling of 'dizziness'. Her eyes were deviated to the left, followed by a similar deviation of the head. No convulsions occurred and she was well within 15 min.

At age 7 and 8 years she had brief diurnal episodes during which she felt dizzy, the environment appearing to move slowly away from her and then come back towards her with increasing speed. Occasionally, this sensation was followed by impairment of consciousness and automatisms. On a few other occasions she complained of rotatory vertigo. She thought that these episodes were precipitated by darkness or eye closure but was unable to reproduce them. She had never experienced generalized convulsions or headache. EEG occipital paroxysms and FOS were demonstrated in all her EEGs up to the age of 16 years (Figs. 7, 8) when she had her first normal EEG. Last follow-up April, 1992: she is well, obtaining her second university degree in mathematics.

One of the best arguments I use in favour of the benign character of BCEOP is the frequent occurrence of BCEOP with BCECTS. This is illustrated in the following Case 4 with multiple foci of occipital paroxysms, centrotemporal spikes, frontal spikes and somatosensory evoked spikes. Her first seizure at age 7 years was typical of the early onset variant BCEOP while the second fit, 1 year later, was typical of BCECTS:

Case 4. M. Sf., was born in 1975. Two febrile convulsions occurred at age 2 and 3 years old. At 7 years, she had a prolonged nocturnal seizure which started with vomiting and impairment of consciousness during sleep. She was taken

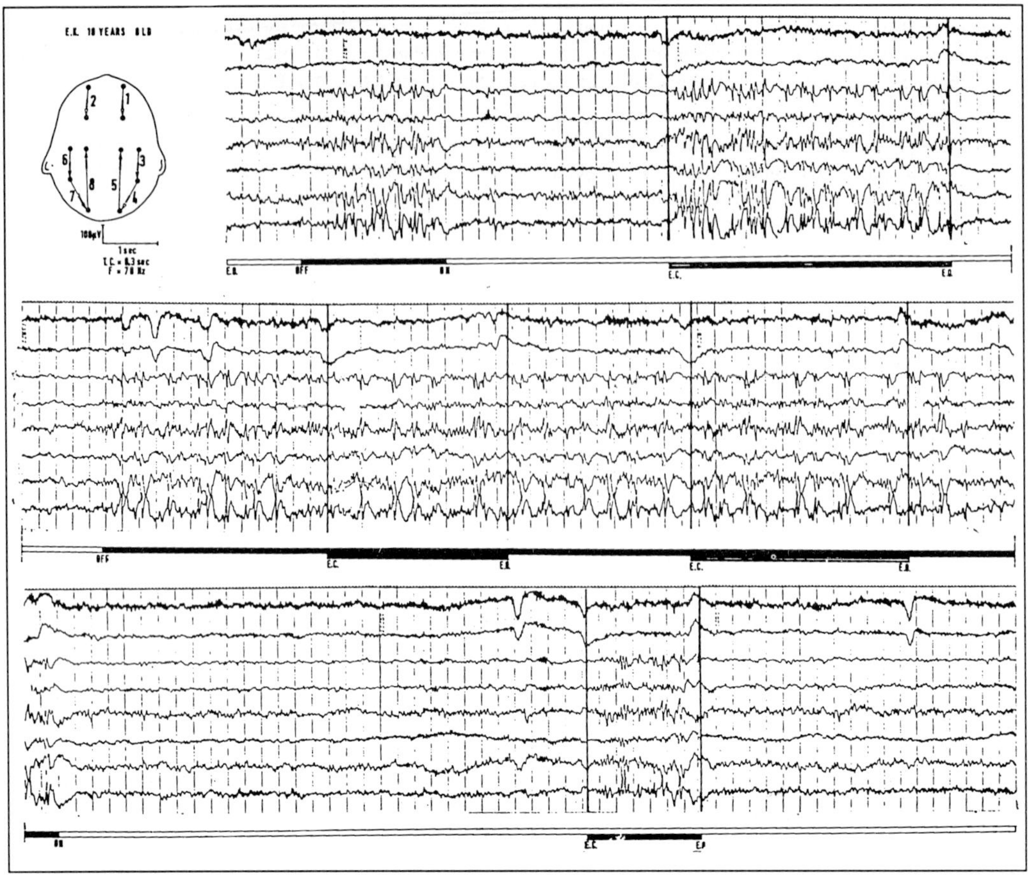

Fig. 7. Case 3. Occipital paroxysms are eyes-closed related (black bar below white bar). In darkness (black bar interrupting the white bar) the occipital paroxysms are induced with eyes opened, i.e. they persist irrespective of whether the eyes are opened or closed (from Panayiotopoulos et al., 1978).

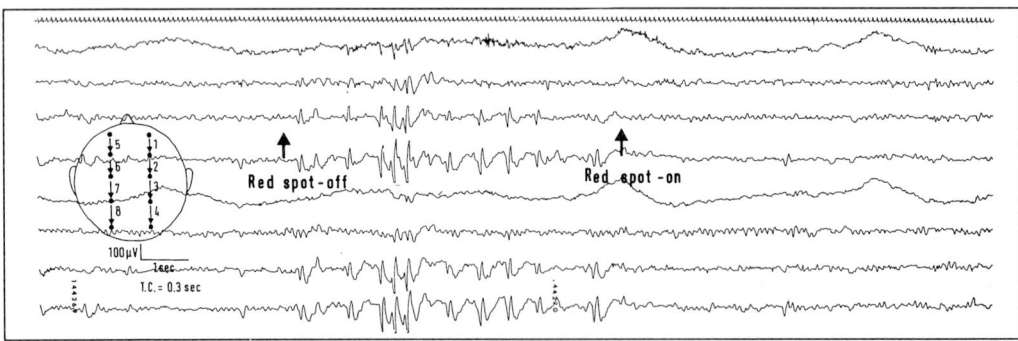

Fig. 8. Case 3. Recording is in complete darkness with eyes opened. Occipital paroxysms are inhibited when the patient looks at a small red spot of light (from Panayiotopoulos (1981), by permission of Neurology).

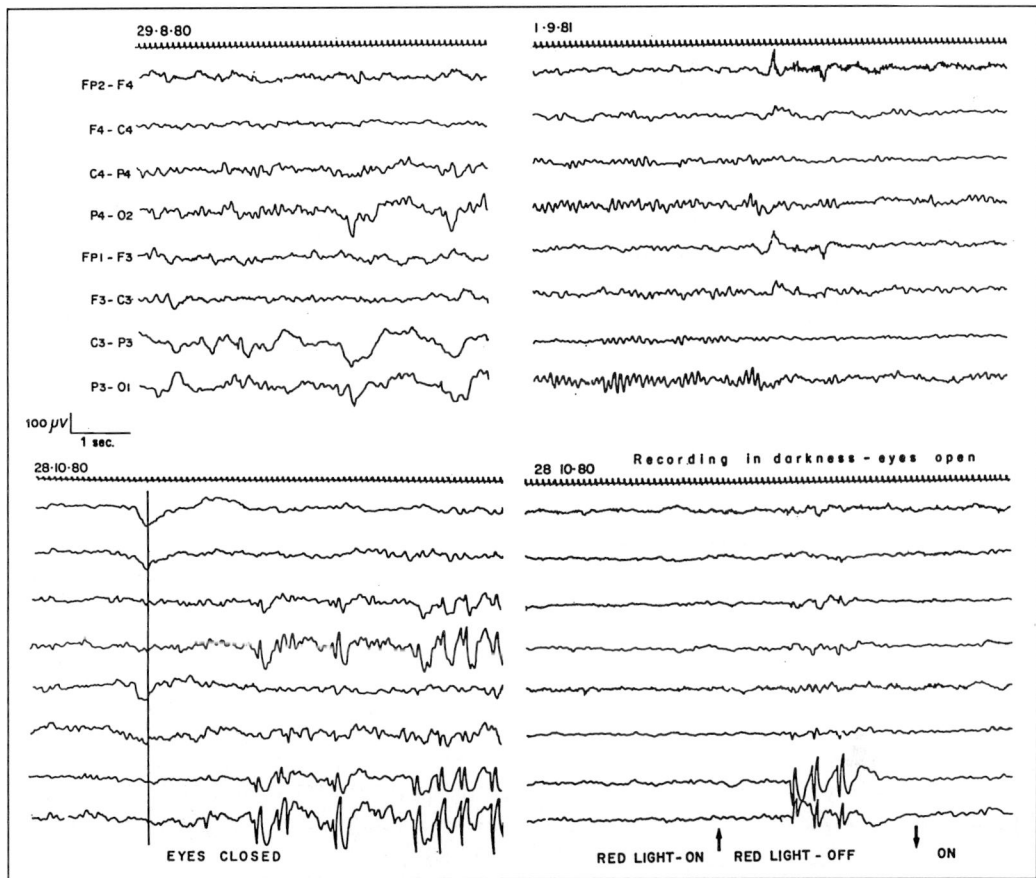

Fig. 9. EEG of a girl with a single, one and a half hour nocturnal partial status epilepticus of early onset BCEOP. Slow delta waves are seen in the posterior regions mainly on the left with unilateral poverty of a-rhythm and scattered small occipital spikes 2 days after the first and only fit in her life (upper left, 29.8.80). A second EEG (lower traces, 28.10.80), 2 months later, demonstrated high amplitude occipital paroxysms which were seen with eyes closed and in darkness. Fixation on a red spot of light inhibited the abnormalities (low right). One year later, her EEG was normal (upper right, 1.9.81) and has remained normal to date (from Panayiotopoulos, 1989b, by permission of Annals of Neurology).

to hospital with vomiting and unresponsiveness; subsequently her eyes deviated to the right followed by right-sided convulsions. The whole episode lasted for more than 3–4 h. She was well the next morning.

An EEG 6 days postictally showed some diffuse slow waves 3–5 Hz, with no spikes. Significant EEG abnormalities appeared 3 months later with long runs of high amplitude spike and slow wave paroxysms in the right occipital electrode which attenuated on opening the eyes. Two additional less active foci of smaller amplitude spikes were recorded from the left occipital and right frontal electrode simultaneously with the right occipital spikes.

Another episode occurred 1 year later, at age 8, during a mild febrile illness. She woke up in the morning with oropharyngeal movements, her eyes turned to the right. She tried but was unable to speak. This lasted for approximately 10 min. No further seizures occurred in the long follow-up.

Her last EEGs in 1988–91 were normal but previous EEGs had shown multiple foci of spikes in the left frontal, left and right central electrodes with no further occipital paroxysms. In one, but no other, EEG tactile stimuli consistently elicited contralateral somatosensory evoked spikes with a delay of the negative peak of 50 ms. The last abnormal EEG in 1986 showed independent high amplitude spikes mainly in the left and less often in the right central electrode. Evoked spikes were not elicited by tactile stimuli. In addition, high amplitude atypical spike and slow wave generalized discharges were recorded with a higher amplitude anteriorly and left.

Last follow-up was in 1991, age 16 years old. She was well, on no medication, with normal EEG, successfully attending high school.

Some children may have the clinical manifestations of BCEOP without EEG documentation of occipital paroxysms. I base this suggestion on the observation that in some children occipital paroxysms may not be detected interictally even when clinical seizures are active (see example of Case 7, Patient P.E. below) or postictally (see Case 4, Fig. 9 and Panayiotopoulos, 1989b). I have seen such case with clinical manifestations but no occipital paroxysms only once:

Case 5. D. MM., born 10.5.88. Had his first episode at age two and a half. He vomited in the back of the car and being taken out was very pale. His eyes were open but not obviously looking at anything and he was unable to stand or sit. He continued to retch. His mother took him to a friend's house, where 30 min later he held his head, cried, rolled on the floor and lost control of his bladder. He returned to his normal self after about 4 h having slept in the interim. A second episode occurred 4 months later when after an hour's sleep in the evening, he woke and became apparently unresponsive to visual stimuli for a period of half an hour despite having eyes wide open, vomited and slept. Three similar nocturnal episodes occurred in the following 4 months. No further attacks after initiation of treatment with carbamazepine. His awake and sleep EEG were entirely normal.

Late onset variant BCEOP and illustrative cases

BCEOP with visual partial seizures, episodes of blindness and frequent postictal headache, i.e. symptoms imposing difficulties in differentiating migraine and epilepsy (Panayiotopoulos, 1980, 1987) have attracted more attention than the early onset variant of BCEOP. Camfield *et al.* (1978) reported four adolescents with clinical manifestations attributed to basilar migraine and seizures interpreted as secondary to brain ischaemia. I questioned the diagnosis of basilar migraine (Panayiotopoulos, 1980) and reported a similar case which I had diagnosed as occipital lobe epilepsy (Figs. 2, 3) (Panayiotopoulos, 1976, 1978, 1980, 1981). However, the dispute regarding the diagnosis of migraine or epilepsy was decisively ended in favour of epilepsy by Gastaut (1982). The work of this great epileptologist has been extensively reviewed and naturally dominated the ILAE definition and the profile of the syndrome in all relevant reports. In my experience, comparing elementary visual illusions of patients with occipital lobe seizures versus classical migraine 'the visual epileptic seizures are predominantly multicoloured and circular/spherical in contrast with the predominantly black and white linear pattern of migraine' (Panayiotopoulos, 1993).

The following is probably the first published case of the late onset BCEOP in which FOS was demonstrated (Panayiotopoulos, 1978, 1980). It is presented because of its characteristic features (which are strikingly different to those of the early onset syndrome), the relatively resistant and frequent seizures, the less favourable outcome than the early onset BCEOP, the long follow-up (15 years) and finally because it has worked as a link (Panayiotopoulos, 1980) between the report of Camfield *et al.* (1978) and Gastaut (1982).

Case 6. D. M., born in 1965, a doctor's son, has had a 15 year regular follow-up from 1976. His clinical and EEG manifestations (Figs. 2 and 3) have been reported extensively (Panayiotopoulos, 1978, 1980, 1981, 1989b). From age 11 years he had:

(a) Frequent diurnal episodes of visual illusions consisting of 'millions of small, very bright, coloured mainly blue and green, circular, spots of light which appeared on the left side and sometimes moved to the right'. Initially, there was no postictal headache or vomiting which occurred later in the course of his disease. Since age 13 years, he has experienced short-lived simple visual hallucinations on three occasions only. The last was at age 23, when he woke from sleep with his familiar simple visual hallucinations on the left visual field which lasted for 20 min. The next morning he had unilateral headache and nausea.

(b) Two episodes of 'eyes turning to the right, right arm rigid and impairment of consciousness' at age 11 years. A further convulsive seizure occurred at age 16 when he once woke from sleep with left visual field simple hallucinations, fell asleep and later was witnessed to have a left motor partial seizure with secondary generalization followed by postictal confusion, vomiting and prolonged headache.

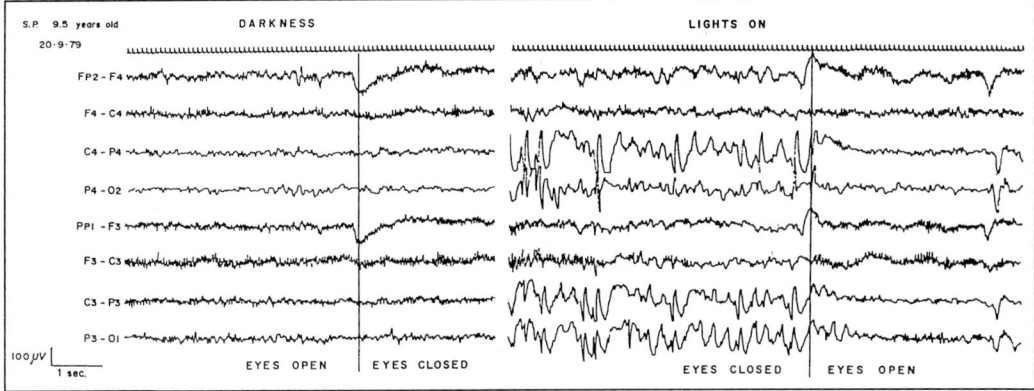

Fig. 10. The EEG of a boy with symptoms of the early onset BCEOP showed high amplitude occipital paroxysms, mainly or exclusively when his eyes were closed (right). This was the only patient in whom darkness inhibited, instead of inducing occipital paroxysms (left) (from Panayiotopoulos, 1989b, by permission of Annals of Neurology).

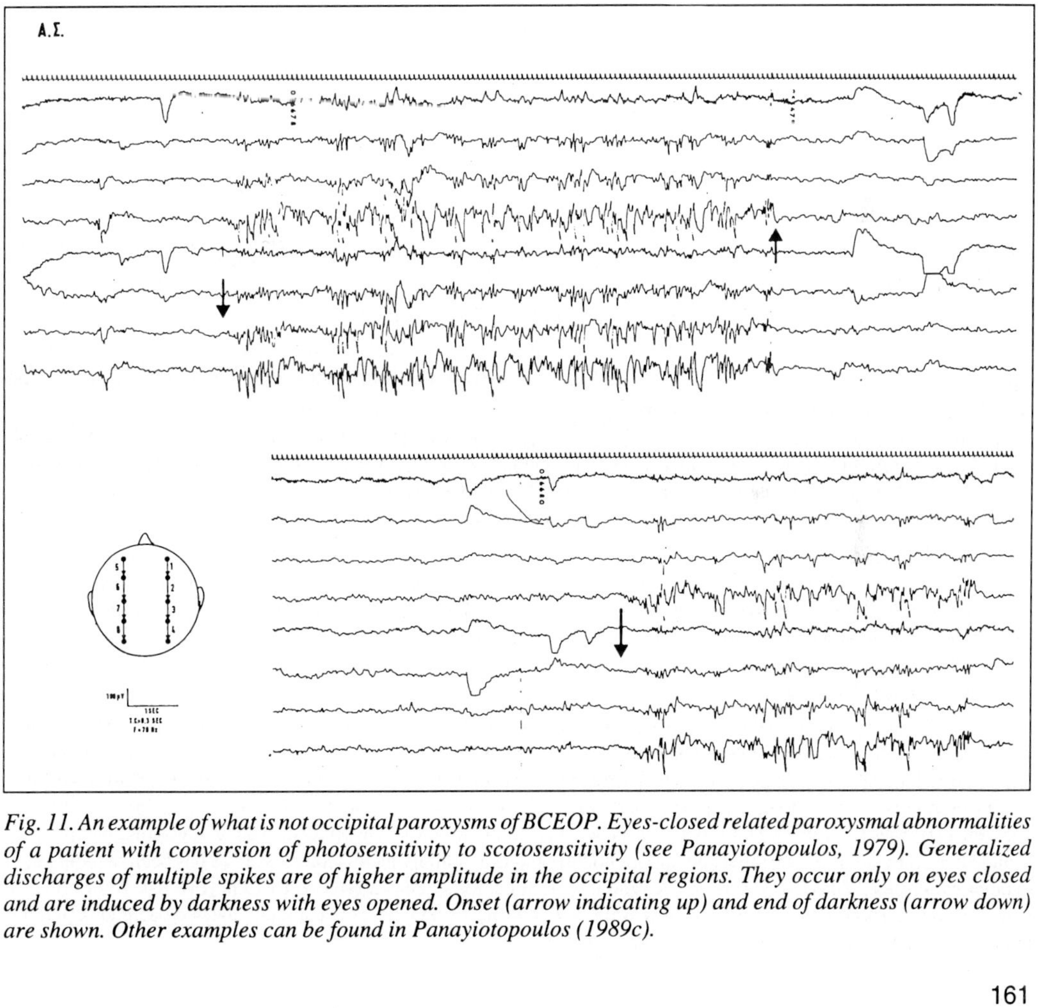

Fig. 11. An example of what is not occipital paroxysms of BCEOP. Eyes-closed related paroxysmal abnormalities of a patient with conversion of photosensitivity to scotosensitivity (see Panayiotopoulos, 1979). Generalized discharges of multiple spikes are of higher amplitude in the occipital regions. They occur only on eyes closed and are induced by darkness with eyes opened. Onset (arrow indicating up) and end of darkness (arrow down) are shown. Other examples can be found in Panayiotopoulos (1989c).

(c) Three episodes of blindness at age 11–12.

No further such episodes occurred. His EEG (Figs. 2, 3) (Panayiotopoulos, 1978, 1980) has been normal since the age of 13 years. By April 1992 he had become a solicitor, recently suffering a manic-depressive illness.

The following case is also presented because of the characteristic clinical features and his consistent 'fixation-off sensitivity' which have been recorded in video-EEG studies. Three hours of video-EEG recording showed bilateral, high amplitude sharp-slow wave occipital paroxysms when eyes were closed or open provided that central vision was eliminated binocularly (patient 'looking' through +10 spherical lenses, underwater goggles fixed with semi-transparent tape, darkness). However, his EEG (one week later, with no medication) and all subsequent EEGs (alert and asleep) were normal, indicating that BCEOP may occur without documented occipital paroxysms:

Case 7. P. E., born 24.1.80, has from age 10:

(a) Brief episodes of complete blindness without warning or impairment of consciousness.

(b) Frequent (1–3 per week), transient visual disturbances lasting for 10–30 s. He is unable to define his visual experiences which he calls 'visions' (impairment of consciousness?): 'It looked like a rectangle filled with coloured small circles. This time I saw the colours. They were blue, green, red and yellow. While I was reading I started seeing the words stuck all together. I blink a lot to see more clearly. It is a familiar vision, sometimes bright or dark. It replaces, obscures the real images. They are large objects, probably people, which I cannot identify.' 'They are always in my right eye and draws my right eye and my head to the right' (secondary motor partial seizures?).

(c) Four brief (1–2 min) episodes of loss of consciousness without convulsions whilst sitting or standing. He falls down and becomes unresponsive, but there are no postictal symptoms. One episode was witnessed in hospital as 'clumsiness, vacant, unresponsive for a minute or so'. No convulsions. Another one was witnessed by his parents: 'He was next to us in a shop. We heard a bang and saw him on the ground. Colour white not blue. He was out for a few seconds.'

No further episodes occurred 6 months after initiation of treatment with carbamazepine.

Occipital paroxysms

Occipital paroxysms consist of high amplitude, long runs of repetitive occipital spikes/sharp and slow wave complexes which are often bilateral and attenuate on eyes open. Their shape and amplitude are similar to the centrotemporal spikes. Fixation-off sensitivity is frequently demonstrated. This definition is proposed to emphasize the similarities between the occipital and the centrotemporal spikes so as to avoid further confusion in their recognition and evaluation. The following clarifications should be made:

(a) Occipital paroxysms are closely associated with the syndrome of BCEOP but even in their most typical form are not diagnostic of BCEOP, Like centrotemporal spikes, occipital spikes have been described in association with structural lesions, in symptomatic and cryptogenic epilepsies. Occipital paroxysms have also been described in children who do not suffer from seizures (see Beaumanoir, Chapter 12 in this volume).

(b) Occipital paroxysms may persist for years after remission of clinical seizures (see Case 3), but they may also not be detected interictally even when clinical seizures are active (see example of Case 7) or postictally (see Case 4 of this report and Fig. 9). In the postictal state, unilateral slow waves rather than occipital paroxysms were recorded in three of the 16 children with the early variant of BCEOP (within hours to 1 week). This incidence may be higher because not all children had a postictal EEG. It is also conceivable that in some patients these EEG abnormalities may exist but are never documented (Case 5 of this report).

(c) Occipital paroxysms are 'eyes-closed' related which is mainly due to fixation-off sensitivity (Figs. 2, 5–9). They are induced by elimination of central vision (vision through +10 spherical lenses, underwater goggles covered with semi-transparent tape and darkness) which appears to be the critical factor for their excitation and inhibition. Darkness is not a prerequisite for inducing occipital paroxysms as shown by their excitation in the presence of light (underwater goggles, +10 spherical lenses). This is why I proposed the term fixation-off sensitivity instead of scotosensitive epilepsy. Monocular elimination of central vision and monocular fixation inhibits them. However, FOS has been demonstrated in other epilepsies (Panayiotopoulos, 1989c) and FOS is not always demonstrable in BCEOP (Fig.10). Some children may have the characteristic spike/sharp slow wave in the posterior regions, not accurately located occipitally and not always consistently associated with eyes being closed.

(d) Intermittent photic stimulation has an inhibitory effect particularly at high flash frequencies. Photo-paroxysmal reponses were never induced in children with BCEOP described in my reports. This is expected in view that FOS and photosensitive epilepsies have opposite reactions to light, darkness, fixation and central vision (see review Panayiotopoulos, 1989c).

(e) Ten per cent of the patients may have additionally to the occipital paroxysms, in the same or subsequent EEGs, centrotemporal and/or frontal and/or somatosensory evoked spikes (Panayiotopoulos, 1988, 1989b, 1992, 1993).

Patients also may have generalized discharges in addition to the occipital paroxysms (see Case 4 and Panayiotopoulos, 1989a).

What are not occipital paroxysms?

Erroneous arguments against the existence of BCEOP are based on populations of children who have any type of EEG abnormality (spikes, multiple spikes, slow waves with abortive small spikes) in the posterior regions which appear mainly with eyes closed and attenuate with eyes open (Fig. 11). These, in accordance with the definition of this report, are not occipital paroxysms. Polyspikes, tiny spikes intermixed with slow waves, scattered occipital spikes as seen in photosensitive patients or slow waves which happen to attenuate with eyes open, are not occipital paroxysms and should not be confused with the syndrome of BCEOP.

Conclusions

The two variants of BCEOP and particularly 'early onset BCEOP' have unique clinical and EEG manifestations which make them easy to diagnose and treat (carbamazepine appears to be the drug of choice if treatment is needed), and to predict accurately a benign course despite dramatic initial attacks of partial status epilepticus. It is strange that the syndrome of early onset BCEOP, with the most striking, characteristic and often dramatic clinical symptoms and EEG abnormalities, has not been previously described. It is even more strange that recognition has met with such resistance and that it is not yet included in the ILAE classification (1989) although the description of the occipital paroxysms with their fascinating response to fixation and darkness as well as the clinical manifestations of the early onset variant have pre-dated that recognized by the ILAE as CEOP. It is hoped that this book will provide conclusive support for its long-awaited recognition.

Acknowledgements

I am grateful to the children of this study and their parents who all these years have kept me informed about their progress. I am indebted to Mr. P. Nastas, biomedical engineer, who performed all the EEGs, Dr A. Goumas-Kartalas, neurologist-psychiatrist, who referred four cases and drew my attention to the ictal vomiting of Case 4, Prof R.O. Robinson, consultant in paediatric neurology, Guy's Hospital, London, for showing me Case 5 and allowing me to present it in this report. My wife Thalia and my children Sophia and Paris have very generously and without complaint accepted my additional time commitment and preoccupation with the study of these syndromes over the last 20 years.

References

Aicardi, J. (1989): Commentary: benign epileptic syndromes. *Child. Neurol.* **4**, 48–49.

Beaumanoir, A. (1983): Infantile epilepsy with occipital focus and good prognosis. *Eur. Neurol.* **22**, 43–52.

Camfield, P.R., Metrakos, K. & Andermann, F. (1978): Basilar migraine, seizures, and severe epileptiform EEG abnormalities. *Neurology* **28**, 584–588.

Commission on Classification and Terminology of the International League Against Epilepsy (1989): Proposal for classification of epilepsies and epileptic syndromes. *Epilepsia* **30**, 389–399.

Gastaut, H. (1982): A new type of epilepsy: benign partial epilepsy of children with occipital spike focus. *Clin. Electroencephalogr.* **13**, 13–22.

Panayiotopoulos, C. P. (1974): Effectiveness of photic stimulation on various eyes states in photosensitive epilepsy. *J. Neurol. Sci.* **23**, 165–173.

Panayiotopoulos, C.P. (1976): EEG paroxysmal abnormalities after closing the eyes in epileptic patients. *Archives of Greek Association of EEG and Clin. Neurophysiology*, pp. 169–179.

Panayiotopoulos, C.P. (1977): 'Eye closure' and 'eyes closed' EEG abnormalities: discrimination and effectiveness of light and dark. *Electroencephalogr. Clin. Neurophysiol.* **43**, 523.

Panayiotopoulos, C.P., Hatziconstantinou, M. & Scarpalezos, S. (1978) Clinical and EEG observations in occipital epilepsy. *Archives of the 4th Panhellenic Medical Symposium*, pp. 98–100

Panayiotopoulos, C.P. (1978): Occipital epilepsy. *Materia Medica Greca* **30**, 557–564.

Panayiotopoulos, C.P. (1979): Conversion of photosensitive to scotosensitive epilepsy. *Neurology* **29**, 1550–1555.

Panayiotopoulos, C.P. & Siafacas, A. (1980): Triggering factors in occipital lobe epilepsy. *Acta Neurol. Scand. Suppl.* **79**, 112.

Panayiotopoulos, C.P. (1980): Basilar migraine? seizures and severe epileptiform E.E.G. abnormalities. *Neurology* **30**, 1122–1125.

Panayiotopoulos, C.P. (1981): Inhibitory effect of central vision on occipital lobe seizures. *Neurology* **31**, 1331–1333.

Panayiotopoulos, C.P. (1987): Difficulties in differentiating migraine and epilepsy based on clinical and electroencephalographic findings. In: *Migraine and epilepsy*, eds. F. Andermann & E. Lugaresi., pp. 31–46. London, Boston: Butterworth.

Panayiotopoulos, C.P. (1988): Vomiting as an ictal manifestation of epileptic seizures and syndromes. *J. Neurol. Neurosurg. Psychiatry* **51**, 1448–1451.

Panayiotopoulos, C.P. (1989a): Benign nocturnal childhood occipital epilepsy: a new syndrome with nocturnal seizures, tonic deviation of the eyes, and vomiting. *J. Child. Neurol.* **4**, 43–48.

Panayiotopoulos, C.P. (1989b): Benign childhood epilepsy with occipital paroxysms: a 15 year prospective study. *Ann. Neurol.* **26**, 51–56.

Panayiotopoulos, C.P. (1989c): Fixation-off-sensitive epilepsies. In: *Reflex seizures and reflex epilepsies*, eds. A. Beaumanoir, H. Gastaut, R. Naquet. pp. 203–217. Genève: Editions Médicine and Hygiène.

Panayiotopoulos, C.P. (1991): Benign age and localisation-related idiopathic epilepsies: a 17 years study of 94 patients. *J. Neurol. Neurosurg. Psychiatry* **55**, 245.

Panayiotopoulos, C.P. & Igoe, D.M. (1992): Cerebral insult-like partial status epilepticus in the early onset variant of benign childhood epilepsy with occipital paroxysms. *Seizure* **1**, 99–102.

Panayiotopoulos, C.P. (1993): Benign childhood partial epilepsies: benign childhood seizure susceptibility syndromes (Editorial). *J. Neurol. Neurosurg. Psychiatry* **56**, 2–5.

Chapter 19

Outcome of idiopathic childhood epilepsy with occipital paroxysms

Renzo Guerrini*, Agatino Battaglia*, Charlotte Dravet[†], Michelle Bureau[†] and Pierre Genton[†]

*INPE University of Pisa-IRCCS Stella Maris, Pisa, Italy; and †Centre Saint Paul, Marseille, France

Summary

The clinical and evolutive spectrum of benign childhood epilepsy with occipital paroxysms is wider than is recognized in the best known epilepsy with rolandic spikes. Two groups of patients stand at the extremes of this spectrum. Infrequent or isolated seizures may occur in some children where treatment might not be necessary. This seems the case in patients presenting with the seizure pattern of tonic deviation of the eyes and vomiting, even when prolonged, or when typical occipital EEG paroxysms are only captured in postictal recordings. Some of these children could remain undiagnosed if postical EEGs are not performed. Periods of seizure recurrence, often in clusters, seem to represent the wrong evolution in spite of treatment in a minority of patients, in which, however, no worsening of the clinical picture occurs over time. Between these two groups stands a greater number of patients in which AED monotherapy is effective in controlling seizures. Treatment duration is, however, hard to establish because the period of active epilepsy is variable and difficult to predict. Onset age does not seem to influence disease severity. Seizures might continue until 16–18 years, although, in the majority of patients, they cease earlier. No definite data from long term follow-up of a big series of patients are available and the ultimate rate of remission is unknown.

Introduction

A syndrome of childhood epilepsy with occipital paroxysms (CEOP) was recognized after studies by Gastaut (1982a, b) and Beaumanoir (1983); it was initially described as a benign epilepsy in analogy to benign childhood epilepsy with centrotemporal spikes (BCECTS).

Ictal visual phenomena, followed or not by motor and psychomotor manifestations and by frequent postictal migrainous headache, were considered the distinctive clinical picture. Repetitive occipital paroxysms appearing after eye closure represented the electroencephalographic (EEG) marker.

Further studies dealing with CEOP (Gastaut, 1985; Gastaut & Zifkin, 1987; Nalin et al., 1989; Kivity & Lerman, 1989; Panayiotopoulos, 1989) have provided additional data about both clinical presentation and outcome, despite scanty long-term clinical and EEG follow-up. In the majority of the studies, adopting different inclusion and exclusion criteria has probably made the data biased and information on outcome difficult to interpret.

It has proved difficult to recognize the same clinical homogeneity and uniformly benign prognosis in CEOP as found in BCECTS. As a consequence, the latest classification of epilepsies and epileptic syndromes (Commission, 1989) recognizes CEOP as a clinical and EEG age- and localization-related syndrome in which 'no definite statement on prognosis' is still possible.

With an analysis of both literature data and from our study of 18 patients, we have attempted to establish what can be pointed out concerning the prognosis of CEOP.

Clinical data

The uncertainty about the prognosis of CEOP is probably due to a number of factors. It is undoubtedly difficult to make a firm diagnosis of this condition. Various studies have shown how the classical interictal EEG picture described by Gastaut (1982a, b), i.e. high voltage occipital paroxysms blocked by opening of the eyes, can be frequently seen even in symptomatic epilepsy (Newton & Aicardi, 1983; Aicardi & Newton, 1987; Gobbi et al., 1988; Fois et al., 1988; Nalin et al., 1989; Cooper & Lee, 1991). Therefore, in CEOP we do not observe an EEG marker of such a high diagnostic value as in BCECTS.

Clinically, CEOP presents a certain polymorphism (Lerman & Kivity, 1991) which is due to the variability of seizure types. Furthermore, the presence of migrainous symptoms, which can be both ictal and postictal, makes CEOP sometimes difficult to distinguish from other conditions associating migraine, seizures and occipital epileptiform EEG abnormalities (Andermann, 1987a, b; Beaumanoir & Grandjean, 1987).

The recent clarification of CEOP and the low prevalence of the syndrome (Panayiotopoulos, 1989) have meant that long follow-ups of great series of patients are scanty. In addition, the interpretation of data from literature proves difficult. The criteria adopted in the recruitment of patients vary so widely in the different series that it is often necessary to 'look for' patients with CEOP within case studies that are not homogeneous from an aetiological point of view.

Beaumanoir (1983) called our attention to a form of childhood epilepsy with occipital EEG paroxysms and good prognosis, selecting 18 patients who had not had seizures for 3 years or more. All the patients were free from neurological signs but half of them had visual deficits. This author concluded on the existence of a benign occipital epilepsy accompanied by a disappearance of seizures before the age of 13. However, the study had been designed in such a way to make it impossible to know whether patients with idiopathic epilepsy but bad prognosis had been excluded.

Gastaut (1985) recruited a series of 63 patients on the basis of clinical, EEG or electroclinical patterns consistent with occipital epilepsy. The author observed a 'generally good prognosis,' with seizure control during the active period of the disease in 60 per cent of patients and persistence of seizures after age 19 in 5 per cent. Two major problems exist regarding the interpretation of these data: follow-up duration is not provided; some symptomatic cases were included in this series without clarifying if their prognosis was different from that of idiopathic ones.

Aicardi & Newton (1987) selected a series of children on the basis of the interictal EEG pattern of reactive occipital paroxysms. Among their patients it is possible to recognize seven idiopathic and 21 symptomatic cases with good and variable prognosis respectively. These authors concluded that the EEG pattern described by Gastaut (1982a, b) is not a marker of benign epilepsy.

Terasaki et al. (1987) reported 23 patients with 'non-organic' occipital epilepsy and favourable prognosis. Of the 14 patients with a follow-up of more than 2 years, 10 were seizure free and no patient was uncontrolled.

Nalin et al. (1989) selected a group of children who had an ictal clinical pattern of visual seizures. Nine of them had idiopathic occipital lobe epilepsy and were followed from 1 to 7 years; seizures were controlled with antiepileptic drugs (AEDs) in all of them.

Kivity & Lerman (1989) followed up 62 children for 2 to 17 years with clinical and EEG findings suggesting idiopathic occipital epilepsy. The authors described the variable ictal patterns and stressed the polymorphism of the syndrome. They affirmed that this type of epilepsy is of varying severity during the active phase but long-term prognosis is consistently good. Nevertheless, they did not supply analytical data.

The prospective study by Panayiotopoulos (1989), in which criteria for idiopathic epilepsy were strictly applied, led to the delineation of two subsets of CEOP patients, whose clinical picture and outcome were somewhat different from those described in previous reports. Sixteen of them presented a homogeneous syndrome of mainly nocturnal seizures marked by deviation of the head and vomiting, with onset between ages 2 and 8, and remission before 12. A worse outcome was observed in two other patients who had identical EEG findings, but late seizure onset, mainly diurnal and frequent ictal visual phenomena, followed by hemiclonic seizures, or automatisms and migrainous headache.

In our experience, based upon 18 CEOP patients (11 male, seven female) aged 4 years 5 months – 18 years 6 months (mean age, 11 years 6 months), clinical presentation and outcome coincided partially with those reported both by Gastaut (1985) and Panayiotopoulos (1989). Follow-up ranged from 1 year to 12 years 5 months (mean 4 years 2 months). Age at the first seizure ranged from 3 to 14 years (mean 7 years) coming to a peak around the third year (Fig. 1).

The seizure types observed are reported in Table 1. Eleven patients had had one seizure type only, six patients two types and one patient three types. The most frequent ictal pattern was tonic deviation of the eyes. This occurred without other signs in four patients and was accompanied by ictal vomiting in another four. Both these and unilateral seizures could last as long as 30 min in some children. Generalized tonic–clonic seizures are probably overestimated because the parents are not able to describe the asymmetric shaking that might occur during unilateral seizures. In addition, as Beaumanoir (1983) has already pointed out, secondary generalization is probably more frequent than can be shown, but seizure onset cannot often be observed, particularly if nocturnal; no more can a small child report the early seizure symptomatology. In fact, a focal onset was evident in all three patients whose seizures occurred during wakefulness; this was never recognizable in the four patients with nocturnal seizures. We observed ictal visual phenomena with relative frequency. On this point, our experience differs from that of Panayiotopoulos (1989) in that we observed this seizure type also in small children and in patients with excellent outcome.

Table 1. Seizure patterns in 18 patients with idiopathic childhood epilepsy with occipital paroxysms (note that ictal vomiting always occurred together with tonic deviation of the eyes)

Clinical seizure patterns	No. of patients
Tonic deviation of the eyes	8
Generalized tonic–clonic S	8
(evolving to)	(3)
Visual seizures	6
Blurred vision, blindness	5
Phosphenes	3
Hallucinations	1
Ictal headache	4
Ictal vomiting	4
Clear cut unilateral seizures	4
Seizures evolving to complex partial seizures	2
Dysarthria	2
Oculoclonic seizures	1
Simple partial somatosensory seizures	1

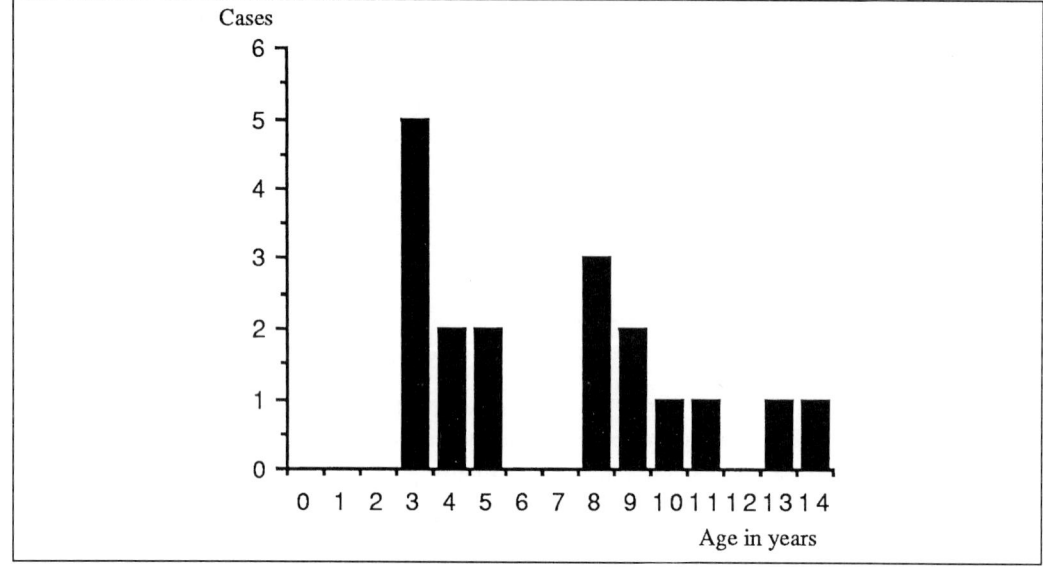

Fig. 1. Histogram of the age at seizure onset in 18 patients with idiopathic childhood epilepsy with occipital paroxysms.

Figure 2 shows the relationships between seizure occurrence and drug monotherapy. Six patients suffered an isolated seizure (Cases 3, 5, 7, 11, 12, 16) two of which received no treatment. Clusters of seizures are frequent, especially at the beginning of disease, and do not seem to be influenced by treatment (see Patients 1, 2, 13, 17, 18). None of the AEDs seem to be more effective than the other. Relapses do not seem to be predictable on a clinical basis because patients with more than a 2-year seizure remission under treatment can relapse at drug withdrawal (see Patients 2 and 13). On the other hand, long spontaneous remissions could be not definitive (see Patient 18). Seizure duration and age of onset were not indicators of disease severity. The ictal pattern of tonic deviation of the eyes and vomiting more often occurred in patients who suffered isolated seizures.

Overall six patients (33 per cent) suffered an isolated seizure and three others (16 per cent) had two attacks. Three patients (16 per cent) were not treated and in 86 per cent of treated patients, seizure control was achieved by monotherapy.

Clusters of seizures appeared in five patients (27 per cent), two of which were under treatment. In no patient could epilepsy be considered so severe as to influence school achievement or social adjustment. The treatment was successfully withdrawn before the age of 16 in 33 per cent of patients.

EEG data

When dealing with the problem of AEDs withdrawal, the prognostic value of EEG is obviously taken into consideration. It has been reported that in CEOP, seizure remission parallels EEG normalization, or, on the other hand, typical EEG abnormalities can outlast seizure remission (Lerman & Kivity, 1991). Nevertheless, this topic has never been an object of systematic study.

The relationships between seizure occurrence and EEG abnormalities in our patients are shown in Fig. 3; the accuracy in collecting EEG data varies from patient to patient depending on the number of recordings. In all our patients the EEG abnormalities were apparent during waking and activated during slow wave sleep. Two possibilities can be observed in the majority of patients: (a) seizures disappear spontaneously or are controlled medically and the EEG abnormalities persist (see Cases

Chapter 19 Outcome of idiopathic childhood epilepsy with occipital paroxysms

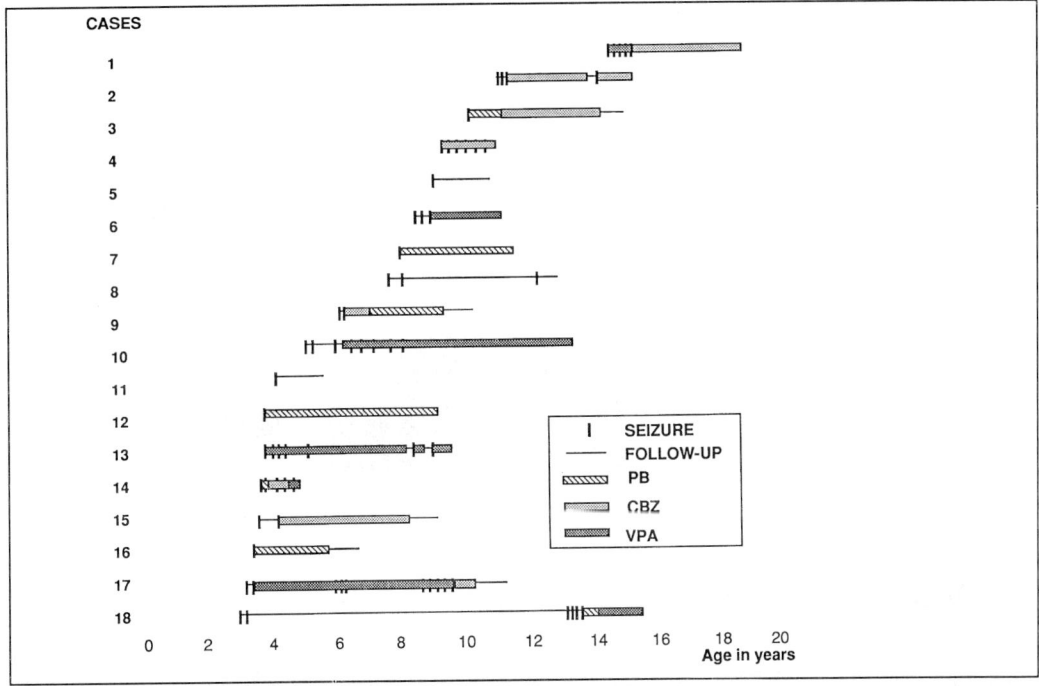

Fig. 2. Diagram showing the relationships between seizure occurrence and antiepileptic drug treatment during follow-up.

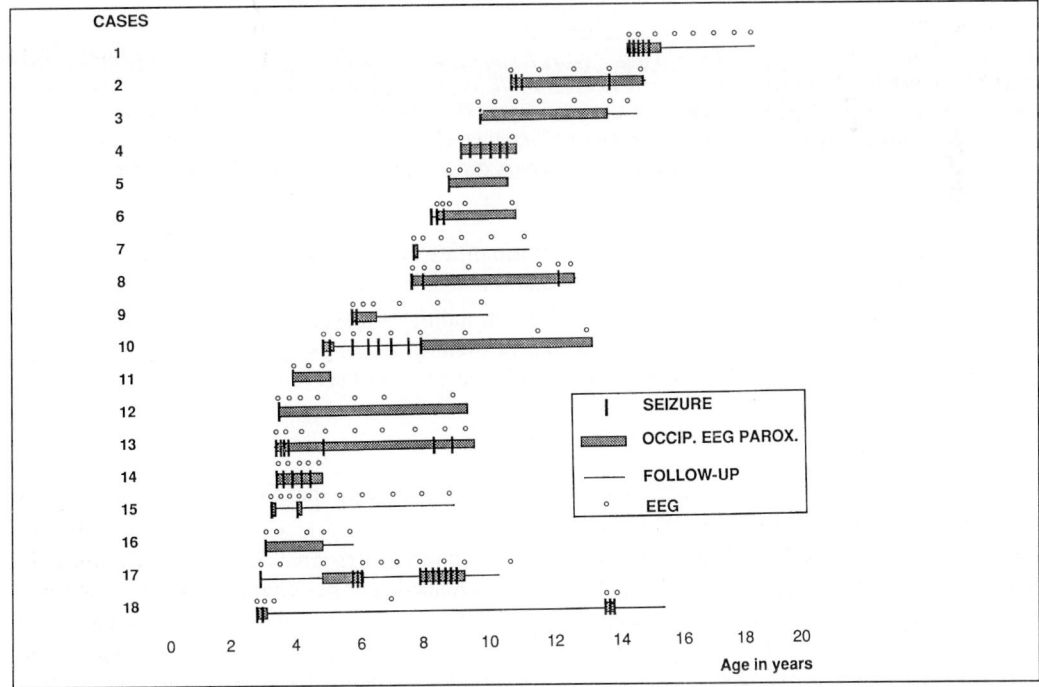

Fig. 3. Diagram showing the relationships between seizure occurrence and appearance of occipital EEG paroxysms during follow-up.

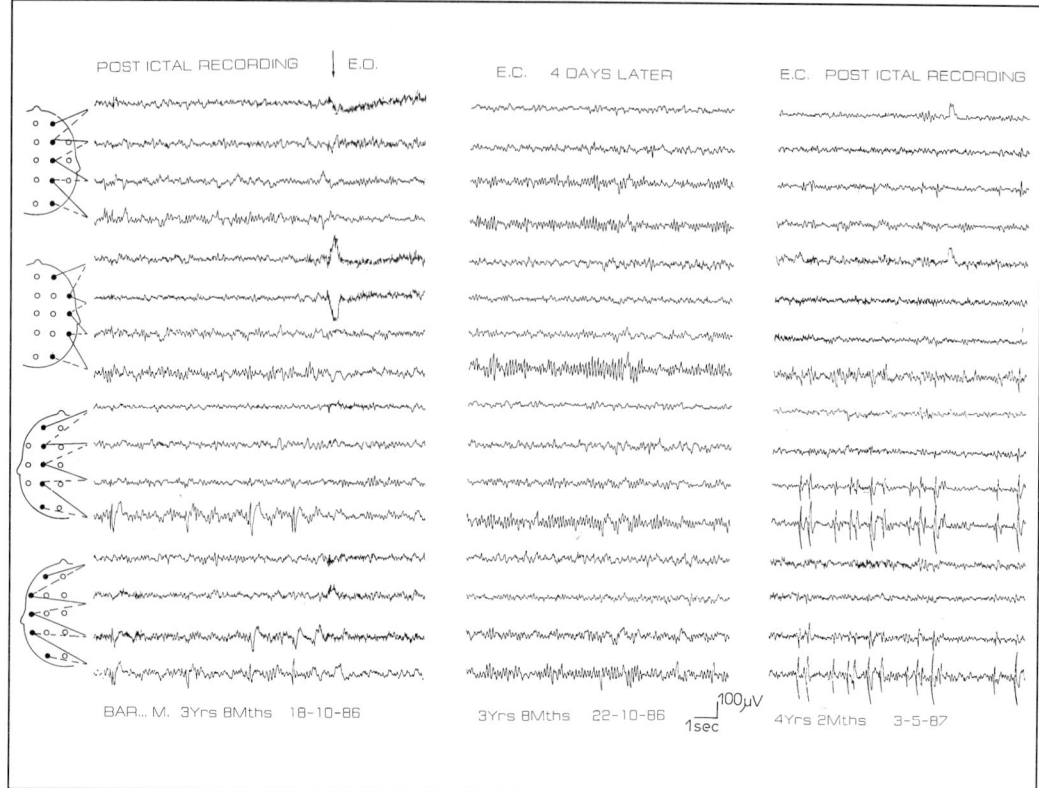

Fig. 4. (Patient 15) This boy presented at age 3 years 8 months with a typical seizure of tonic deviation of the eyes, vomiting and loss of consciousness. EEG recording, performed about 2 h after the seizure, discloses typical spikes in the left occipital region on eye closure. No treatment was given and no abnormalities were found on a control EEG 4 days later. At age 4 years 2 months another identical seizure occurred and was followed by transient reappearance of typical posterior paroxysms. Follow-up EEGs were normal (see Fig. 3).

2, 3, 5, 6, 10, 12, 16); (b) both seizures and abnormalities persist (Cases 4, 13, 14). Nevertheless sporadic seizure recurrence after EEG normalization can also be observed (Case 18).

In some patients the possibility to detect EEG abnormalities is restricted to time, namely in the seizure period (Cases 17 and 18) or only in the postictal recordings (Cases 7 and 15) (Fig. 4). Outcome was good in the patients where the latter instance was observed.

Conclusions

The data from literature taken together with our experience indicate that the evolutive spectrum is wider in CEOP than recognized in BCECTS.

Two groups of patients stand at the extremes of this spectrum. Infrequent or isolated seizures may occur in a few, very benign, cases, where treatment is not needed or no longer required. This seems particularly true for patients with seizure patterns of tonic deviation of the eyes and vomiting, or when typical EEG paroxysms are only captured in postictal recordings. Some of these children remain undiagnosed if postictal EEG recordings are not performed. Periods of seizure recurrence, often in clusters, in spite of treatment, seem to represent the wrong evolution in a minority of patients, in which, however, no worsening of the clinical picture occurs over time. Between these two groups stands a greater number of patients where AED monotherapy is effective in controlling seizures. Treatment duration is, however, hard to assess because the period of active epilepsy is variable and difficult to predict. Classic warnings of a possible severe evolution, such as prolonged seizures or clusters of seizures do not preclude a very good outcome. The age of onset, which varies from 3 to 14 years, does not seem to influence the severity of the disease. Seizures might continue until 16–18 years although, in the majority of patients, they cease earlier. No definite data from long term follow-up of a big series of CEOP patients are available and the ultimate rate of remission is unknown.

References

Aicardi, J. & Newton, R. (1987): Clinical findings in children with occipital spike wave complexes suppressed by eye opening. In: *Migraine and epilepsy*, eds. F. Andermann & E. Lugaresi, pp. 111–124. Boston, London: Butterworths.

Andermann, F. (1987a) Clinical features of migrain-epilepsy syndromes. In: *Migraine and epilepsy* eds. F. Andermann & E. Lugaresi, pp. 47–81. Boston, London: Butterworths.

Andermann, F. (1987b) Migraine and epilepsy: an overview. In: *Migraine and epilepsy*, eds F. Andermann & E. Lugaresi, pp. 405–422. Boston, London: Butterworths.

Beaumanoir, A. (1983): Infantile epilepsy with occipital focus and good prognosis. *Eur. Neurol.* **22**, 43–52.

Beaumanoir, A. & Grandjean, E. (1987): Occipital spikes, migraine, and epilepsy. In: *Migraine and epilepsy*. eds. F. Andermann & E. Lugaresi, pp. 97–110. Boston, London: Butterworths.

Cooper, G.W. & Lee, S.I. (1991): Reactive occipital epileptiform activity: is it benign? *Epilepsia* **32**, 63–68.

Commission on Classification and Terminology of the International League Against Epilepsy. (1989) Proposal for revised classification of epilepsies and epileptic syndromes. *Epilepsia* **30**, 389–399.

Fois, A., Malandrini, F. & Tomaccini, D. (1988): Clinical findings in children with occipital paroxysmal discharges. *Epilepsia* **29**, 620–623.

Gastaut, H. (1982a): L'épilepsie bénigne de l'enfant à pointe-ondes occipitales. *Rev. EEG Neurophysiol. Clin.* **12**, 179–201.

Gastaut, H. (1982b): A new type of epilepsy: benign partial epilepsy of childhood with occipital spike-waves. *Clin. Electroencephalogr.* **13**, 13–22.

Gastaut, H. (1992): Benign epilepsy of childhood with occipital paroxysms. In: *Epileptic syndromes in infancy, childhood and adolescence* (second edition), eds. J. Roger, M. Bureau, C. Dravet, F.E. Dreifuss, A. Perret & P. Wolf, pp. 137–149. London: John Libbey.

Gastaut, H. & Zifkin, B.G. (1987): Benign epilepsy of childhood with occipital spike and wave complexes. In: *Migraine and epilepsy*, eds. F. Andermann & E. Lugaresi, pp. 47–81. Boston, London: Butterworths.

Gobbi, G., Sorrenti, G., Santucci, M., Giovanardi Rossi, P., Ambrosetto, P., Michelucci, R. & Tassinari, C.A. (1988): Epilepsy with bilateral occipital calcifications: a benign onset with progressive severity. *Neurology* **38**, 913–920.

Lerman, K. & Kivity, S. (1991) The benign partial nonrolandic epilepsies. *J. Clin. Neurophysiol.* **8**, 275–287.

Kivity, S. & Lerman, P. (1989): Benign partial epilepsy of childhood with occipital discharges. In: *Advances in epileptology*. Vol. XVII. eds J. Manelis, E. Bental, J.N. Loeber & F.E. Dreifuss, pp. 371–373. New York: Raven Press.

Nalin, A., Ruggerini, C., Ferrari, E., Galli, V., Ferrari, P. & Finelli, T. (1989): Clinique, diagnostic différentiel et évolution des crises épileptiques visuelles de l'enfant. *Neurophysiol. Clin.* **19**, 25–36.

Newton, R. & Aicardi, J. (1983): Clinical findings in children with occipital spike wave complexes suppressed by eye opening. *Neurology* **33**, 1526–1529.

Panayiotopoulos, C.P. (1989): Benign childhood epilepsy with occipital paroxysms. A 15 year prospective study. *Ann. Neurol.* **26**, 51–56.

Terasaki, T., Yamatogi, Y. & Ohtahara, S. (1987): Electroclinical delineation of occipital lobe epilepsy in childhood. In: *Migraine and epilepsy*, eds. F. Andermann & E. Lugaresi, pp. 125–137. Boston, London: Butterworths.

Chapter 20

The partial occipital epilepsies in childhood

Bernardo Dalla Bernardina, Elena Fontana, Ornella Cappellaro, Emanuele Zullini, Francesca Darra, Vito Colamaria and *Roberto Caraballo

*Servizio di Neuropsichiatria Infantile, Università di Verona, Policlinico Borgo Roma, 37134 Verona; *Hospital General de Pediatria Juan P. Garrahan, Buenos Aires, Argentina*

Summary

In order to clarify the electroclinical features permitting the differential diagnosis between symptomatic and cryptogenic cases and the recognition of the idiopathic cases, the authors studied longitudinally a population of 64 children aged between 3 years 8 months and 22 years 2 months suffering from partial occipital epilepsy. On the basis of only the neurological and neuroradiological picture at onset, the cases have been divided in cryptogenic (C) (45 cases) and symptomatic (S) (19 cases). The most important differences are constituted by the predominance in the cryptogenic group of the seizures with occipital semeiology (C: 51 per cent – S: 31.5 per cent) or showing a spreading to the motor areas (C: 24.5 per cent – S: 10.5 per cent), often accompanied by vomiting (C: 53.5 per cent – S: 21 per cent). In the symptomatic group, the seizures with spreading to the temporal regions (S: 42 per cent – C: 20 per cent), the very brief, less than 30 s seizures (S: 31.5 per cent – C: 9 per cent) and the polymorphous seizures (S: 21 per cent – C: 4.5 per cent) predominate. In the S group the background EEG abnormalities (S: 47.5 per cent – C: 9 per cent) and the slow paroxysmal abnormalities (S: 89 per cent – C: 22 per cent) predominate. Moreover, a morphological modification of the paroxysmal abnormalities induced by sleep is observed more frequently in the S (58 per cent) than in C (13.5 per cent) group. Excluding all cases showing neuropsychological and neuroradiological abnormalities, polymorphous seizures, very brief (less than 30 s) and/or persistently very frequent seizures, EEG background abnormalities, slow EEG paroxysmal abnormalities, and EEG paroxysmal abnormalities morphologically modified by sleep, the authors obtained a group of 33 idiopathic cases. Analysing their different electroclinical features, the authors have had the possibility to recognize and better define the different features of benign occipital epilepsies as previously reported.

Introduction

In spite of their frequency and variability, the studies concerning the occipital epilepsies in childhood are relatively rare (Deonna & Ziegler, 1984; Gastaut & Zifkin, 1987; Terasaki *et al.*, 1987; Nalin *et al.*, 1989) and the only recognized form (Commission, 1989) is constituted by the benign epilepsy of childhood with occipital paroxysms (BEOP) (Gastaut 1982a, b, 1985; Beaumanoir, 1983; Giroud *et al.*, 1986; Niedermeyer *et al.*, 1988; Panayiotopoulos, 1989). However its existence is still debated by several authors (Newton & Aicardi, 1983; Deonna & Ziegler,

1984; Aso *et al.*, 1987; Luders *et al.*, 1987; Aicardi & Newton, 1987; Fois *et al.*, 1988; Cooper & Lee, 1991).

In order to clarify the elements leading to a better distinction between symptomatic and idiopathic cases and to recognize possible electroclinical entities other than BEOP, 64 children suffering from an occipital epilepsy have been electroclinically studied.

Materials and methods

The study concerns 64 subjects: 36 (56 per cent) males and 28 (44 per cent) females, aged between 3 years 8 months and 22 years 2 months (mean age, 10 years 10 months 5 days). We considered as occipital epilepsies those characterized by seizures with clinical phenomena peculiar to the occipital cortex. All subjects have been longitudinally followed at the Neuropediatric Service of the Verona University, by repeated clinical and EEG-polygraphic records both while awake and during sleep for a mean period of 6 years 9 months (range 5 months – 20 years). All cases have been neuroradiologically investigated by CAT and 10 by NMR too. The following parameters have been analysed:
 – age at onset;
 – familial antecedents for epilepsy and febrile convulsions;
 – neurological picture at onset;
 – semiology, duration and frequency of seizures;
 – morphology, topography, reactivity of the paroxysmal interictal EEG abnormalities when awake and during sleep;
 – electroclinical evolution.

On the basis of the neurological and neuroradiological data, the cases have been divided at onset in 19 symptomatic (S) (29.5 per cent) and 45 cryptogenic (C) (70.5 per cent) and the different parameters have been compared in both groups.

Results

Familial antecedents

A positive family history for epilepsy is present in 21 per cent of symptomatic cases and in 18 per cent of the cryptogenic; but in this last group there is also a positive family history for febrile convulsions in 11 per cent of the cases.

Sex

No significant differences exist between the two groups. The males are 58 per cent in the C group and 52.5 per cent in the S group; females 42 per cent in the C and 47.5% per cent in the S group.

Age at onset

The mean age does not show any difference between the two groups (3 years 9 months 14 days in C group and 3 years 10 months 23 days in S group).

Neuropsychological picture at onset

Absent for definition in cryptogenic cases, neuropsychological deficits are present in 11/19 (58 per cent) of symptomatic cases (neurological deficits in six and intellectual impairment in eight).

Neuroradiological findings

Negative by definition in cryptogenic cases, the neuroradiological investigations are positive in 16

(84 per cent) of the symptomatic group (poroencephalic lesion in five, more or less focal atrophic lesion in seven, focal cortical dysplasia in two and cerebral calcifications in two).

Ictal semiology

The ictal manifestations have been divided into occipital, occipital spreading to motor areas, occipital spreading to temporal areas, occipital leading to generalized tonic–clonic seizures. Autonomic symptoms as vomiting, vertigo and headache have been considered too.

Finally the cases with very polymorphous seizures have been considered. As shown in Table 1 there is no significant difference between C group and S group concerning the incidence of the occipital seizures. A spreading to motor areas and autonomic symptoms is more frequent in C group whilst the spreading to temporal areas and polymorphous seizures predominate in the S group.

Seizure duration and frequency

As shown in Table 1 the very brief (lasting less than 30 s) and the long lasting seizures (more than 30 min) have been considered separately. The first predominate in the S group and the second in the C group. Concerning the frequency rare seizures predominate in the C group, while the very frequent (several a week or a day) predominate in the S group.

Table 1. Comparison of cryptogenic and symptomatic groups.

		Cryptogenic 45 (70.5%)	Symptomatic 19 (29.5%)	Total 64
Mean age at onset		3 y 10 m	3 y 9 m	
Occ		23 (51%)	6 (31.5%)	45%
Occ →R		11 (24.5%)	2 (10.5%)	20.5%
Occ → T		9 (20%)	8 (42%)	26.5%
Vomiting		24 (53.5%)	4 (21%)	44%
Vertigo		2 (4.5%)	1 (5%)	4.5%
Headache		12 (26.5%)	6 (31.5%)	28%
Polymorphous		2 (4.5%)	4 (21%)	9.5%
Seizure duration:	> 30 min	12 (26.5%)	3 (16%)	23.5%
	< 30 s	4 (9%)	6 (31.5%)	15.5%
Frequency:	Very frequent	12 (26.5%)	14 (73.5%)	40.5%
	Rare	33 (77%)	5 (26.5%)	59.5%

Occ: Occipital seizures; Occ →R: Occipital spreading to motor areas; Occ → T: Occipital spreading to temporal areas.

Associated seizures

Simple partial motor seizures have been observed during sleep in four subjects of the C group. Tonic–clonic generalized seizures are reported in five cases of the C group and in three of the S group. Typical absences appeared during the evolution in three cases of the C group.

Polymorphous seizures associating long-lasting partial complex seizures, atypical absences, tonic seizures and drop attacks have been observed in two cases (4.5 per cent) of the C group and in four (21 per cent) of the S group.

EEG findings

Background activity and sleep organization are normal in 41 cases (91 per cent) of the C group and only in 10 cases (52.5 per cent) of the S group.

Interictal abnormalities

These have been divided into the following:

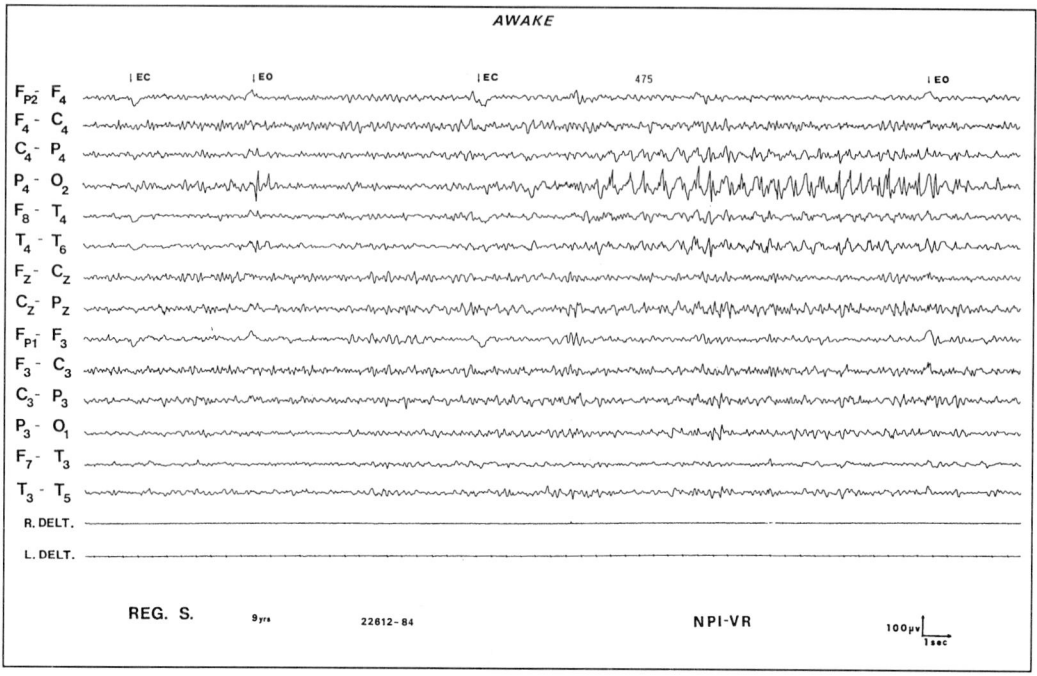

Fig. 1. REG. S. Girl 9 years old, suffering from partial occipital seizures with visual onset followed by complex automatisms and consciousness impairment, since the age of three. At the age of 7 years partial complex seizures with drop attacks and long lasting atypical absences appear in spite of different treatments. The neurological and neuroradiological picture at onset are normal, but an important neuropsychological impairment during the evolution appears. On the EEG it is possible to see the presence of focal theta waves mixed with slow spikes sometimes evoking a biphasic theta wave, frequently elicited by eyes-closing, involving the temporo-occipital right regions.

- Focal spike-wave complexes (S–W) of great amplitude involving one or both occipital regions; often they are frequent and pseudorythmic when the eyes are closed;

- Slow spike-slow wave complexes, often isolated (SS–SW), similar to those observed in benign rolandic epilepsy involving the parieto-occipital or the temporo-occipital regions;

- Sharp waves (ShW) often mimicking biphasic theta waves involving the temporo-occipital regions in very long bursts (Fig. 1);

- Polymorphous slow waves (PSW) associated with more or less frequent fast spikes variable in morphology and amplitude involving the temporo-occipital regions (Fig. 2). As shown in Table 2 the first two types predominate in the C group and the others in the S group.

Finally the suppression by eye-opening of the occipital discharges (EOS) and their modifications (increase in frequency of paroxysms and their morphological modification) induced by sleep have been analysed.

EOS and frequency increase during sleep (Table 2) are more or less equally present in the two groups. The only significant difference is constituted by a frequent modification of the morphology in the S group (58 per cent group S; 13.3 per cent group C). The most common are the appearance of fast spikes and polyspikes associated with an increase of the slow component often showing a brief 'suppression' following the spike.

Chapter 20 The partial occipital epilepsies in childhood

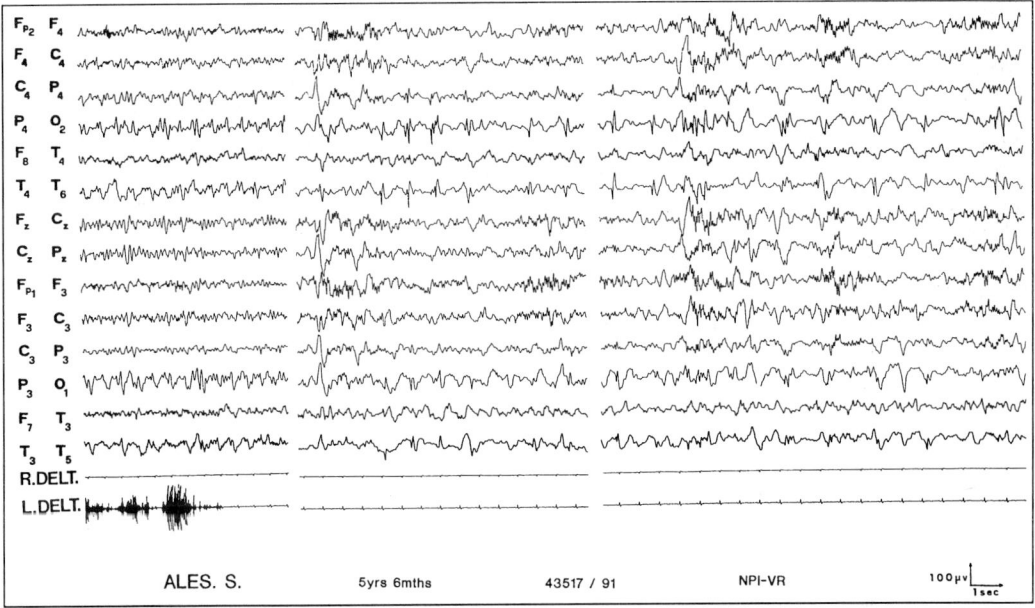

Fig. 2 ALES. S. Girl 5 years 6 months old suffering from partial occipital seizures with visual symptomatology, often followed by fear and consciousness impairment, appeared at the age of 4 years 3 months. CAT and MNR show a right occipital poroenchephalic lesion. On the EEG it is possible to see on the right temporo-occipital regions polymorphous theta waves mixed with slow spikes becoming more rapid during sleep. Note the appearance during sleep of a brief 'flattening' following the focal spikes.

Table 2. EEG findings in cryptogenic and symptomatic groups.

	Cryptogenic 45 (70.5%)	Symptomatic 19 (29.5%)
Spike wave complexes	23 (51%)	1 (5%)
Slow spike–slow wave complexes	11 (24.5%)	–
Sharp waves (biphasic theta waves)	7 (15.5%)	12 (63%)
Polymorphous slow waves	3 (6.5%)	5 (26.5%)
Associated slow spike–slow wave complexes	18 (40%)	2 (10.5%)
Eye opening suppression	21 (46%)	6 (31.5%)
Paroxysmal abnormalities: sleep increase	24 (53.5%)	8 (42%)
Paroxysmal abnormalities: sleep morphological modification	6 (13.5%)	11 (58%)

Evolution

Seizures have stopped for at least 2 years (2 years) (9 years 5 months) in 22 cases (49 per cent) of the C group and in one (5 per cent) of the S group. On the contrary they are drug resistant in 5 cases (11 per cent) of the C and in 13 (68.5 per cent) of the S group. At this point we considered separately the cases showing the following parameters:

* neuropsychological integrity at onset;
* neuroradiological normality;
* absence of polymorphous seizures;
* absence of seizures with significant involvement of the temporal regions;
* absence of very brief seizures;

* absence of seizures persistently very frequent;
* normal background activity;
* absence of slow EEG paroxysmal abnormalities (ShW and PSW);
* absence of paroxysmal abnormalities significantly modified in morphology by sleep.

In this way we obtained from the C group a population of 33 probably idiopathic (I) cases.

In Table 3 and 4 the parameters considered above are compared for the three groups I, C and S. Concerning the ictal semiology (Table 3) the most striking differences between groups I and S are constituted by the predominance of pure occipital seizures, the possible spreading to motor areas and the incidence of vomiting in the first group, while polymorphous seizures, the spreading to the temporal lobe and very brief seizures predominate in the second group. The seizure frequency also appears higher in group S than C.

Table 3. Comparison of idiopathic, cryptogenic and symptomatic groups.

	Idiopathic 33 (51.5%)	Cryptogenic 12 (19%)	Symptomatic 19 (29.5%)
Neurological deficits	–	–	11 (58%)
Neuro-Rx abnormalities	–	–	16 (84%)
Occ	21 (63.5%)	2 (16.5%)	6 (31.5%)
Occ →R	10 (30.5%)	1 (8.5%)	2 (10.5%)
Occ → T	3 (9%)	6 (50%)	8 (42%)
Vomiting	21 (63.5%)	3 (25%)	4 (21%)
Vertigo	–	2 (16.5%)	1 (5%)
Headache	10 (30.5%)	2 (16.5%)	6 (31.5%)
Polymorphous seizures	–	2 (16.5%)	4 (21%)
Seizure duration: > 30 min	10 (30.5%)	2 (16.5%)	3 (16%)
< 30 s	–	4 (33.5%)	6 (31.5%)
Frequency: very frequent	3 (9%)	9 (75%)	14 (73.5%)
rare	30 (91%)	3 (25%)	5 (26.5%)

Occ: Occipital seizures; Occ →R: Occipital spreading to motor areas; Occ → T: Occipital spreading to temporal areas.

Table 4. EEG findings in idiopathic, cryptogenic and symptomatic groups.

	Idiopathic 33	Cryptogenic 12	Symptomatic 19
Spike wave complexes	22 (66.5%)	1 (8.5%)	1 (5%)
Slow spike–slow wave complexes	10 (30.5%)	1 (8.5%)	–
Sharp waves (biphasic theta waves)	–	7 (58.5%)	12 (63%)
Polymorphous slow waves	–	3 (25%)	5 (26.5%)
Associated slow spike–slow wave complexes	10 (30.5%)	8 (66.5%)	2 (10.5%)
Eye opening suppression	14 (42.5%)	3 (25%)	6 (31.5%)
Paroxysmal abnormalities: sleep increase	17 (51.5%)	7 (58.5%)	8 (42%)
Paroxysmal abnormalities: sleep morphological modification	–	6 (50%)	11 (58%)

From the EEG point of view (Table 4) in spite of the possible presence of associated paroxysmal abnormalities evoking a more or less typical slow spike–slow waves, the polymorphous paroxysmal discharges morphologically modified by sleep that are absent by definition in the group are frequently present in both S and C groups. The remaining cryptogenic cases appear more similar to the S than to the I group.

Considering the idiopathic cases only, it is possible recognize three quite different electroclinical entities. Their most striking features are listed in Table 5.

Table 5.

EEG	Visual occ seizures occ. S–W	Eye deviation occ seizures TO SS–SW	Occ – Motor seizures O/PO SS–SW
N. patients	14	8	11
Mean age at onset	4 y 4 m	3 y 9 m	3 y 4 m
Visual occipital seizures	10 (71.5%)		2 (18%)
Occ seizures eye deviation	2 (14%)	8 (100 %)	
Occ →R	3 (21.5%)		9 (82%)
Occ → T	2 (14%)		2 (18%)
Vomiting	9 (64%)	8 (100%)	4 (36.5%)
Headache	6 (43%)	2 (25%)	2 (18%)
Long lasting		7 (87.5%)	5 (45.5%)
Awake	10 (71.5%)	1 (12.5%)	4 (36.5%)
Sleep	4 (28.5%)	7 (87.5%)	7 (63.5%)
EOS	12 (85.5%)	4 (50%)	2 (18%)

TO = temporo-occipital; O = occipital; PO = parieto-occipital; Occ →R = occipital spreading to motor areas; Occ →T = occipital spreading to temporal areas, EOS – eye opening suppression; S–W = spike-waves complexes; SS SW = slow spike-slow waves complexes.

The first entity is characterized by the association between occipital seizures with visual symptomatology and occipital focal S–W complexes on the EEG. In this group the spreading from the occipital areas is rare, vomiting and headache relatively frequent and seizures recur preferentially when awake.

The second entity is characterized by the association of long-lasting occipital seizures marked by deviation of the eyes and vomiting and temporo-occipital SS–SW. The spreading is absent. In this group headache is rare and the seizures recur mainly during sleep.

The third entity is characterized by the association of seizures frequently spreading to motor areas associated with isolated occipital or parieto-temporal SS–SW. The seizures, sometimes accompained by vomiting and very rarely by headache, preferentially recur during sleep.

Discussion and conclusions

Following the descriptions of BEOP published by Gastaut (1982a, b, 1985) and Beaumanoir (1983) many authors maintained that the electroclinical picture described by them can be observed in different clinical entities variable from the aetiological and evolutive point of view.

In fact the electroclinical elements indicated by Gastaut as indispensable for diagnosis are relatively poor; on the other hand the studies of Newton & Aicardi (1983), Deonna & Ziegler (1984), Aso *et al.* (1987), Luders *et al.* (1987), Aicardi & Newton (1987), Fois *et al.* (1988) and Cooper & Lee (1991), have been performed choosing the patients only on the basis of the presence of epileptic visual seizures and/or the presence of occipital paroxysmal discharges suppressed by eye opening.

The extreme variability of the clinical situations in which it is possible to observe occipital electroencephalographic foci is well known from the papers of Smith & Kellaway (1964), Huott *et al.* (1974) and Ludwig & Ajmone Marsan (1975). Analogously it is well known (Nalin *et al.*, 1989; Terasaki *et al.*, 1987) that the suppression of the occipital paroxysmal discharges by eye opening can be absent in some idiopathic cases too. So it is not surprising that by utilizing only a few and unspecific parameters it will be impossible to identify any homogeneous entity.

Cooper & Lee (1991) and Terasaki *et al.* (1987) have already demonstrated how by utilizing some more electroclinical criteria it is possible to recognize the cases having a benign course and good prognosis.

Our study firstly confirms that:

> Partial occipital epilepsies in childhood can be very variable from the aetiological and evolutive point of view;
>
> The suppression of the occipital paroxysmal discharges by eye opening has a non-specific meaning.

By dividing the cases only on the basis of the neurological and neuroradiological features at onset into cryptogenic and symptomatic, it is possible to recognize two subsets of patients having a statistically different course (the stopping of seizures is observed in 48.8 per cent of the C group and in 5.2 per cent of the S group). Utilizing only these parameters, an early recognition of the idiopathic cases having a benign course remains impossible.

Nevertheless if all electroclinical parameters are correctly analysed from the onset, the idiopathic cases can be recognized. In fact, in order to recognize the idiopathic cases all subjects showing the features incompatible with this diagnosis must be excluded (Dalla Bernardina *et al.*, 1985, 1992):

- Neuropsychological and neuroradiological abnormalities;
- Polymorphous seizures;
- Very brief (less than 30 s) and/or persistently very frequent seizures;
- EEG background abnormalities;
- Slow EEG paroxysmal abnormalities;
- EEG paroxysmal abnormalities morphologically modified by sleep;

Finally the idiopathic cases can be divided in the three following subsets:

- Cases with partial visual seizures with focal occipital S-W often suppressed by eye-opening, more or less increased in frequency during sleep. Headache is relatively frequent; vomiting less frequent. These cases appear very similar to those described by Gastaut (1982a, b, 1985), Nalin *et al.* (1989), Giroud *et al.* (1986) and some of those described by Beaumanoir (1983).
- Cases with long-lasting seizures frequently appearing during sleep characterized by tonic deviation of the eyes and vomiting and, in some cases only, with focal occipital SS–SW complexes suppressed by eyes-opening. These cases are very similar to those described by Panayiotopoulos (1988, 1989), Vigevano *et al.* (1989) and Dalla Bernardina *et al.* (1992).
- Cases with partial occipital seizures often spreading to motor areas and frequently associated with rolandic or hemiconvulsive seizures and with EEG focal SS–SW similar to those of the rolandic epilepsy, dramatically increasing in frequency during sleep. These last cases evoke some of Beaumanoir's (1983) cases and the electroclinical picture described by Dalla Bernardina *et al.* (1984, 1991) under the name of 'benign partial epilepsy with occipital spikes' (BPEOS).

References

Aicardi, J & Newton, R. (1987): Clinical findings in children with occipital spike-wave complexes suppressed by eye opening. In: *Migraine and epilepsy*, eds. F. Andermann & E. Lugaresi, pp. 111–124. Boston, London: Butterworths.

Aso, K., Watanabe, K., Negro, T., Takaesu, E., Furune, E., Furune, A., Takahashi, I., Yamamoto, N. & Nomura, K. (1987): Visual seizures in children. *Epilepsy Res.* **1**, 246–253.

Beaumanoir, A. (1983): Infantile epilepsy with occipital focus and good prognosis. *Eur. Neurol.* **22**, 43–52.

Commission on Classification and Terminology of the International League Against Epilepsy (1989): Proposal for revised classification of epilepsies and epileptic syndromes. *Epilepsia* **30**, 389–399.

Cooper, G.W. & Lee, S.I. (1991): Reactive occipital epileptiform activity: is it benign? *Epilepsia* **32**, 63–68.

Dalla Bernardina, B., Colamaria, V., Capovilla, G. & Bondavalli, S.(1984): Sleep and benign partial epilepsies of childhood. In: *Epilepsy, sleep and sleep deprivation*, eds. R. Degen & R. Niedermeyer, pp. 119–133. Amsterdam: Elsevier.

Dalla Bernardina, B., Sgro, V., Caraballo, R., Fontana, E., Colamaria, V., Zullini, E., Simeone, M. & Zanetti, R. (1991): Sleep and benign partial epilepsies of childhood: EEG and evoked potentials study. In: *Epilepsy, sleep and sleep deprivation* (2nd edn.), eds. R. Degen & E.A. Rodin, pp. 83– 96. Amsterdam: Elsevier.

Dalla Bernardina, B., Chiamenti, C., Capovilla, G. & Colamaria, V. (1985b): Benign partial epilepsies in childhood. In: *Epileptic syndromes in infancy, childhood and adolescence*, eds. J. Roger, M. Bureau, Ch. Dravet, F.E. Dreifuss & P. Wolf, pp. 137–149. London: John Libbey.

Dalla Bernardina, B., Sgro, V., Fontana, E., Colamaria, V. & La Selva, L. (1992): Idiopathic partial epilepsies in children. In: *Epileptic syndromes in infancy, childhood and adolescence* (2nd edn.), eds. J. Roger, M. Bureau, Ch. Dravet, F.E. Dreifuss, A. Perret & P. Wolf, pp. 173–188. London: John Libbey.

Deonna, T. & Ziegler, A. (1984): Paroxysmal visual disturbances of epileptic origin and occipital epilepsy in children. *Neuropediatrics* **15**, 131–135.

Fois, A., Malandrini, F. & Tomaccini, D. (1988): Clinical findings in children with occipital paroxysmal discharges. *Epilepsia* **29**, 620–623.

Gastaut, H. (1982a): L'épilepsie bénigne de l'enfant à pointe-ondes occipitales. *Rev. EEG Neurophysiol.* **12**, 179–201.

Gastaut, H. (1982b): A new type of epilepsy: benign partial epilepsy of childhood with occipital spike-waves. *Clin. Electroencephalogr.* **13**, 13–22.

Gastaut, H. (1985): Benigne epilepsy of childhood with occipital paroxysms. In: *Epileptic syndromes in infancy, childhood and adolescence.* eds. J. Roger, M. Bureau, Ch. Dravet, F.E. Dreifuss & P. Wolf, pp. 159–170. London: John Libbey.

Gastaut, H. & Zifkin, B.J. (1987): Benign epilepsy of childhood with occipital spike and wave complexes. In: *Migraine and epilepsy*, eds. F. Andermann & E. Lugaresi, pp. 47–81. Boston, London: Butterworths.

Giroud, M., Soichot, P., Weyl, M., Dauvergne, M., Alison, M. & Dumas, R. (1986): L'épilepsie a pointe-ondes occipitales. *Ann. Pediatr.* **33**, 131–135.

Huott, A.D., Madison, D.S. & Niedermeyer, E. (1974): Occipital lobe epilepsy. A clinical and electroencephalographic study. *Eur. Neurol.* **11**, 325–339.

Luders, H., Lesser, R.P., Dinner, D.S. & Morris, H.H. III (1987): Benign focal epilepsy of childhood. In: *Epilepsy: electroclinical syndromes*, eds. H. Luders & R.P. Lesser, pp. 342–343. London: Springer-Verlag.

Ludwig, B.I. & Ajmone Marsan, C. (1975): Clinical ictal patterns in epileptic patients with occipital electroencephalographic foci. *Neurology* **25**, 463–471.

Nalin, A., Ruggerini, C., Ferrari, E., Galli, D., Ferrari, D. & Finelli, T. (1989): Clinique, diagnostic différentiel et évolution des crises épileptiques visuelles de l'enfant. *Neurophysiol. Clin.* **19**, 25–36.

Newton, R. & Aicardi, J. (1983): Clinical findings in children with occipital spike-wave complexes suppressed by eye opening. *Neurology* **33**, 1526–1529.

Niedermeyer, E., Riggio, S. & Santiago, M. (1988): Benign occipital lobe epilepsy. *J. Epilepsy* **1**, 3–11.

Panayiotopoulos, C.P. (1988): Vomiting as an ictal manifestation of epileptic seizures and syndromes. *J. Neurol. Neurosurg. Psychiatry* **51**, 1448–1451.

Panayiotopoulos, C.P. (1989): Benign childhood epilepsy with occipital paroxysms: a 15 year prospective study. *Ann. Neurol.* **26**, 51–56.

Smith, J.B. & Kellaway, P. (1964): The natural history and clinical correlates of occipital foci in children. In: *Neurological and electroencephalographic correlative studies in infancy*, eds. P. Kellaway & I. Peterson, pp. 230–249. New York: Grune & Stratton.

Terasaki, T., Yamatogi, Y. & Ohtahara, S. (1987): Electroclinical delineation of occipital lobe epilepsy in childhood. In: *Migraine and epilepsy*, eds. F. Andermann & E. Lugaresi, pp. 125–137. Boston, London: Butterworths.

Vigevano, F., Ricci, S., Di Capua, M., Claps, D. & Fusco, L. (1989): Vomito, deviazione oculare, emiconvulsione: una particolare forma di stato epilettico nel bambino. *Boll. Lega. It. Epil.* **66/67**, 315–316.

Chapter 21

Occipital symptomatic epilepsy: epidemiological aspects

Giorgio Capizzi, Piernanda Vigliano, Anna Maria Pengo and Maria Baiona

Cattedra di NPI, Ospedale Infantile Regina Margherita, Piazza Polonia 94, Torino

Summary

We have studied 263 symptomatic epileptic children. According to Hauser *et al.*'s (1991) criteria, patients were excluded from this series if they had only one seizure, if the CT-scan was positive and with persistent focal EEG abnormalities, independent of whether they were undergoing treatment or not. 168 had the partial symptomatic form and in 19 cases (11.3 per cent) occipital epilepsy was found. In 20 per cent of cases there is cerebrovascular pathology, while malformative pathology is less frequent in our series (two phakomatosis, one lissencephaly) compared with data in literature.

As concerns clinical evolution, seizure semiology and EEG show occipital lobe involvement also in terms of follow-up. Therapeutic control is possible in 42.1 per cent of our cases. A good response to therapy was usually found in patients with acute vascular disease outcome and cryptogenetic epilepsy. Clinical evolution is unfavourable but with differentiating features in 4/9 patients who showed occipital calcifications.

Introduction

Epidemiological studies reported in the literature relating epilepsy to population characteristics (age range, geographic location, social and health levels), and the lack of similar criteria in inclusion or exclusion of cases and grouping of patients based on symptomatology, show the differences in percentages, at times significant, demonstrated by the widest ranging series, making any comparison difficult. For example, the percentage of partial seizure epilepsy ranges from 9.21 per cent (Matsumoto *et al.*, 1983) to 76.6 per cent (Danesi, 1982) and nosographic grouping varies in relation to the age ranges considered. In studies carried out on children less than 1 year old (Cavazzuti *et al.*, 1984; Chevrie & Aicardi, 1977, 1978, 1979), infantile spasms, status epilepticus and partial seizures were mainly found. Among the latter both unilateral and elementary seizures with focal onset and head and eye deviation seizures are reported (Chevrie & Aicardi, 1978). If a population older than 1 year is considered, partial seizures are divided into simple, complex or secondarily generalized, by most authors. Hauser *et al.* (1991) consider focal onset as an indispensable element in partial seizure definition, independent of a possible generalization.

The following division of simple or complex partial seizures depends on the presence or not of a confusional state. If research is carried out on a paediatric aged series, the simple or complex subjective clinical manifestation may be lost in the collection of data, especially when onset is at an early age. In such cases part of the symptomatology will be disregarded and/or the patient will be classified only on the basis of objective phenomenology of seizures, as pointed out by Oller-Daurella et al. (1989). For this reason only 23 per cent of their patients with partial epilepsy or seizures beginning before the age of 3 would have started with partial seizures. Data selected from partial epileptic patients give more precise results, even if the subdivision into symptomatic, idiopathic and/or cryptogenetic cases is not always verifiable and based on criteria not always comparable. Moreover, it is not constantly possible to deduce the rate of occipital seizures or occipital epilepsy within nosographic groups. 46 patients without preceding neonatal pathologies and with partial seizures started before the age of 4, were retrospectively studied by Blume et al. (1989) with a finding of occipital epilepsy in 13 per cent. From an EEG point of view they were able to give a significant localizing value, when present, to a focal delta polymorphic activity. Aetiology reported was of a malformative type, as already described by Chevrie & Aicardi (1977). Yamamoto et al. (1988) reported occipital seizures which later became periodic seizures in severely cerebrally injured infants. In a selected group of symptomatic partial epileptic patients Gobbi et al. (1989) have shown the presence of posterior abnormalities exclusively within a group of patients with poor therapeutic response. While in their series seizure semiology seems to change clinically over time, electroencephalographic data are rather stereotypic. Therefore it can be hypothesized that clinical polymorphism does not imply a different starting point of the seizure.

Semiology varies according to modifications of cerebral maturation and multidirectional propagation with successive activation of the involved functional systems. Oculoclonic seizures seem to be due to the involvement of peri- and parastriatal areas and of the geniculostriatal pathway. In hemiclonic seizures, propagation takes place in the frontocentral region, in complex seizures in the temporal and olfactory lobe. However, also in idiopathic forms, a polymorphism of seizures typically oriented from the nyctomeral cycle is present (seizures are usually sensorial while awake and motor during sleep). Detailed descriptions of semiology, with many documented seizures in presurgical patients, show that if there is a head and eye tonic deviation, it is always contralateral to the epileptic discharge (Takeda et al., 1969, 1970). In many patients visual symptomatology is absent, but when present it is at onset of the discharge, with retained consciousness. When there are variations in the level of consciousness, the discharge has already spread into the temporal lobe. The eye deviation has been considered by some to be a sensorial symptomatological epiphenomenon and by others an independent tonic phenomenon. Seizure semiology with symptoms involving both the visual function and consciousness level, linked in part to a migraine with vertebrobasilar aura and in part to epilepsy of the occipital and temporal lobe, complicate nosographic grouping.

Bickerstaff (1961, 1962) in his by now classic works has given two possible mechanisms in explaining the loss or change in consciousness level during a migraine attack: (a) brainstem transitory ischaemic attacks, including reticular formation, and (b) ischaemic effect on a potentially epileptic brain. All his patients were however without EEG alterations. Only subsequently has the frequent coexistence of severe posterior abnormalities, typically blocked or dramatically reduced by central vision (ROEA = reactive occipital epileptic activity) been underlined in idiopathic occipital epileptic patients. A common feature is the contrast between the intensity and persistence of EEG abnormalities in connection with good clinical state. These abnormalities make up an electroencephalographic pattern different from the little- or non-reacting posterior anomalies typical of occipital lesional epilepsy.

The presence of ROEA is not in itself sufficient to give a clear syndromic picture, as is shown by Cooper & Lee's (1991) data. In a group of 348 occipital paroxysm patients they found the presence of ROEA in 10.9 per cent. A study on treatment sensitivity and clinical evolution showed a response to therapy in 36.4 per cent and total recovery only in 9.1 per cent. From a multivariate analysis, antecedent pathological history, neurological damage, or focal or diffused alterations of EEG activity was a very significant prognosis. Aldrich et al. (1989) previously showed the existence of ischaemic complications consistently in permanent cortical blindness, similar to those described in mitochondrial encephalopathy with lactic acidosis and stroke-like episodes (MELAS) in a migraine patient with epilepsy and ROEA.

Longitudinal studies which follow foci evolution are rare and do not permit a distinction between symptomatic and idiopathic forms. Sofijanov (1982) considered EEG of the abnormality evolution in his study centred on evolution and prognosis of infantile epilepsy. Normalization takes place in 19 per cent of cases and in particular in patients with posterior focal and centro-temporal abnormalities, without a tendency to generalize, whereas in 8 per cent of cases a temporary generalization or migration of foci can be seen in an average period of 5 years. Konishi et al. (1987) have faced the problem of foci migration in a longitudinal study carried out on 116 patients between 10 months and 12 years of age. Series were divided according to the initial site of anomalies. A site change was observed in 32.8 per cent of cases. In patients with occipital and frontal localization there was a migration of 56 and 67 per cent in longitudinal sense, while in those with rolandic localization, migration was in a horizontal sense toward the temporal lobe.

Personal series

We have studied 263 symptomatic epileptic children. According to the criteria of Hauser et al. (1991), patients who had only one seizure were excluded from this series as also were those whose CT-scan was positive and those with persistent focal EEG abnormalities, independent of whether they were undergoing treatment or not. In 19 cases (11.3 per cent of partial symptomatic form) occipital epilepsy was found (Table 1). There were 10 males and nine females with an average follow-up of 4.5 years. In our group, age at onset of symptoms was early in 5/19 cases (less than 2 years of age in one vascular pathology, three cerebral malformations, one with bilateral occipital calcifications).

Table 1. Inpatients and outpatients examined in three years in the Clinic of Child Neuropsychiatry of Turin

All symptomatic epilepsies	Partial symptomatic epilepsies	Occipital epilepsies*
263	168/263 = 64%	19/263 = 7.2%
		19/168 = 11.3%

*Male/female ratio = 10/9.

Table 2. Clinical features of personal cases

Aetiology		Age of onset of seizures	Seizure control*	Migraine
Cerebrovascular disease	4	3 m; 2 y; 6 y; 7 y	3	1
Trauma	1	6 y	1	1
Cerebral malformations	1	3 m	–	
Phakomatoses	2	6 m; 18 m	1	
Infections	1	2 y	1±	
Bilateral calcifications	2	15 m; 13 y	–	1
Prenatal injury	2	3 y; 4 y	–	
Other	3	3 m; 2 y; 4 y	–	2
Cryptogenetic	3	3 y; 4 y; 10 y	2	1

*Follow-up: 4.5 years.

In 17/19 patients (89.4 per cent) seizure origin (confirmed by many records as shown in Figs. 1 and 2) was in the posterior lobes. Semiology was sensorial in six cases, oculocephalogyric and/or oculoclonic in eight cases. In the remaining two (in which seizure recording was not possible) symptomatology was motor at onset. In all cases, during evolution, seizure symptomatology became complicated due to the involvement of other structures (temporal lobe, motor cortex) despite

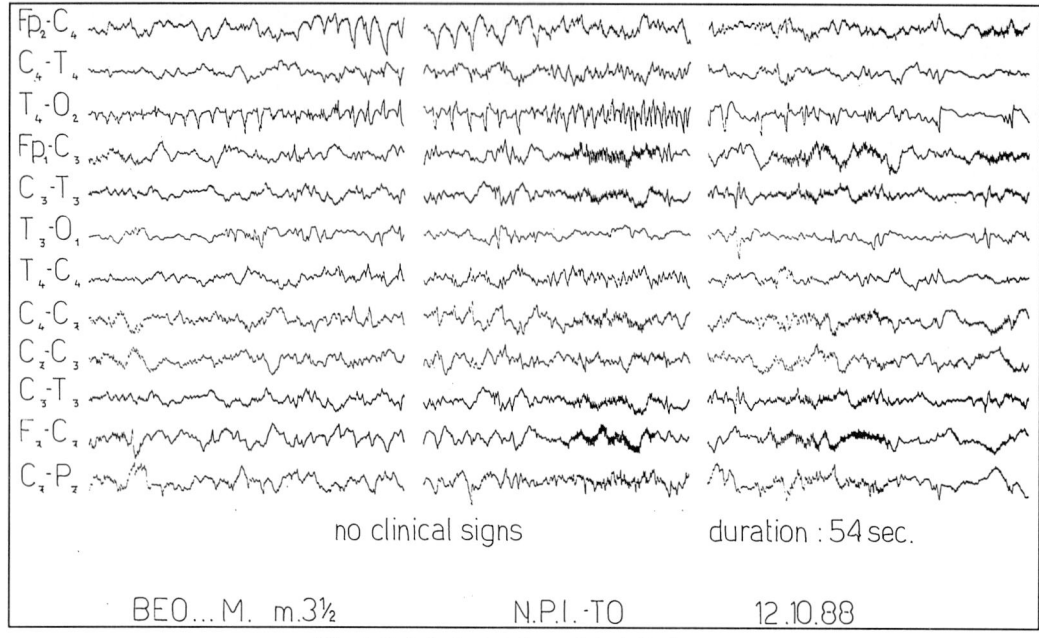

Fig. 1. Subclinical right occipital discharge.

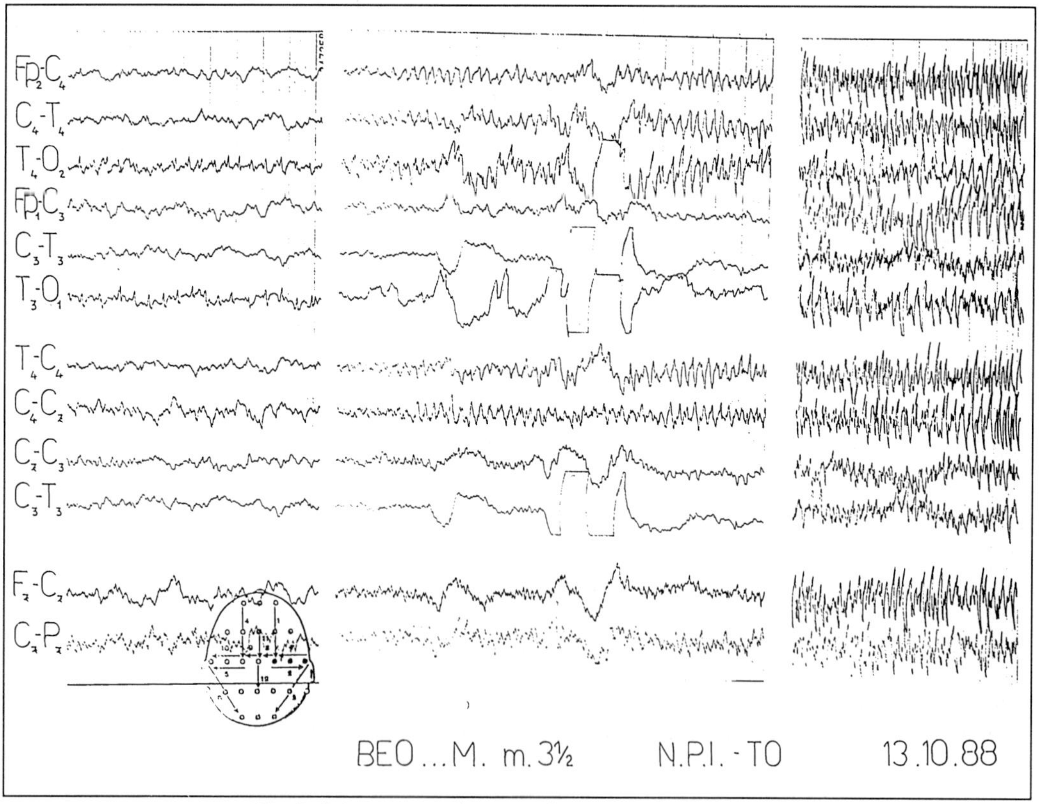

Fig. 2. Seizure generalization after right posterior onset.

demonstrating a posterior beginning even at the end of follow-up. Focal neurological signs were present in four patients (one vascular damage, one perinatal damage and two phakomatoses) while severe global motor damage was seen in lissencephaly. Mental deficiency was present in two cases of vascular damage, one patient with posterior calcification, one phakomatosis and one encephalopathy associated to malabsorbtion. The main features of our group are shown in Table 2. Patients with cerebrovascular aetiology included two cases with damage following cardiac surgery or catheterism, and two outcomes of intraparenchymal haemorrhage due to vascular pathology. The malformation was lissencephaly, one of the phakomatoses was a Bourneville Syndrome and another was a Sturge–Weber syndrome, incomplete, without flat facial angioma. Grouped under the heading 'other' included one vascular malformation of the 'capillary telangiectasis' type, one febrile state and one encephalopathy with malabsorption without posterior calcification. Symptomatology management was good in 42.1 per cent of cases and poor in those suffering from severe malformations with perinatal damage and early seizures. Patients with acute vascular disease, including one who was 3 months old at seizure onset and cryptogenetic epileptic cases generally respond well to therapy.

Conclusions

In our patient sample, aetiopathogenical and clinical features are difficult to compare to those found in literature, confirming that inclusion criteria play a large part in groups made up of small numbers. Data from our series was particularly compared with Blume's (1987) study, utilizing Hauser *et al.*'s (1991) aetiological classification (Table 3).

Table 3. Aetiology of personal series compared with literature data

	Hauser (1991)	Blume (1987)		Personal cases
		All cases	Posterior cases	Posterior cases
Idiopathic	76%	–	–	–
Cerebrovascular	6%	–	–	4
Trauma	5%	–	–	1
Malformations	5%	12	3	1
Infections	4%	4	–	1
Tumour	2%	8	–	–
Degenerative	1%	–	–	–
Other	1%	22	3	12
Total		46	6/46	19

As can be seen, 50 per cent of our and Blume's cases are grouped under the heading 'other' showing the necessity of more detailed definition. It is significant in our series that in 20 per cent of cases there is a cerebrovascular pathology. This is remarkable when compared to 6 per cent for all symptomatic forms in Hauser (1991) and complete absence in Blume (1989). The latter has instead seen a net prevalence of malformative pathology (phakomatosis, hemimegalencephaly) which was less noted in our series. In clinical evolution, the apparent polymorphism, seizure semiology and EEG show an occipital lobe involvement also at follow-up. This agrees with what is expressed by Gobbi *et al.* (1989). In particular therapeutic control data, possible in 42 per cent of our cases, is far from that of both Blume *et al.* (1989) and Gobbi *et al.* (1989) whereas it is close to that of Cooper & Lee (1991). We feel that such a difference can be explained by the presence of a fair number of cryptogenetic epilepsies or cases following acute cerebral pathology in which a good therapeutic control has been easy to obtain. Clinical evolution is unfavourable but with differentiating features in 4/9 patients who showed occipital calcifications. In one case, included among those with phakomatosis, we put forward the atypical Sturge–Weber diagnosis due to its clinical and arteriographic picture. EEG was always asymmetrical during the course of evolution, with poor intercritical abnormalities. Seizures were almost daily. In another patient, listed under 'others', calcification was related to a vascular malformation of a capillary telangiectasis type. This was evidenced by an arteriographic study carried out at 4 years of age, when seizures first began. Posterior calcification unilaterally appeared soon after. This patient also had frequent seizures. The two bilateral calcification cases, one associated to malabsorbtion, have non-homogeneous clinical evolutive features, as reported by various authors (Gobbi *et al.*, 1988; Magaudda *et al.*, 1988).

References

Aldrich, M.S., Vanderzant C.W., Alessi, A.G., Abou-Khalil, B. & Sackellars, J.C. (1989): Ictal cortical blindness with permanent visual loss. *Epilepsia* **30**, 116–120.

Bickerstaff, E. (1961): Basilar artery migraine. *Lancet* **i**, 15–17.

Bickerstaff, E. (1962): The basilar artery and migraine epilepsy syndrome. *Proc. R. Soc. Med.* **55**, 167.

Blume, W.T. (1989): Clinical profile of partial seizures beginning at less than four years of age. *Epilepsia.* **30**, 813–819.

Cavazzuti, G.B., Ferrari, P. & Lalla M. (1984): Follow-up study of 482 cases with convulsive disorders in the first year of life. *Dev. Med. Child Neurol.* **26**, 425–437.

Chevrie, J.J. & Aicardi, J. (1977): Convulsive disorders in the first year of life: aetiological factors. *Epilepsia* **18**, 489–498.

Chevrie, J.J. & Aicardi, J. (1978): Convulsive disorders in the first year of life: neurological and mental outcome and mortality. *Epilepsia.* **19**, 67–74.

Chevrie, J.J. & Aicardi, J. (1979): Convulsive disorders in the first year of life: persistence of epileptic seizures. *Epilepsia* **20**, 643–649.

Cooper, G.W. & Lee, S. (1991): Reactive occipital epileptiform activity: is it benign? *Epilepsia* **32**, 63–68.

Danesi, M.A. (1985): Classification of the epilepsies. An investigation of 945 patients in a developing country. *Epilepsia* **26**, 131–136.

Gobbi, G., Sorrenti, G., Santucci, M, *et al.* (1988): Epilepsy with bilateral occipital calcifications: a benign onset with progressive severity. *Neurology* **38**, 913–920.

Gobbi, G., Tassinari, C.A., Roger, J., Bureau, M., Dravet, C. & Salas-Puig, X. (1989): Particularités électroencéphalographiques des épilepsies partielles symptomatiques sévères de l'enfant. *Neurophysiol. Clin.* **19**, 209–218.

Hauser, W.A., Annegers, J.F. & Kurland, L. (1991): Prevalence of epilepsy in Rochester, Minnesota: 1940–1980. *Epilepsia.* **32**, 429–445.

Konishi, T., Murakami, M., Yamatani, M., Konda, M. & Okada, T. (1987): Longitudinal study of epileptic foci in childhood. *No To Shinkei* **39**(3), 267–271.

Oller-Daurella, L. & Oller F-V., L. (1987): Partial epilepsy with seizures appearing in the first three years of life. *Epilepsia* **30**(6), 820–826.

Magaudda, A., Colamaria, V., Narbone, M.C., Capizzi, G., Landre, E., De Domenico, P. & Dalla Bernardina, B. (1990): Calcificazioni occipitali bilaterali senza nevo flammeo: studio di 8 casi. *Boll. Lega. It. Epil.* **70/71**, 251–254.

Matsumoto, A., Watanabe, K., Sugiura, M., *et al.* (1983): Long-term prognosis of convulsive disorders in the first year of life: mental and physical development and seizure persistence. *Epilepsia* **24**, 321–329.

Sofijanov, N.G. (1982): Clinical evolution and prognosis of childhood epilepsies. *Epilepsia* **23**, 61–69.

Takeda, A., Bancaud, J., Talairach, J., Bonis, A. & Bordas-Ferrer, M. (1969): A propos des accès épileptiques d'origine occipitale. *Rev. Neurol.* **121**, 306–315.

Takeda, A., Bancaud, J., Talairach, J., Bonis, A. & Bordas-Ferrer, M. (1970): Concerning epileptic attacks of occipital origin. *Electroencephalogr. Clin. Neurophysiol.* **28**, 647–648.

Yamamoto, N., Watanabe, K., Negoro, T., Furune, S., Takahashi, I., Nomura, K. & Matsumoto A. (1988): Partial seizures evolving to infantile spasm. *Epilepsia* **29**, 34–40.

Chapter 22

Coeliac disease, epilepsy and cerebral calcifications: a multicentric study

Italian Working Group on coeliac disease and epilepsy
Coordinators: Furio Bouquet[1], Giuseppe Gobbi[2*], Luigi Greco[3], Andrea Lambertini[4], Carlo Alberto Tassinari[5], Alessandro Ventura[6] and Maria Gilda Zaniboni[4]

[1]*Divisione di Neuropsichiatria Infantile, Istituto per l'Infanzia, Trieste, Italy;*
[2]*Servizio di Neuropsichiatria Infantile, U.S.L. 9, Via Amendola, 2, 42100 Reggio Emilia, Italy*
(* for reprints request);
[3]*Clinica Pediatrica, II Facoltà di Medicina e Chirurgia, Università di Napoli, Italy;*
[4]*Divisione di Pediatria, Ospedale Maggiore, Bologna, Italy;*
[5]*Divisione di Neurologia, II Cattedra di Neurologia, Ospedale Bellaria, Università di Bologna, Italy;*
[6]*Clinica Pediatrica dell'Università, Istituto per l'Infanzia, Trieste, Italy*

Participants: P. Ambrosetto, Clinica Neurologica, Università di Bologna; F. Balli & V. Galli, Clinica Pediatrica, Università di Modena; P.A. Battistella, C. Boniver & F. Donzelli, Dipartimento di Pediatria, Università di Padova; P.A. Bianchi, N. Molteni & M.T. Bardella, Patologia Medica III, Università di Milano; E. Del Giudice & F. Correale, Clinica Pediatrica, Università di Napoli; G. Della Cella, Divisione Pediatrica Ospedali Riuniti di Chiavari; P.G. Garofalo, C. Durisotti & C. Filati, Divisione Neurologica, Ospedale Civile di Vicenza; A.M. Giunta, Clinica, Pediatrica II, Università di Milano; A. Miano, Divisione Pediatrica, Ospedale Bufalini di Cesena; A. Pascotto & G. Coppola, Istituto Neuropsichiatria Infantile, Università di Napoli; L. Piattella & N. Zamponi, Divisione di Neuropsichiatria Infantile, Ospedale Salesi di Ancona; P. Santanelli, Clinica Neurologica, Università di Napoli; E. Veneselli, Divisione Neuropsichiatria Infantile, Istituto Gaslini, Università di Genova; F. Viani & A. Van Lierde, Centro Regionale Studio Epilessia, Milano.

Summary

Forty-three patients (15 males) were selected from two different series. Thirty-one cases with cerebral calcifications of unexplained origin and epilepsy (series 'a') underwent intestinal biopsy. Twelve patients with coeliac disease and epilepsy (series 'b') underwent CT scan. HLA typing was also studied. Twenty-four cases (77.4 per cent) from series 'a' were identified as coeliac disease patients on the basis of a flat intestinal mucosa. Five cases from series 'b' showed cerebral calcifications. Consequently, 29 cases presented the association of coeliac disease, epilepsy and cerebral calcifications (CEC group), seven cases epilepsy and coeliac disease without cerebral calcifications (Group 2) and seven cases epilepsy and cerebral calcifications without coeliac disease (Group 3).

In 27 cases of the CEC group the cortical and/or subcortical cerebral calcifications were serpiginous and located in the parieto-occipital regions. The epilepsy was studied in 16 patients of the CEC group and it is constituted of partial occipital epilepsy in all cases. The evolution was benign in two cases, drug-resistant in six, with progressive severity in eight.

In conclusion we believe that: (1) the association of cerebral calcifications and epilepsy with coeliac disease is much more frequent than expected and so it does not appear to be casual; (2) the cases labelled in the past as atypical Sturge Weber syndrome may belong to this group; (3) the child neurologist must rule out coeliac disease in all cases of occipital epilepsy and cerebral calcifications of unexplained origin.

Introduction

There has been considerable interest in the association of neurological disorders with coeliac disease (CD) (Morris et al., 1970). A high incidence of epilepsy among patients with coeliac disease (Laidlow et al., 1977; Chapman et al., 1978) and in patients with low folic acid levels has been found in a number of studies (Norris & Pratt, 1971; Dennis & Taylor, 1969; Reynolds, 1973; Grant et al., 1965). Moreover, anecdotal reports have described an association of CD with epilepsy and cerebral calcifications, mimicking those of the Sturge Weber syndrome (SWS) (Ciccarone et al., 1987; Sammaritano et al., 1988; Garwicz & Mortensson, 1976; Molteni et al., 1988; Della Cella et al., 1991).

We reported a severe type of progressive epilepsy in patients with bioccipital cortico-subcortical calcifications resembling those found in the SWS without a port-wine facial nevus (Gobbi et al., 1988), and reviewed similar anecdotal cases reported in the neurological literature. Unfortunately, no investigation for CD was ever attempted in these patients and no clear explanation of the consistency of 'atypical SWS' is currently available.

An unexpected series of cases of cerebral calcifications with epilepsy in which CD was casually observed (Molteni et al., 1988; Zaniboni et al., 1989; Ventura et al., 1991) and prompted the organization of an Italian Multicentric Study by neurologists and gastroenterologists to determine the association between CD and epilepsy (Italian Working Group, IWG).

The study aimed to evaluate the frequency of CD in patients with epilepsy and unexplained cerebral calcifications and to describe a large series of patients in order to report the clinical and laboratory findings of patients with coeliac disease, epilepsy and cerebral calcifications.

Materials and methods

Forty-three patients (15 males, 28 females) were identified by members of the IWG. Ages ranged from 4.6 to 30.7 years (mean 16.44, SD 6.61).

The patients were selected from two different series:

> *Series a:* 31 patients with epilepsy and cerebral calcifications of unexplained origin attending neurological departments.
>
> *Series b:* 12 patients with confirmed CD (according to the 1979 ESPGAN criteria) (McNeish et al., 1979) and epilepsy attending paediatric and gastroenterological departments. No patient with other known cause of cerebral calcifications was included (namely encephalitis, purulent meningitis, ossifying meningoencephalitis, leukaemia, chemotherapy, neonatal haemorrhage, congenital infections – TORCH group diseases – calcium and phosphorus metabolism disturbances). Tuberous sclerosis and SWS with port-wine facial nevus were also excluded, but three patients with complete SWS underwent intestinal biopsy as control cases.

The 31 patients from 'series a' underwent a full gastrointestinal evaluation to identify CD including a small intestinal biopsy. Nineteen had a xylose load test and 28 had antigluten antibody assessment. Serum folic acid was determined in 26 cases. HLA typing was available for 22 patients. Individuals with unequivocal flat mucosal biopsy were prescribed a gluten-free diet (GFD).

The 12 patients from 'series b' underwent neurological testing, including CT scan and electroencephalography. Written informed consent was obtained before the study from all patients or their parents.

Small bowel biopsy was performed with a Watson–Crosby capsule at the Treitz ligament. Morphological evaluation was scored according to Dunill & Whithead's criteria (1972). Crypts hyperplasia and unequivocal flat mucosa were accepted as markers of CD. Antigliadin IgG and IgA antibodies were assessed by an Elisa method with a commercial kit (Alfa-Gliatest, Eurospital Pharma). Cerebral CT scan was performed according to standard techniques: images were re-assessed by a Peer Review Committee of the Italian Working Group. EEG recordings agreed with the 10–20 International System. Psychosocial development was assessed by the Wechsler Scale for children or adults, or other methods (i.e. Brunet Lezine adapted for age test), as appropriate to the age of subject. Epilepsy was classified according to the 1981 and 1989 ILAE criteria. The SPSS-PC+ package was used for statistical analysis.

Results

Twenty-four out of 31 patients from 'series a' were identified as unequivocal CD cases, while five out of the 12 in 'series b' showed cerebral calcifications on the CT scan. Consequently, three groups of cases were identified:

Group 1 (29 cases): Coeliac disease, epilepsy and cerebral calcifications (CEC).

Group 2 (seven cases): Coeliac disease and epilepsy without cerebral calcifications.

Group 3 (seven cases): Epilepsy and cerebral calcifications without coeliac disease.

In the three complete SWS patients the intestinal biopsy showed a normal mucosa, and no gastrointestinal complaints were present. At present we will refer only to Group 1 (CEC). The CEC group comprised 29 cases (eight males and 21 females; F/M ratio: 2.62) with a mean age of 15.5 years (range 4.4–30; SD 6.2).

Cerebral calcifications

Impressive calcifications on CT scan were identified in all cases at a mean age of 12.9 years (range 4–20; SD 3.6). They were located in the parieto-occipital regions in 27 cases (23 bilateral, four extended to the frontal region). Two cases presented calcifications with different morphology and located in other regions, the first in the latero-sellar and the second at the lenticular nuclei level. Nevertheless the clinical characteristics of early onset epilepsy and severely impaired psychomotor development do not rule out another diagnosis. Fig. 1 illustrates the typical pattern of calcifications.

Coeliac disease

Mean age at diagnosis of coeliac disease was 14.8 years (range 4–32) in the 24 patients from 'series a' and 19.2 years in the five of 'series b' (range 8–28).

The distribution of weight and height centiles at diagnosis did not differ between the two series: 17 per cent were underweight and 27 per cent were short in stature.

All five cases from 'series b' showed significant gastroenterological symptoms at the time of biopsy (i.e. chronic diarrhoea, failure to thrive, abdominal distension and mild to severe anaemia). On the contrary, only two of 'series a' cases had mild recurrent diarrhoea at the time of biopsy. Nevertheless the great majority of this series recalled significant complaints in the early years of life. Nineteen reported recurrent diarrhoea in the first 3 years of life, 14 meteorism, seven anaemia and three recurrent aphthous stomatitis. In nine the diagnosis of coeliac disease had been clearly suggested in infancy, but the GFD was not started or was discontinued after a short period.

Antigluten IgA and IgG antibodies were above normal in 16 and 10 respectively out of 24 CEC tested cases. Xylose afterload was below normal range in 10 out 16 tested cases. Serum folate level was below normal in 17 out of 19 tested cases. Table 1 reports the HLA typing in 16 CEC cases and in seven Group 3 cases.

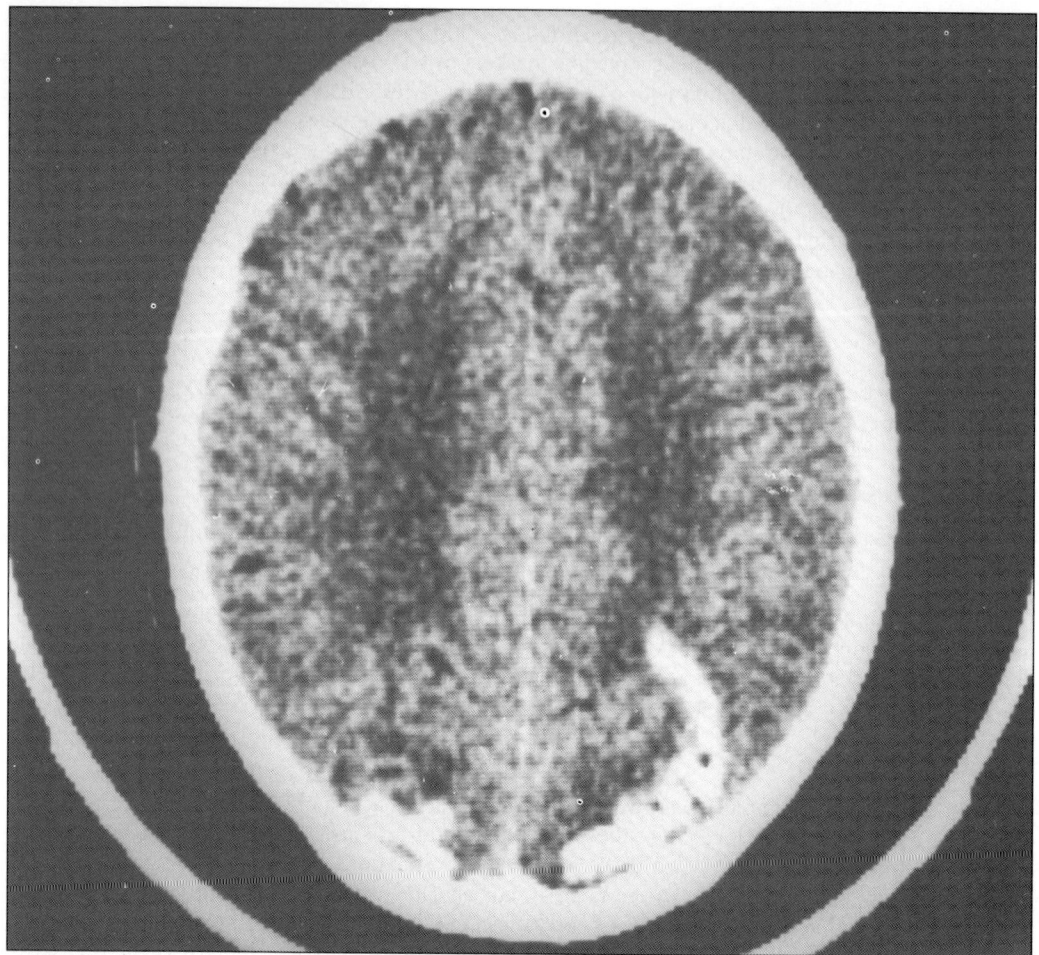

Fig. 1. Typical pattern of cerebral calcifications in CEC patients is characterized by impressive bilateral occipital cortical-subcortical calcifications.

Table 1. HLA antigens in CEC group and in Group 3

	Total cases	Evaluated cases	DR3	DR7	DQw2	DR5
Group 1 (CEC)	29	16	12	8	15	1
Group 3	7	6	3	2	4	1

Epilepsy

At present the clinical history of the epilepsy is available in 16 CEC cases.

The seizures started in childhood at a mean age of 6.25 years (range 2–14 years) and consisted of simple visual (six cases), complex visual (two cases), motor adversive with or without secondary generalization (eight cases), hemiclonic (three cases), oculoclonic (two cases), absences (three cases) and nocturnal generalized tonic–clonic (two cases). The seizure frequency ranged from one per year to more than one per day. At the onset of the epilepsy mental development was normal in all but two patients.

The interictal EEG records during wake showed normal background activity in all patients. The paroxysmal abnormalities comprised rhythmic high amplitude spike and wave discharges localized in both occipital regions or in one side of the occipital region and occurring only when the eyes were closed; independent multifocal discharges, generalized 2 to 4 Hz spike and slow wave complexes were also found.

After a mean follow-up of 14.5 years (range 2–29 years), three distinct features were identified in the evolution. The epilepsy was benign with disappearance of the seizures and normalization of the EEG in only two cases. The seizures persisted unchanged, without mental deterioration, despite antiepileptic therapy in six cases. In these patients the EEG abnormalities also remained unchanged. The evolution was severe with appearance of atypical absences, frequently with an atonic component, and tonic seizures during wake and sleep and with progressive mental impairment associated with a decline in school performance in the remaining patients. In these cases at the last control the EEGs showed a slowing of the background activity, while the occipital interictal discharges were more frequent and diffused anteriorly. The reactivity on eye opening persisted, although to a lesser degree. During non-REM sleep, fast polyspike bursts and rapid rhythm discharges, often diffuse but always with greater prominence in the posterior regions, were observed. These sleep EEG findings did not differ from those of the onset period in the same patients.

Discussion

The most significant result is the biopsy-proven coeliac disease in 24 out of 31 patients affected by epilepsy with posterior cerebral calcifications of unknown origin (77.4 per cent). Four of these 31 cases have already been discussed within the 'SW-like syndromes', without considering the gastrointestinal involvement (Del Giudice et al., 1984; Gobbi et al., 1988) and CD was found in one of them (Del Giudice et al., 1984). The frequency of CD in patients with cerebral calcifications and epilepsy was much higher than expected. As there is no reason for a higher frequency of CD in subjects with cerebral calcifications than in the normal population, it is no coincidence that 77.4 per cent of patients with epilepsy and cerebral calcifications had CD.

The second most important finding is that the diagnosis of CD was established only because of the association of epilepsy and posterior cerebral calcifications at an epoch of life when the typical signs of malabsorption had disappeared. In fact, CD may be asymptomatic in teenagers and young adults. Our series had a mean age at biopsy of 14.8 years and many of these cases could be labelled as asymptomatic coeliac disease. Nevertheless, most of these patients may well be missed coeliac diagnoses, since in their past personal histories significant gastrointestinal complaints (i.e. recurrent diarrhoea, anaemia) were reported. Moreover, in nine cases the diagnosis of coeliac disease had been suggested by the paediatricians during infancy, but the patients did not undergo intestinal biopsy and a definitive GFD.

In our series the epilepsy was severe. In fact, even though at onset the clinical and EEG findings suggested a diagnosis of benign occipital epilepsy (Gastaut, 1982) in all cases, the seizures were resistant to antiepileptic drugs in 14 out of 16 cases. In six patients the seizures persisted unchanged over the years and in eight the evolution was characterized by progressive severity. This severe prognosis of epilepsy with mental impairment in patients with serpiginous occipital calcifications has already been suggested by Gobbi et al. (1988) and recently confirmed by Giroud et al. (1990) in a review of 21 cases, albeit without mention of CD.

It is difficult to establish whether our CEC cases had Sturge Weber syndrome or not. The clinical course of the disease and epilepsy in our cases differed from those of SWS (Alexander, 1972).

None of our patients underwent cerebral biopsy, but the two literature cases with histological examination cannot solve this problem (Ito et al., 1990: Taly et al., 1987). Even though histological findings appear to be typical of the Sturge Weber syndrome in Case No. 3 of Ito *et al.*'s series, leptomeningeal angiomatosis was not observed in Taly *et al.*'s case, in accordance with a report by other authors (Giroud *et al.*, 1990).

We can speculate on whether or not posterior cerebral calcifications and epilepsy are the result of coeliac disease and, in particular, of a folate deficiency. Some cases have been reported in the literature in which posterior calcifications were detected in patients with a folic acid deficiency: in one case it was due to a congenital condition (De Marchi *et al.*, 1983), and in others to methotrexate therapy (Tosi *et al.*, 1983) or radiotherapy (Corazza *et al.*, 1985). The calcifications in our series could be related to chronic persistent folic acid deficiency due not only to unrecognized coeliac disease but also to the effect of antiepileptic drugs (Reynolds, 1973). Drug influence, however, seems less probable, since antiepileptic-induced folate deficiency is rare and in some of our cases therapy was started after discovery of the calcifications.

As CD may be associated with different autoimmune disorders and/or autoantibodies (Copper *et al.*, 1978; Burgin-Wolff *et al.*, 1991; Maki *et al.*, 1991), we cannot rule out that cerebral calcifications depend on autoimmune or immunocomplex-related endothelitis. In this case the particular cerebral location of the calcifications, which remains unexplained, could be related to a selective vulnerability of the occipital lobe (Hauser *et al.*, 1988). Finally, a genetically related disorder might be implicated.

An additional finding emerging from this study was the presence of some class II antigens (DQw2, DR3 and/or DR7) in all 16 CEC cases in which the HLA test was performed. As recently noted (De Marchi *et al.*, 1984; Tosi *et al.*, 1986; Zaniboni *et al.*, 1988), the presence of some class II HLA (DQw2, DR3 and/or DR7) allows the identification of the majority of patients with coeliac disease. In our study, the presence of class II antigens was found even in cases with posterior cerebral calcifications and epilepsy without CD (patients of Group 3). The presence of the same HLA in both groups, i.e. with and without coeliac disease, might imply that some Group 3 patients are affected by latent (or potential) coeliac disease with mucosal patchiness, as recently described by Maki *et al.* (1990).

In conclusion, our results suggest that the association of coeliac disease, posterior cerebral calcifications and epilepsy is not a mere coincidence. For this reason we believe that child neurologists should rule out CD in all cases of epilepsy and cerebral calcifications of unexplained origin, particularly when the epilepsy is characterized by occipital seizures and the calcifications are located in the posterior regions bilaterally. Because gastrointestinal signs are often missing, child neurologists might be the only ones to discover CD in these patients.

Even though the role of malabsorption in the pathogenesis of epilepsy and posterior cerebral calcifications has yet to be established, there is no doubt that a correct diet leads to overall physical improvement.

Acknowledgements

The authors wish to thank Mrs Serena Nannini for her kind cooperation. They are grateful to Mrs Anne Collins for revising the English text.

References

Alexander, G.L. (1972): Sturge–Weber syndrome. In: *Handbook of clinical neurology*, eds. P.J. Vinken & G.W. Bruyn, pp. 223–239. Amsterdam: Elsevier.

Burgin-Wolff, A., Gaze, H., Hadziselimovic, F. *et al.* (1991): Antigliadin and antiendomysium antibody determination for coeliac disease. *Arch. Dis. Child.* **66**, 941–947.

Chapman, R.G., Lailow, J.M., Colin Jones, D.G., Eade, O.E. & Smith, C.L. (1978): Increased prevalence of epilepsy in coeliac disease. *Br. Med. J.* **2**, 250–251.

Ciccarone, V., Rozzi, N., Balli, F. & Galli, V. (1987): Calcificazioni endocraniche simulanti la malattia di Sturge–Weber in una bambina con malattia celiaca. *Riv. Ital. Ped.* (I.J.P.) **13** (suppl. 1), 186.

Commission on Classification and Terminology of the International League Against Epilepsy (1981): Proposal for revised clinical and electroencephalographic classification of epileptic seizures. *Epilepsia* **22**, 489–501.

Commission on Classification and Terminology of the International League Against Epilepsy (1989): Proposal for revised classification of epilepsies and epileptic syndromes. *Epilepsia* **30**, 389–399.

Copper, B.T., Holmes, G.K.T. & Cooke, W.T. (1978): Coeliac disease and immunologic disorders. *Br. Med. J.* **1**, 537–542.

Corazza, G.R., Tabacchi, P., Frisoni, M., Prati, C. & Gasbarrini, G. (1985): DR and non-DR Ia allotypes are associated with susceptibility to coeliac disease. *Gut* **26**, 1210–1213.

Della Cella, G., Beluschi, C. & Cipollina, F. (1991): Intracranial calcifications – epilepsy – coeliac disease: description of a case. *Med. Surg. Ped.* **13**, 427–430.

Del Giudice, E., Pelosi, L., Romano, A., De Bellis, P., Licenziati, M.R., Pastore, I. & Andria, G. (1984): Unexplained bilateral occipital calcifications and reduced vision. *Neuropediatrics* **15**, 218–219.

De Marchi, M., Carbonara, A., Ansaldi, N., Santini, B., Barbera, C., Borelli, I., Rossino, P. & Rendine, S. (1983): HLA–DR3 and DR7 in coeliac disease: immunogenetic and clinical aspects. *Gut* **24**, 706–712.

De Marchi, M., Carbonara, A., Ansaldi, N., Hetzel, P.A.S., Koskimies, S., Werkasalo, M. & Woodrow, J.C. (1984): HLA–DR3 and DR7 – negative coeliac disease. In: *Histocompatibility testing*, ed. E.D. Albert, pp. 359–362. Berlin, Heidelberg: Springer-Verlag.

Dennis, J. & Taylor, D.C. (1969): Epilepsy and folate deficiency. *Br. Med. J.* **4**, 807–808.

Dunnill, M.S. & Whitehead, R. (1972): A method for the qualification of small intestinal biopsy specimen. *J. Clin. Pathol.* **25**, 243–245.

Garwicz, S. & Mortensson, W. (1976): Intracranial calcification mimicking the Sturge–Weber syndrome (a consequence of cerebral folic acid deficiency?). *Pediat. Radiol.* **5**, 5–9.

Gastaut, H. (1982): A new type of epilepsy: benign partial epilepsy of childhood with occipital spike-waves. *Clin. Electroencephalogr.* **13**, 13–22.

Giroud, M., Borsotti, J.P., Michiels, R., Tommasi, M. & Dumas, R. (1990): Epilepsie et calcifications occipitales bilatérales: 3 cas. *Rev. Neurol.* **4**, 288–292.

Gobbi, G., Sorrenti, G., Santucci, M., Giovanardi Rossi, P., Ambrosetto, P., Michelucci, R. & Tassinari, C.A. (1988): Epilepsy with bilateral occipital calcifications: a benign onset with progressive severity. *Neurology* **38**, 913–920.

Grant, H.C., Hoffbrand, A.V. & Wells, D.G. (1965): Folate deficiency and neurological disease. *Lancet* **ii**, 763–767.

Hauser, R.A., Lacey, M. & Knight, M.R. (1988): Hypertensive encephalopathy: magnetic resonance imaging demonstration of reversible cortical and white matter lesions. *Arch. Neurol.* **45**, 1078–1083.

Ito, M., Sato, K., Ohnuki, A. & Uto, A. (1990): Sturge-Weber disease: operative indications and surgical results. *Brain. Dev.* **12**, 473–477.

Laidlow, J.M., Chapman, R.G., Colin Jones, D.G., Eade, O. & Smith, C.L. (1977): Increased prevalence of epilepsy in coeliac disease. *Gut* **18**, A–943.

Maki, M., Holm, K., Kosmies, S., Hallstrom, O. & Visakorpi, J.K. (1990): Normal small bowel biopsy followed by coeliac disease. *Arch. Dis. Child.* **65**, 1137–1141.

Maki, M., Hallstrom, O. & Marttinen, A. (1991): Reaction of human non collagenous polypeptides with coeliac disease autoantibodies. *Lancet* **338**, 724–725.

McNeish, A.S., Harms, H.K., Rey, J., Shmerling, D.H., Visakorpi, J.K. & Walker Smith, J.A. (1979): The diagnosis of coeliac disease. *Arch. Dis. Child.* **54**, 783–786.

Molteni, N., Bardella, M.T., Baldassarri, A.R. & Bianchi, P.A. (1988): Coeliac disease associated with epilepsy and intracranial calcifications: report of two patients. *Am. J. Gastroent.* **83**, 992–994.

Morris, J.S., Ajdukiewicz, A.B. & Read, A.E. (1970): Neurological disorders and adult coeliac disease. *Gut* **11**, 549–554.

Norris, J.W. & Pratt, R.F. (1971): A controlled study of folic acid in epilepsy. *Neurology* **21**, 659–664.

Reynolds, E.H. (1973): Anticonvulsants, folic acid and epilepsy. *Lancet* **i**, 1376–1378.

Sammaritano, M., Andermann, F., Melanson, D., Guberman, A., Tinuper, P. & Gastaut, H. (1988): The syndrome of intractable epilepsy, bilateral occipital calcifications and folic acid deficiency. *Neurology* **38** (suppl. 1), 239.

Taly, A.B., Nagaraja, D., Das, S., Shankar, S.K. & Pratibha, N.G. (1987): Sturge–Weber–Dimitri disease without facial nevus. *Neurology* **37**, 1063–1064.

Tosi, R., Vismara, D., Tanigaki, N., Ferrara, G.B., Cicimarra, F., Buffolano, W., Follo, D. & Auricchio, S. (1983): Evidence that coeliac disease is primarily associated with DC locus allelic specificity. *Clin. Immunol. Immunopathol.* **28**, 395–404.

Tosi, R., Tanigaki, N., Polanco, I., De Marchi, M., Woodrow, J.C. & Hetzel, P.A.S. (1986): A radioimmunoassay typing study of non-DQw2 associated coeliac disease. *Clin. Immunol. Immunopathol.* **39**, 168–172.

Ventura, A., Bouquet, F., Sartorelli, C., Barbi, E., Torre, G. & Tommasini, G. (1991): Coeliac disease, folic acid deficiency and epilepsy with cerebral calcifications. *Acta Paediatr. Scand.* **80**, 559–562.

Zaniboni, M.G., Mantovani, V., Lambertini, A., Romeo, N., Finelli, F. & Valentini, S. (1988): Fenotipo HLA e malattia coeliaca: analisi di una casistica pediatrica. In: *Recenti progressi in gastroenterologia e nutrizione pediatrica*, ed. S. Guandalini, pp. 187–192, Roma: CIC Edizioni Internazionali.

Zaniboni, M.G., Lambertini, A., Gobbi, G., Romeo, R., Conti, G., Ambrosioni, G., Ambrosetto, P., Santucci, M., Michelucci, R. & Tassinari, C.A. (1989): Coeliac disease and epilepsy with occipital calcifications: an uncasual association. In: *Proceedings of the 1st British Italian paediatric gastroenterology meeting*, 22–23 September 1989, eds. G. Banchini, S. Guandalini, G.L. De Angelis & J.A. Walker-Smith, p. 54, Parma.

Chapter 23

Medical management of occipital epilepsies

Margherita Santucci, Giuseppe Gobbi*, Lorella Minotti[†], Emanuela Donati, Daniele Giovanni Poggioli, Elisabetta Tarsi and Paola Giovanardi Rossi

*Department of Child Neurology and Psychiatry, Neurological Institute, University of Bologna; *Service of Child Neurology and Psychiatry, USL 9, Reggio Emilia, Italy; †Chair of Clinical Neurophysiology, S.Paolo Hospital, University of Milano, Italy*

Summary

We assessed seizure evolution in relation to administered antiepileptic drugs in 29 children and adolescents with an electroclinical picture of partial occipital epilepsy. Following the Proposal for Classification of Epilepsies and Epileptic Syndromes, we divided the patients into two main groups: (1) idiopathic childhood epilepsy with occipital paroxysms: nine cases; (2) symptomatic occipital lobe epilepsy: 18 cases. Separately, we considered two patients with photosensitive occipital seizures. In the group of symptomatic patients we identified a subgroup of six cases showing a clinical and EEG evolution compatible with an epileptic encephalopathy and called 'occipital epileptic encephalopathy' in agreement with the literature.

Seizure evolution was good in all idiopathic cases irrespective of the drug administered: two cases with poor response to PB were controlled with CBZ. In the two boys with reflex photosensitive occipital fits, the visual seizures ceased on treatment with VPA in one case, CBZ and clobazam in the other. Prognosis was more severe in the symptomatic cases: only in five of the 18 cases was seizure control achieved with pharmacological treatment. In particular, the outcome was very severe in the six patients with occipital epileptic encephalopathy. In all cases the advanced stages of the disease were characterized by polymorphous and frequent seizures resistant to all antiepileptic drugs used in various associations. In four of these six patients a diagnosis of coeliac disease was made at 15 and 18 years of age: a gluten-free diet begun at this time has failed to improve clinical symptoms to date (follow-up on gluten-free diet: 1–2 years).

In 1982 Henry Gastaut identified a new epileptic syndrome termed 'benign partial epilepsy of childhood with occipital spike-waves' (Gastaut, 1982a, b). The author reported a good evolution, but not as good as for 'benign epilepsy of childhood with rolandic spikes'. Treatment suppressed seizures in 53 per cent of cases. Almost all antiepileptic drugs have been used with uniformly good results apart from clobazam which suppressed seizures and spike-waves after a few days in some patients.

The syndrome was finally recognized in the Proposal for Classification of Epilepsies and Epileptic Syndromes in 1985 and 1989 under the term of 'childhood epilepsy with occipital paroxysms' (CEOP) and included in the idiopathic localization related group of epilepsies.

Numerous studies on CEOP have been published since 1982 and the efficacy of different antiepileptic drugs has been confirmed by different authors (Giroud *et al.*, 1986; Kuzniecky & Rosenblatt,

1987; Niedermeyer et al., 1988; Nalin et al., 1989). However, other studies have described patients affected by an epilepsy with EEG features similar to CEOP (spike-wave complexes suppressed by eye-opening) with a poor response to antiepileptic treatment and persistent seizures (Newton & Aicardi, 1983; Aicardi & Newton, 1987; Cooper & Lee, 1991). The frequent finding of neurological, CT and/or MRI abnormalities, associated with unfavourable prognosis, suggests a symptomatic or cryptogenic focal epilepsy following the division of the Proposal for Classification of Epilepsies and Epileptic Syndromes (1989). The clinical and electroencephalographic features of symptomatic occipital lobe epilepsies have been the object of a study of 25 patients evaluated for resective epilepsy surgery (Williamson et al., 1992).

In 1988 some of us (Gobbi et al., 1988) described a severe form of partial epilepsy in patients with bilateral occipital calcifications, without any sign of phakomatosis. At the onset and early phase of the disease, the electroclinical picture and seizure control by antiepileptic drugs suggested a diagnosis of CEOP. In the advanced stages the disease evolved to a severe 'epileptic encephalopathy' characterized by numerous seizures of different types (absences, sometimes atonic, diurnal and nocturnal tonic seizures, partial seizures), progressive mental impairment, progressive slowing of the background EEG activity, with more frequent bioccipital interictal discharges extending to the anterior regions. Reactivity of the spike-wave discharges on eye opening persisted even when almost continuous and generalized. The seizures remained resistant to antiepileptic drugs despite the use of various combinations. A similar picture of 'occipital epileptic encephalopathy' has been recently described in cryptogenetic patients without bioccipital calcifications (Magaudda et al., 1990).

In a very recent study, Gobbi et al. (1992) reported the presence of coeliac disease in 60 per cent of patients with posterior cerebral calcifications and occipital epilepsy. Our report assesses seizure evolution in relation to antiepileptic drugs in young patients (children and adolescents) with idiopathic or symptomatic partial occipital epilepsy.

Methods and results

We selected children and adolescents attending the Department of Child Neurology and Psychiatry (University of Bologna Medical School) between 1985 and 1990 who showed an electroclinical picture compatible with partial occipital epilepsy.

Table 1. Partial occipital epilepsies: personal cases

Groups	No. of cases	Boys	Girls
Childhood epilepsy with occipital paroxysms	9	6	3
Partial occipital epilepsy with photosensitive occipital seizures	2	2	–
Symptomatic occipital lobe epilepsies	18	10	8
occipital epileptic encephalopathy	(6)	(4)	(2)
Total	29	18	11

The patients were divided into two main groups: Group 1: idiopathic childhood epilepsy with occipital paroxysms = nine cases. Group 2: symptomatic occipital lobe epilepsy = 18 cases. In this second group we distinguished a subgroup of six cases with 'occipital epileptic encephalopathy'.

In a separate group we considered two patients with an occipital epilepsy characterized by photosensitive occipital seizures which did not fall into one of the two previous groups. Table 1 summarizes our cohort.

Idiopathic childhood epilepsy with occipital paroxysms

The main features of the nine cases are listed in Table 2. At the last study (ages between 8 and 18 years, mean 14 years), seizures had been absent for over 2 years in all patients, and in six cases treatment had been suspended for at least 2 years. In three cases therapy was begun after the first seizure and in another four after the second, without recurrence of fits: three patients received phenobarbital (PB), three carbamazepine (CBZ), and one valproic acid (VPA). Two boys presented more seizures, seven and nine respectively over a period of 4 years: in both patients, the seizures ceased with CBZ, whereas they were not controlled by PB or phenytoin (PHT) (very low dosage).

Table 2. Idiopathic childhood epilepsy with occipital paroxysms (nine cases)

Patient no.	Age(yr)/Sex	Age of first seizure (yr)	Age of last seizure (yr)	Active period (yr)	No. of seizures	Effective therapy	Follow-up (yr) from onset/without therapy
1	8½/M	4½	4½	–	1	CBZ	4/2
2	18½/M	14½	14½	–	2	CBZ	4/0
3	17/M	7	11	4	7	CBZ	10/3
4	17/F	9	9½	< ½	2	CBZ	8/2
5	13/M	3½	3½	–	2	PB	10/7
6	8/F	4	4	–	1	PB	4/2
7	12½/M	9½	9½	< ½	2	VPA	2/0
8	15/F	6	6	–	1	PB	9/7
9	15½/M	9½	13½	4	9	CBZ	6/0

Occipital epilepsy with photosensitive occipital seizures

Two boys presented occipital seizures on watching television or induced by intermittent light stimulation (ILS) during EEG recordings: the photosensitive seizures were elementary visual (phosphenes). One patient also presented a seizure with deviation of the eyes followed by vomiting, loss of consciousness and falling on watching TV, the other suffered rare generalized convulsions during sleep.

The photosensitive seizures ceased in one case after a few months on VPA treatment at the age of 15 years; in the second boy the visual seizures persisted for 6 years despite PB therapy and were controlled at 14 years by CBZ combined with clobazam. Both patients, aged 21 and 16 years respectively, still take therapy, the older one for recurrence of nocturnal convulsions on withdrawal of VPA.

Symptomatic occipital lobe epilepsies

For evolution assessment in relation to therapy, this group (18 cases) was divided into two subgroups: the first comprised 12 subjects affected by a typical focal occipital epilepsy with the main features outlined by the Proposal for Classification of Epilepsies and Epileptic Syndromes of 1989. The second subgroup comprised six patients presenting the electroclinical features of the 'occipital epileptic encephalopathy' described in the Introduction.

First subgroup. The clinical findings of the 12 cases are summarized in Table 3. The mean age of epilepsy onset was 8 years (range 1–16 years), and the mean follow-up from onset 8 years. At the last study (ages between 9½ and 26 years, mean 16 years), the seizures were controlled by antiepileptic drugs in only five patients. Three cases were on monotherapy of PHT, CBZ or VPA respectively; two patients were taking three drugs: PB, VPA and CBZ.

The clinical and laboratory variables considered to establish any significant differences between controlled and non-controlled patients are listed in Table 4. Statistical analysis was not performed owing to the small number of patients. An abnormal CT and/or MRI was noted in most patients (all the controlled, and six of seven non-controlled subjects) and polymorphous seizures were present in six of seven non-controlled patients but also in three of five controlled cases. The EEG features differed in the two groups: the non-controlled patients presented more frequent bilateral occipital paroxysms (indeed unilateral), hemispheric diffusion and independent focal abnormalities.

Table 3. Symptomatic occipital lobe epilepsy (12 cases)

Patient no.	Age (yr)/Sex	Age of first seizure (yr)	Follow-up from onset	Seizure control/ free period (yr)	Effective therapy
1	15/M	1	14	No	
2	14½/M	7	7½	Yes/< 1	VPA-PB-CBZ
3	13½/F	10	3½	No	
4	22/F	11	11	No	
5	14/F	6	8	Yes/2	PHT
6	10½/M	1	9½	No	
7	17/M	12	5	Yes/2	CBZ
8	9½/F	3	6½	Yes/1	PB
9	21/F	16	5	No	
10	26/M	13	13	No	
11	18/F	10	8	Yes/< 1	CBZ-PB-VPA
12	15½/M	11	4½	No	

Table 4. Clinical and laboratory variables in controlled and non-controlled patients with symptomatic occipital lobe epilepsy

Variable		Not controlled PTS $n = 7$	Controlled PTS $n = 5$
Age at first seizure/mean (yr)		1–16/9	3–12/7.6
Relevant past medical history		5	2
Mental retardation		1	4
Abnormal CT/MRI		6	5
Polymorphous seizures		6	3
Active period/mean (yr)		3–13/6.5	3–8/7
EEG	bil. occip. parox.	4	1
	hemisph. diff.	3	0
	indep. focal abnormalities	3	1

Second subgroup. Six subjects with symptomatic occipital epilepsy presented the clinical picture of 'occipital epileptic encephalopathy'. These patients have already been reported in previous publications (Gobbi *et al.*, 1988; Ambrosetto *et al.*, 1991; Gobbi *et al.*, 1992a; Ambrosetto *et al.*, 1992). The clinical findings are shown in Table 5. The mean age of epilepsy onset was 7 years, and the mean follow-up from onset 12.7 years.

At the last study at ages between 16 and 22 years (mean 19.7 years) all patients presented frequent polymorphous seizures (often several times a day) with partial and apparently generalized semiology (absences, tonic or atonic seizures).

Five patients had a seizure-free interval lasting 13–60 months in the early phase of the disease, on treatment with different drugs (CBZ, PB, PHT, clonazepam, primidone (PRI) alone or in association); one patient had a significant reduction of seizures treated with PB, ethosuximide (ETS), clonazepam.

In all cases the seizures subsequently recurred very frequently, despite administration of antiepileptic drugs at high doses and in different associations. Hormonal therapy (with adrenocorticotropic hormone or corticosteroids) was given in all cases without significant or prolonged benefit.

In four of six patients coeliac disease was diagnosed at 15 and 18 years in one and three cases respectively. A gluten-free diet begun at that time has failed to improve seizure frequency to date (follow-up after gluten-free diet beginning at 1 year in two cases, 2 years in the other two).

Table 5. Occipital epileptic encephalopathy (six cases)

Patient no.	Age (yr)/sex	Age first seizure (yr)	Coeliac disease	Post. cer. calcif.	Siezure control	Seizure-free interval	Length (mth)	Treatment
1*	20/F	12½	+	−	No	Yes	24	CBZ
2†	19/M	9	+	+	No	No	−	−
3‡	21/M	8½	−	+	No	Yes	26	PB + DPH
4‡	22/M	8	−	+	No	Yes	13	Clonazepam
5†	20/M	2	+	+	No	Yes	48	PB
6†	16/F	2	+	+	No	Yes	60	CBZ + PRI

*Already reported case (Ambrosetto et al., 1991, 1992); †Already reported cases (Gobbi et al., 1992a);
‡Already reported cases (Gobbi et al., 1988, 1992a).

Discussion

Our findings confirm the efficacy of different antiepileptic drugs in childhood epilepsy with occipital paroxysms. In the two boys who presented a longer active epilepsy period, seizures were not controlled by PB but ceased with CBZ. In three cases a pharmacological treatment was begun after the first fit: the seizures never reappeared, but some doubts remain that the therapy was essential.

The patients with symptomatic occipital lobe epilepsies have a much more severe prognosis. In the subgroup of 12 cases that we define as typical focal occipital epilepsy, seizure control was achieved in only five cases after many years. Moreover, two of these five patients were on polytherapy with three antiepileptic drugs.

Owing to the small number of patients, statistical analysis of clinical and laboratory variables between the controlled and non-controlled cases was not performed. Nevertheless, a relevant past medical history and polymorphous seizures were more frequent in the non-controlled group; the contrary was true for mental retardation. Lesions showing on CT and/or MRI were present in almost all patients, whereas the most relevant EEG abnormalities (bilateral occipital paroxysms, hemispheric diffusion, independent focal abnormalities) were usually found in the non-controlled patients.

We confirm a very poor prognosis in the patients with occipital epileptic encephalopathy. In this group, five of six subjects presented posterior cerebral calcifications like the original cases described by Gobbi et al. (1988). Three of these five patients with calcifications on the CT had coeliac disease, while in two patients this disease was excluded by a series of tests including an intestinal biopsy. These results are in line with the very recent data published by Gobbi et al. (1992a). The sixth case was a girl with coeliac disease, but without cerebral calcifications (CT and MRI negative). Unlike the data reported by Magaudda et al. (1990) we had no cryptogenic cases.

In these patients the seizures were controlled by antiepileptic drugs only at the onset and early phase of the epilepsy. In the advanced stage, the polymorphous and frequent seizures became resistant to all antiepileptic drugs used in various combinations and also to hormonal therapy. This course confirms literature data (Gobbi et al., 1988; Magaudda et al., 1990).

None of the four patients with coeliac disease benefited from a gluten-free diet (follow-up on diet: 1–2 years), but diagnosis of coeliac disease was late in all cases (15–18 years of age). Consequently, the gluten-free diet was begun only in late adolescence.

The data recently published by Gobbi et al. (1992b) show that in patients affected by coeliac disease and epilepsy the shorter the duration of epilepsy before the gluten-free diet and the younger the subjects at the beginning of the diet the better the chance of seizures stopping.

In agreement with these authors and with Ambrosetto et al. (1992) we believe that epileptic patients affected by occipital lobe epilepsy of unknown aetiology (especially if there is a history of malabsorption) or associated with cerebral calcifications must be carefully investigated for coeliac disease. Early gluten-free diet might affect the epilepsy whereas it seems to have no effect on seizures in patients with a late diagnosis.

Acknowledgements

The authors are grateful to Miss Silvia Muzzi and Mrs Manuela Zuffi for expert secretarial assistance.

References

Aicardi, J. & Newton, R. (1987): Clinical findings in children with occipital spike-wave complexes suppressed by eye opening. In: *Migraine and epilepsy*, eds. F. Andermann & E. Lugaresi, pp. 111-124. London, Boston: Butterworths.

Ambrosetto, G., De Maria, G. & Antonini, L. (1991): Occipital lobe seizures and coeliac disease without cortico-subcortical calcifications. *Boll. Lega. It. Epil.* **74**, 135-137.

Ambrosetto, G., Antonini, L. & Tassinari, C.A. (1992): Occipital lobes seizures related to clinically asymptomatic celiac disease in adulthood. *Epilepsia* (in press).

Commission on Classification and Terminology of the International League Against Epilepsy (1985): Proposal for classification of epilepsies and epileptic syndromes. *Epilepsia* **26**, 268-278.

Commission on Classification and Terminology of the International League Against Epilepsy (1989): Proposal for revised classification of epilepsies and epileptic syndromes. *Epilepsia* **30**, 389-399.

Cooper, G.W. & Lee, S.I. (1991): Reactive occipital epileptiform activity: is it benign?. *Epilepsia* **32**, 63-68.

Gastaut, H. (1982a): A new type of epilepsy: benign partial epilepsy of childhood with occipital spike-waves. In: *Advances in epileptology*: The XIIIth epilepsy international symposium, eds. H. Akimoto, H. Kazamatsuri & M. Seino, pp. 19-24. New York: Raven Press.

Gastaut, H. (1982b): L'épilepsie bénigne de l'enfant à pointe-ondes occipitales. *Rév. E.E.G. Neurophysiol.* **12**, 179-201.

Giroud, M., Soichot, P., Weyl, M., Dauvergue, M., Alison, M. & Dumas, R. (1986): L'épilepsie à pointes-ondes occipitales. Sa place parmi les épilepsies bénignes. *Ann. Pédiatr. (Paris)* **33**, 131-135.

Gobbi, G., Sorrenti, G., Santucci, M., Giovanardi Rossi, P., Ambrosetto, P., Michelucci, R. & Tassinari, C.A. (1988): Epilepsy with bilateral occipital calcifications: a benign onset with progressive severity. *Neurology* **38**, 913-920.

Gobbi, G., Ambrosetto, P., Zaniboni, M.G., Lambertini, A., Ambrosioni, G. & Tassinari, C.A. (1992a): Coeliac disease, posterior cerebral calcifications and epilepsy. *Brain Dev.* **14**, 23-29.

Gobbi, G., Bouquet, F., Greco, L., Lambertini, A., Tassinari, C.A., Ventura, A. & Zaniboni, M.G. (1992b): Coeliac disease, epilepsy and cerebral calcifications. *Lancet* **340**, 439-443.

Kuzniecky, R. & Rosenblatt, B. (1987): Benign occipital epilepsy: a family study. *Epilepsia* **28**, 346-350.

Magaudda, A., Colamaria, V., Fontana, E., Capizzi, G., Sgrò, G., Caraballo, R., Candela, L. & Dalla Bernardina, B. (1990): Encefalopatia epilettica in epilessia parziale occipitale: studio di 10 casi. *Boll. Lega. It. Epil.* **70/71**, 85-87.

Nalin, A., Ruggerini, C., Ferrari, E., Galli, V., Ferrari, P. & Finelli, T. (1989): Clinique, diagnostic différentiel et évolution des crises épileptiques visuelles de l'enfant. *Neurophysiol. Clin.* **19**, 25-36.

Newton, R. & Aicardi, J. (1983): Clinical findings in children with occipital spike-wave complexes suppressed by eye-opening. *Neurology* **33**, 1526-1529.

Niedermeyer, E., Riggio, S. & Santiago, M. (1988): Benign occipital lobe epilepsy. *J. Epilepsy* **1**, 3-11.

Williamson, P.D., Thadani, V.M., Darcey, T.M., Spencer, D.D., Spencer, S.S. & Mattson, R.H. (1992): Occipital lobe epilepsy: clinical characteristics, seizure spread patterns, and results of surgery. *Ann. Neurol.* **31**, 3-13.

Chapter 24

Occipital seizures with childhood onset in severe partial epilepsy: a surgical perspective

Claudio Munari, Laura Tassi, Stefano Francione, Philippe Kahane, Chariklia Malapani*, Giorgio Lo Russo and Dominique Hoffmann

Neurosciences Department, INSERM U 318, CHRU Grenoble, France;
*Neurology & Neuropsychology Service, INSERM U 294, Pitié-Salpétrière Hospital, Paris, France

Summary

Occipital epilepsies are relatively uncommon, especially in surgical reports (1 to 2 per cent). This paper concerns 16 patients with seizure onset before the age of 16, all suffering from severe drug-resistant partial epilepsy of supposed occipital origin. Five had a visual field deficit. At the admission, initial clinical symptoms were visual in 14 cases, well-lateralized in five, and associated with an early oculocephalic deviation in four. Sensory-motor manifestations (five cases) and auditory hallucinations (three cases) were the most frequently associated symptoms. Late loss of contact (six cases) and secondary generalization (six cases) were also frequently reported. Scalp EEG showed occipital slow waves in all the patients, but only two had well-localized occipital spikes. A unilateral ictal occipital onset was identified in seven patients. Out of the 16 patients studied, 13 underwent stereo-EEG investigation, which demonstrated a clear well-localized initial ictal occipital discharge in eight. In the other three in whom seizures had been recorded, ictal discharge originated in different posterior cortical areas.

On the basis of this limited experience, we want to point out that somatomotor manifestations and consciousness impairment have never been described as initial symptoms. Even in children, visual signs have the most important localizing value mainly when they are well-lateralized. Scalp EEG can be really useful only if ictal recordings are available, but stereo-EEG seems to be necessary to confirm a pure ictal occipital involvement. Since year after year ictal symptomatology becomes more and more 'complex', presurgical evaluation of drug-resistant occipital epilepsies in children seems reasonable, as well as for the other types of epilepsies.

Introduction

Electroclinical studies of occipital seizures are relatively rare, probably because 'seizures originating in the occipital lobe are relatively uncommon' (Williamson *et. al.*, 1992). Until 1988 at Sainte Anne Hospital (Paris), 145/850 investigated patients (17 per cent) presented with extra-frontal and extra-temporal seizures: in 15 of them (less than 2 per cent), we were able to record partial seizures of 'pure' occipital origin (Bancaud *et al.*, 1991). Similarly, the Montreal Neurological Institute experience showed that, in 'non-tumoral' partial epilepsies, occipital epilepsies represented 1.4 per cent of studied patients (Rasmussen, 1975).

Occipital seizures recorded in children are obviously very rare. Moreover, the interpretation of clinical patterns corresponding to discharges of occipital origin is relatively difficult (Ajmone-Marsan & Ralston, 1957). Such difficulties are probably linked to the different possible spread patterns of the initially occipital discharges.

The aim of this short paper is to discuss the electro-clinical symptomatology of occipital seizures with 'childhood onset'.

Patients and methods

All 16 patients (nine male, seven female) included in this study were candidates for surgical treatment of their severe, drug-resistant, partial epilepsy; 13 of them underwent a stereo-EEG investigation (seven to 11 multilead intracerebral electrodes) during presurgical evaluation. A stereotactic and stereoscopic neuroradiological study was performed previously.

Mean age at this time was 19 years (9–37 years). Seizure onset varied between 2 days and 14 years (mean: 6.4 years). The first admission for surgical therapy occured 4 to 37 years after the first seizure, and mean duration of the epilepsy was 12.4 years. Seizure frequency was daily in 13 patients and monthly in 3. Neurological examination showed a visual field deficit in five, associated with a motor deficit in two. Four other patients presented with only a sensory-motor deficit.

Presurgical investigations were performed according to the original methodology of the Sainte Anne school, partially modified at the Neurosciences Department and the INSERM Unit 318 of the Centre Hospitalier Régional et Universitaire of Grenoble (Table 1).

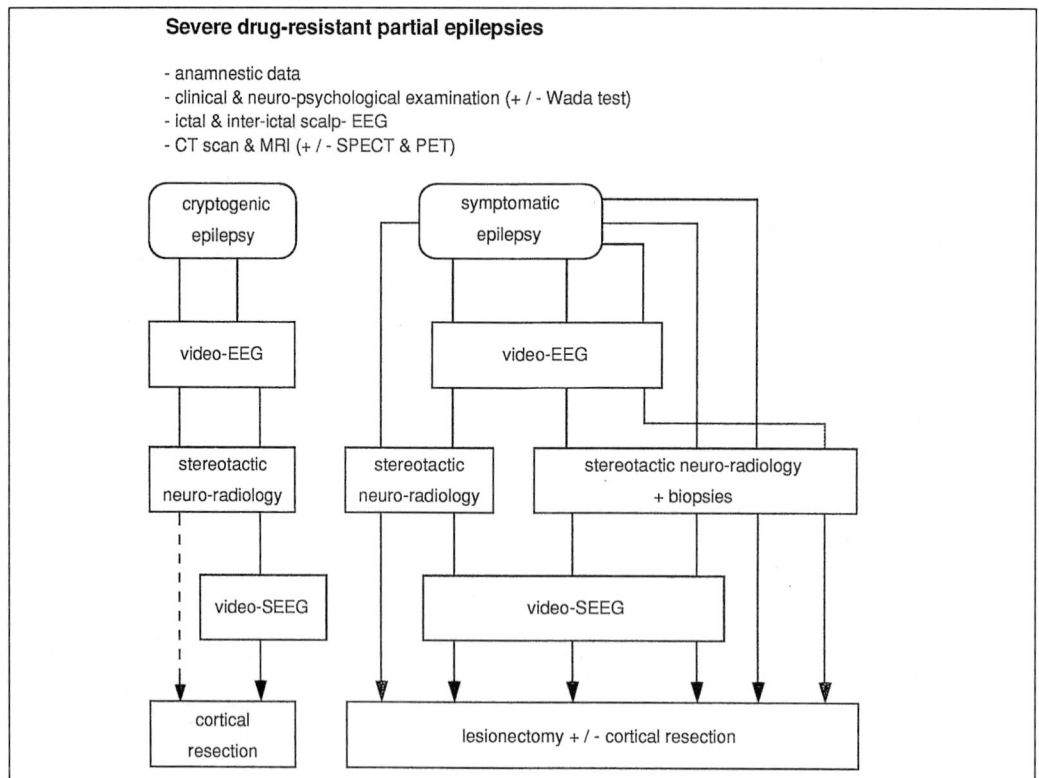

Table 1. Methodology of presurgical evaluation

Three patients did not undergo stereo-EEG investigations:
- A 31-year-old patient refused to take the risk of a postoperative, non pre-existing, hemianopia, in spite of the duration of the epilepsy (onset: 8 years). She had a slow growing glioma, confirmed by serial stereotactic biopsies (Munari & Betti, 1989; Lo Russo et al., 1992). Because the anatomical lesion was not located in the calcarinian cortex (Fig. 1a, b), a simple lesionectomy was performed ;
- In one patient, an occipital progressively expanding cystic lesion was treated by stereotactic endocavitary β-emitter irradiation (Munari et al., 1988a b; Musolino et al., 1989) without any other procedure and the cyst completely disappeared (Fig. 2a, b, c);
- The last patient died, probably during a nocturnal secondarily generalized seizure.

Results

Initial ictal clinical symptomatology (Table 2)

Visual hallucinations were clearly described by six patients, in spite of their sometimes very young age. Such hallucinations could be very simple (white or coloured lights, flashing circles, etc.), or very elaborated (terrifying people, ants, musical instruments, parents' silhouettes, flowers, etc.). A 'black out' was clearly described by one patient.

Table 2. Initial clinical ictal symptoms

	No. of patients
Lateralized visual simple hallucinations	4
Complex visual hallucinations	2
Black out	1
Lateral tonic (clonic) eye deviation	1
Loss of contact	2
Apparently generalized tonic-clonic seizures	6

An initial lateralized eye deviation was clearly described by the parents in one case; they believed that their 9-year-old child had suddenly presented a strabismus. A loss of contact, apparently without any other associated symptoms, was described in two patients.

Clinical evolution

Initial clinical symptomatology was stable for 6 years in one patient. The seizure frequency and severity improved in another one. One patient died (see above). In the remaining 13 patients, ictal symptomatology became more and more 'complex' during the evolution.

Ictal clinical symptoms at admission

Fourteen patients clearly described initial visual manifestations, well lateralized in five, non lateralized in six. An associated early oculocephalic deviation was clearly evident in four. Five patients, whose early clinical symptoms were not described at the fit onset, were later able to describe visual, sometimes inconstant, illusions and/or hallucinations. The boy presenting a 'black out' at the onset of his epilepsy retained this symptom throughout the evolution (7 years). Three patients had initial metamorphopsia.

Lateralized paraesthesia occurred in two patients, associated with auditory hallucinations in one. Auditory hallucinations were also frequently reported by two other patients. Three other patients could have had late somatomotor lateralized manifestations. None of the patients had impairment or loss of contact at the onset of most seizures. A late loss of contact could occur in six. Six others might have had secondarily generalized seizures.

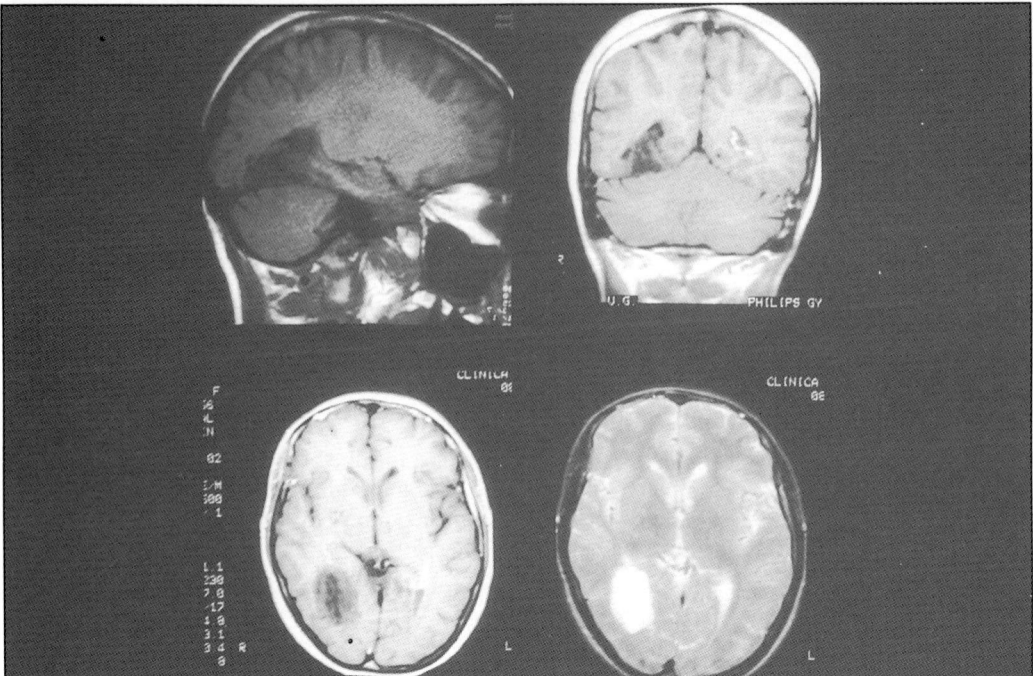

Fig. 1(a). Right occipital astrocytoma in a 31-year-old patient whose seizures began at the age of 8, and were characterized by right complex visual hallucinations. Preoperative MRI.

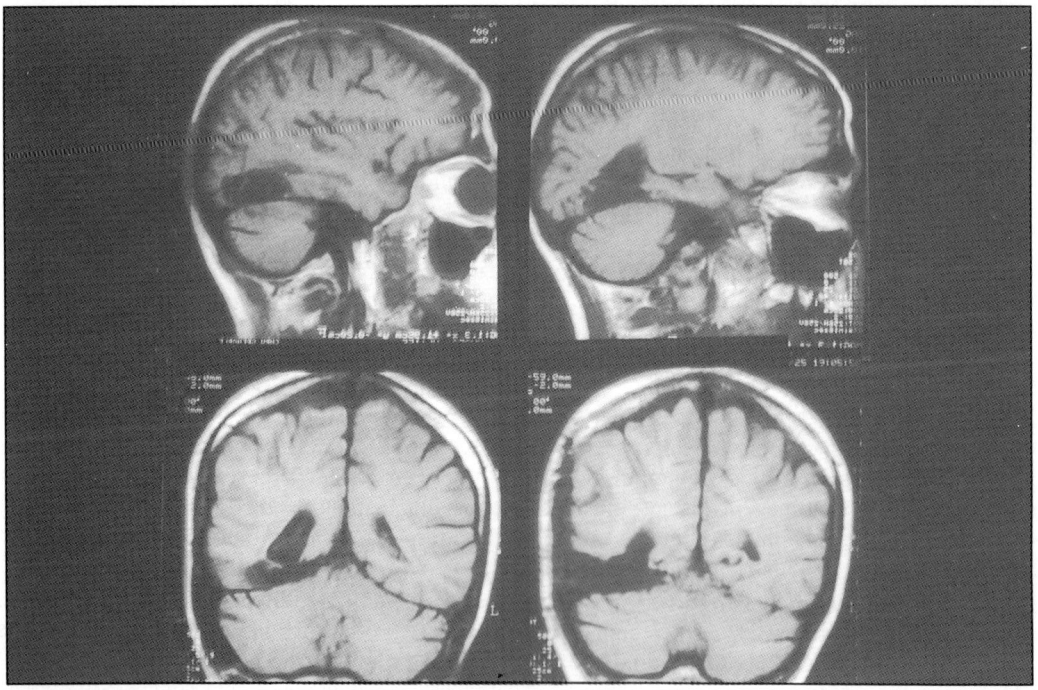

Fig. 1(b). Postoperative MRI: a simple lesionectomy was performed.

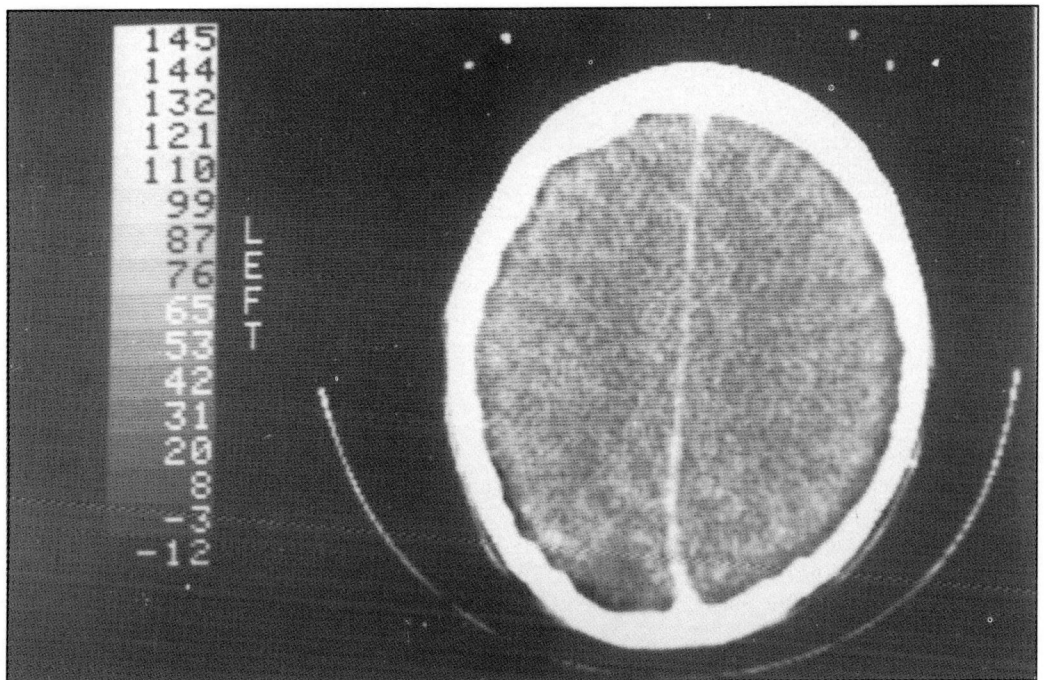

Fig. 2(a). This 18-year-old patient experienced her first seizure (right simple visual hallucinations) at the age of 15. Initial CT-scan showed a small hypodensity on the left occipital region.

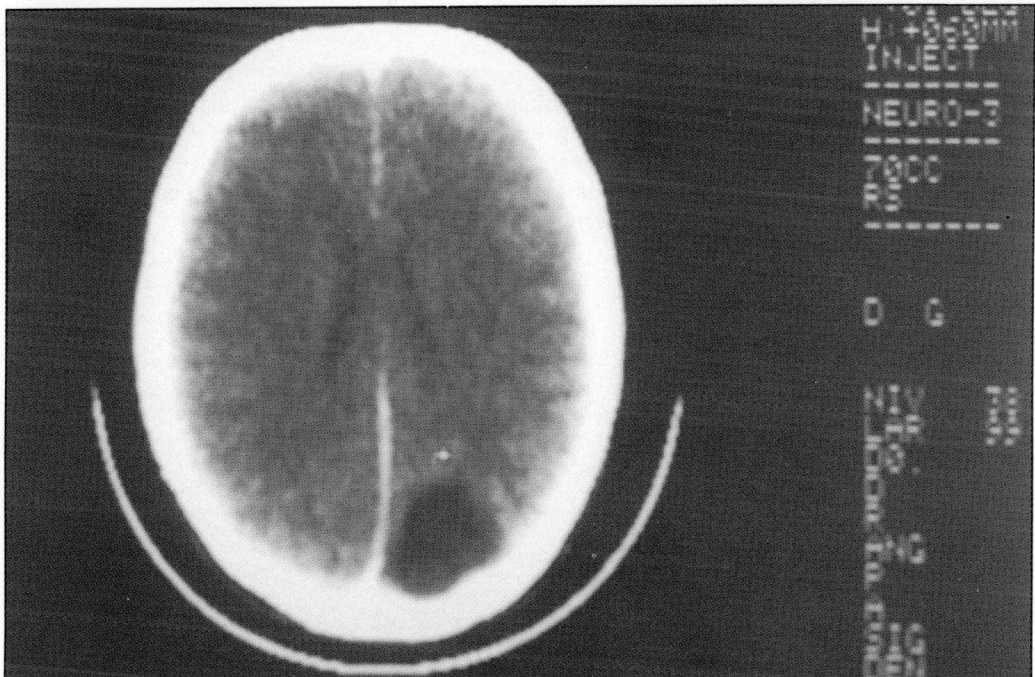

Fig. 2(b). Three years later there was a major increase of the cystic lesion, while the patient presented a right inferior quadrantanopia. A stereotactic endocavitary beta-emitter irradiation treatment was performed.

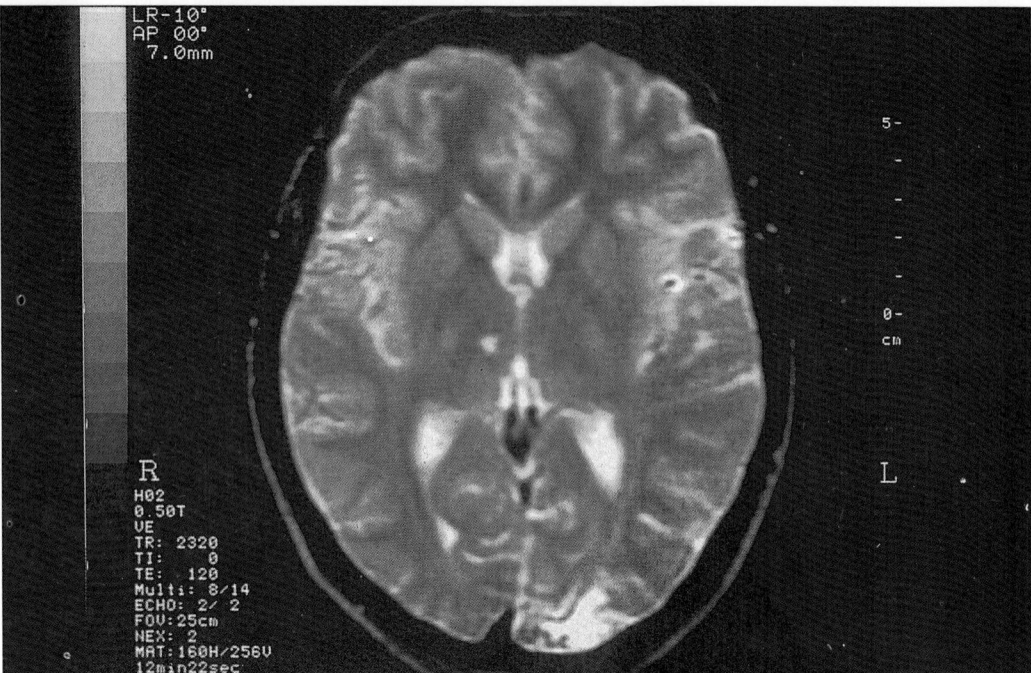

Fig. 2(c). MRI showed a virtual disappearance of the cystic lesion, while the patient became seizure free, but the field deficit remained the same.

Neurophysiological findings

Interictal scalp EEG (Table 3)

All patients had subcontinuous, often high voltage, theta delta activity on the occipital regions, bilateral and asynchronous in two. Such slow abnormalities also involved several extra-occipital regions in 12. Well-localized occipital spikes and/or spike and waves were recorded in two. In eight, spikes were multilobar but unilateral and in two, hemispheric. In two patients (one of those with bilateral slow waves), spikes and waves were bilateral.

Table 3. Interictal scalp EEG

		No. of patients
Theta-delta:		
	Occipital	16
	Occipito-temporal	6
	Occipito-parietal	2
	Occipito-temporo-parietal	4
	Bioccipital	2
Spikes and/or spikes and waves:		14
	Occipital	2
	Occipito-temporal	4
	Occipito-parietal	2
	Occipito-temporo-parietal	2
	Hemispheric	2
	Bilateral	2

Ictal scalp EEG

In the 13 patients later investigated by stereo-EEG, a clearly occipital, well-lateralized onset of the discharges was evident in three patients: in these cases, a low voltage fast activity was identified. A similar low voltage fast activity started in the occipito-temporal regions in three, and in occipito-parietal areas in one. A 'vague posterior onset' was the only possible statement in one patient. In two, ictal discharge was apparently straight off bilateral. In the last patient, we considered that the recorded ictal discharges could originate in different brain regions.

Strategy of stereo-EEG investigations

In all these patients, an occipital onset of the ictal discharges was strongly suspected on the basis of the preliminary clinical, electrical and anatomical investigations. According to this hypothesis, the pericalcarinian cortex was investigated in all patients, by at least two multi-lead electrodes: one above, and one below the calcarine fissure, spatially located by stereoscopic angiography. According to electroclinical characteristics of each individual patient, other cortical areas were also investigated, mostly temporal, or parietal, or both (Fig. 3). In one patient, the occipital, parietal and frontal lobes were explored.

The main aim of stereo-EEG recordings was to try to correlate the chronological sequence of clinical symptoms with the spatial and temporal trajectory of the intracerebral discharges.

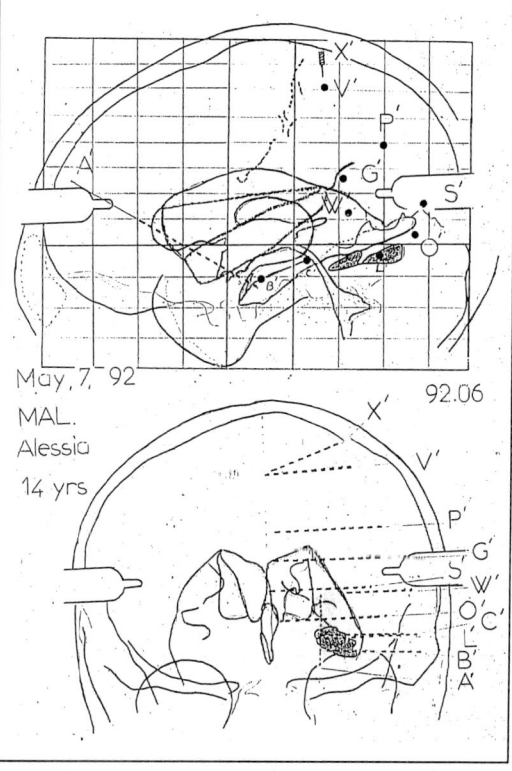

Fig. 3. Stereotactic scheme of a 13-year-old patient suffering from seizures since the age of 2 months. Despite a well-delimited left internal temporo-occipital lesion, ictal electroclinical symptomatology suggested a temporo-parieto-occipital origin of ictal discharges. Thus 11 electrodes have been implanted to explore both the lesion (electrode L'), the temporal (electrodes A', B', C', W'), occipital (S', O') and parietal (P', V', X', G') regions.

Ictal stereo-EEG

Among the 13 patients who underwent stereo-EEG, six were investigated before the age of 16, and spontaneous seizures were recorded in 11.

An initial ictal occipital involvement was clearly demonstrated in eight. A low voltage fast activity was well localized in the mesial, pericalcarinian, occipital cortex in two. In four, the discharges immediately involved the mesial temporal structures. In the other two, the occipital (mesial and lateral) and parietal cortex (mesial and lateral) were simultaneously affected.

In two patients, seizures originated in either occipital or in extra-occipital (parietocentral, temporal) cortical areas.

In one patient, seizure onset was proved to be temporal, even if discharges rapidly spread from the posterior hippocampus and parahippocampal gyrus to the mesial subcalcarinian occipital cortex.

Discussion

Severe, drug-resistant, occipital epilepsies in children seem to be at least as rare as in adults, but their clinical evolution, in our relatively limited experience, seems to indicate that the electro-clinical symptomatology may progressively worsen, as partial epilepsies frequently do (Lindsay et al., 1984).

Concerning clinical symptomatology, Williamson and co-workers (1992) recently described 'two basic types' of seizures in patients with seizures of occipital origin: (a) complex partial with automatisms (temporal lobe type); (b) asymmetrical tonic or clonic motor (frontal lobe type). These clinical observations are completely in contrast with those of our patients: only three of our investigated patients presented late, somatomotor lateralized manifestations. Several reasons can explain such a discrepancy. The first one is that in our preliminary selection of patients, those presenting with early somatomotor symptoms are generally excluded, excepting some particular cases (Bossi et al., 1984). Another possibility is that Williamson's cases have seizures characterized by a very frequent and/or rapid spread of the discharges from the occipital areas to the motor cortex. The same kinds of difference are found concerning the so-called 'complex partial seizures' of temporal type (and of occipital origin): our patients had never presented an initial loss of contact, and less than one half of them had a late impairment of consciousness. Discussions of temporal lobe origin, or responsibility, concerning contact impairment do not find a place here, but we must recall that there is evidence that this loss of contact is not due to the involvement of temporal lobe structures, but is linked to both duration and extension of discharges (Munari et al., 1980).

Clinical patterns of seizures proved to be of occipital origin can vary as a function of the different modes of spreading of the discharges (Bancaud, 1969; Takeda et al., 1970).

There is general agreement concerning the high occipital localizing value of early visual lateralized simple hallucinations. Children are perfectly able to describe this kind of subjective manifestation, mainly if they are questioned during the seizures. Some children clearly describe lateralized visual hallucinations only when the discharges are relatively short and well localized in the pericalcarinian areas. They can also remember and describe such visual phenomena when the initially occipital localized discharge spreads later to other extra-occipital areas. These same children do not describe any visual phenomena when the discharge is occipito-temporal at the onset. Better than concluding that these children can or cannot have visual hallucinations, one can hypothesize that visual manifestations cannot be recalled because of the initial extension of ictal discharges.

The localizing value of an early eye deviation (Gastaut, 1960) has been discussed in opposite ways (Ochs et al., 1984; Robillard et al., 1983). Our data suggest that, in children as in adults, a documented 'tonic' (low voltage fast activity) occipital discharge is often associated with a 'tonic' contralateral eye deviation; according to Williamson et al. 1987). Eye deviation becomes clonic when the occipital discharge becomes clonic too (Munari et al., 1984).

The diagnostic help allowed by scalp EEG recordings is also largely discussed (Williamson et al., 1992). This is probably due to the large utilization of interictal EEG and to the poor number of recorded seizures. We have had the opportunity to record seizures, clearly showing an early involvement of an occipital lobe (alone or in association with other lobes), in one half of the cases.

Ictal intracerebral recordings (stereo-EEG) may be very useful in proving the occipital origin (8/11 cases in this series). But this is true only if the strategy of implantation of the electrodes is correctly adapted to the individual characteristics of each patient, thus avoiding misleading 'falsely proved' locations.

The differential diagnosis between severe, drug-resistant, occipital epilepsies and benign occipital epilepsies in children was not the aim of this study. Considering only severe epilepsies, we could probably state that there are not very important clinical differences between occipital seizures in adults and in children older than 3–4 years. Since a progressive increase of 'complexity' of electroclinical symptoms probably will appear (with all the associated inconvenience), it seems reasonable to evaluate, in a surgical perspective, the drug-resistant childhood occipital epilepsies as well as the other types (Lo Russo et al., 1991).

References

Ajmone-Marsan, C. & Ralston, B.L. (1957): *The epileptic seizure. Its functional morphology and diagnostic significance.* Springfield, IL: Charles C. Thomas.

Bancaud, J. (1969): Les crises épileptiques d'origine occipitale (étude stéréo-électroencéphalographique). *Rev. Oto. Neuro. Opthalmol.* **41**, 299–315.

Bancaud, J., Talairach, J., Munari, C., Giallonardo, A.T. & Brunet, P. (1991): Introduction à l'étude clinique des crises épileptiques rétro-rolandiques. *Can. J. Neurol. Sci.* **18**, 566–569.

Bossi, L., Munari, C., Stoffels, C., Bonis, A., Bacia, T., Talairach, J. & Bancaud, J. (1984): Somatomotor manifestations in temporal lobe seizures. *Epilepsia* **25**, 70–76.

Gastaut, H. (1960): Un aspect méconnu des décharges neuroniques occipitales: la crise oculo-clonique ou 'nystagmus épileptique'. In: *Les grandes activités du lobe occipital*, ed. T. Alajouanine, pp. 169–185. Paris: Masson.

Lindsay, J., Ounsted, C. & Richards, P. (1984): Long-term outcome in children with temporal lobe seizures. V: Indications and contra-indications for neurosurgery. *Dev. Med. Child. Neurol.* **26**, 25–32.

Lo Russo, G., Munari, C., Betti, O.O., Musolino, A., Turak, B., Hamasaki, T., Rosler, R., Hoffmann, D. & Benabid, A.L. (1992): Stereotaxic approach to intracranial lesions. *Ital. J. Neurol. Sci.* **13**, 17–44.

Lo Russo, G., Tassi, L., Francione, S., Kahane, P., Hoffmann, D., Galli, R., Lorenzi, A., Joannard, A., Baudain, P. & Munari, C. (1991): Indicazioni alla chirurgia delle epilessie parziali nei bambini. *Riv. Ped. Siciliana.* **1–2**, 397–398.

Munari, C., Bancaud, J., Bonis, A., Stoffels, C., Szikla, G. & Talairach, J. (1980): Impairment of consciousness in temporal lobe seizures: a stereo-electro-encephalographic study. In: *Advances in epileptology*, eds. R. Canger, F. Angeleri & J.K. Penry, pp. 111–114. New York: Raven Press.

Munari, C. & Betti, O.O. (1989): The stereotactic biopsy of brain lesions : a critical review. In: *Cerebral gliomas*, eds. G. Broggi & M.A. Gerosa, pp. 179–206. Amsterdam: Elsevier.

Munari, C., Bonis, A., Kochen, S., Pestre, M., Brunet, P., Bancaud, J., Chodkiewicz, J.P. & Talairach, J. (1984): Eye movements and occipital seizures in man. *Acta Neurochirurgica Suppl.* **33**, 47–52.

Munari, C., Musolino, A., Betti, O.O., Clodic, R., Askienazy, S. & Chodkiewicz, J.P. (1988a): An advanced therapeutic approach of actively expanding intracranial cysts: stereotactic beta endocavitary irradiation of craniopharyngiomas and gliomas. In: *Advanced technology in neurosurgery*, eds. F. Pluchino & G. Broggi, pp. 120–131. New York, Berlin, Heidelberg: Springer Verlag.

Munari, C., Rosler, J.R., Musolino, A., Franzini, A., Daumas-Duport, C., Missir O. & Chodkiewicz, J.P. (1988b): Stereotactic approach of intracranial lesions in children (report of 134 cases and review of the literature). *J. Paediatr. Neurosci.* **4**, 257–273.

Musolino, A., Merckaert, P., Munari, C., Daumas-Duport, C. & Chodkiewicz, J.P. (1989): Stereotactic endocavitary treatment of cysts and pseudocysts of gliomas. Preliminary report. *J. Neurosurg. Sci.* **33**, 107–114.

Ochs, R., Gloor P., Quesney F., *et al.* (1984): Does head-turning during a seizure have lateralizing or localizing significance? *Neurology* **34**, 884–890.

Rasmussen, T. (1975): Surgery of epilepsy associated with brain tumors. In: *Advances in neurology*, Vol. 8, Neurosurgical management of the epilepsies, eds. D.P. Purpura, J.K. Penry & R.D. Walter, pp. 227–239. New York: Raven Press.

Robillard, A., Saint-Hilaire J.M., Mercier M., *et al.* (1983): The lateralizing and localizing value of adversion in epileptic seizures. *Neurology* **33**, 1241–1242.

Takeda, A., Bancaud, J., Talairach, J., *et al.* (1970): Concerning epileptic attacks of occipital origin. *Electroencephalogr. Clin. Neurophysiol.* **28**, 644–649.

Williamson, P.D., Wieser, H.G. & Delgado-Escueta, A. (1987): Clinical characteristics of partial seizures. In: *Surgical management of the epilepsies*, ed. J.Jr. Engel, pp.101–120. New York: Raven Press.

Williamson, P.D., Thadani, V.M., Darcey, T.M., Spencer, D.D., Spencer, S.S. & Mattson, R.H. (1992): Occipital lobe epilepsy: clinical characteristics, seizure spread patterns, and results of surgery. *Ann. Neurol.* **31**, 3–13.

Chapter 25

Occipital lobe epilepsy in children – electroclinical manifestations, surgical indications and treatment

Frederick Andermann, Vicenta Salanova, André Olivier and Theodore Rasmussen

Department of Neurology and Neurosurgery, McGill University, and the Montreal Neurological Hospital and Institute, 3801 University St., Montreal, Quebec, Canada H3A 2B4

Summary

Patients with occipital lobe epilepsy have distinctive clinical manifestations, and in almost two-thirds these are lateralized. However, because of the different spread patterns, these patients can have more than one seizure type though onset may be in the occipital region. This can lead to misdiagnosis as some patients may appear to have multiple foci.

Surface EEG evaluation often shows large epileptogenic areas involving the posterior temporo-occipital region. This can also contribute to the misdiagnosis of these patients as they can be difficult to distinguish from patients with temporal lobe epilepsy and posterior temporal foci.

Intracranial evaluation and electrocorticography often show large epileptogenic areas, thus requiring extensive resections. Despite this, as many as 72 per cent of children benefited from surgery.

The presence of a field defect facilitates the surgical decision. In those patients with normal visual fields, producing a field defect may be justified depending on the patient's age and the severity of the epilepsy. As in all patients undergoing epilepsy surgery, possible complications must be discussed (Andermann, 1987) and in particular the patient and the family must be informed of the implications of a post-operative field defect.

Introduction

The clinical manifestations of occipital lobe epilepsy can be divided into two categories: (a) those representing seizure phenomena originating in the occipital lobe including elementary visual hallucinations, ictal blindness, and ocular movements, and (b) those signs and symptoms resulting from ictal spread to adjacent cortical structures like complex visual hallucinations, focal motor activity and automatisms typical of temporal lobe seizures.

Elementary visual hallucinations are the most common occipital manifestations and have been reported in 47 per cent to 68 per cent of patients with occipital lobe epilepsy. These consist of coloured lights, flickering bright colours, cone-shaped lights, gross sensations of light, darkness or colour, at times moving, revolving or rotating (Penfield & Erickson, 1941; Penfield & Kristiansen, 1951; Penfield & Jasper, 1954; Russell & Whitty, 1955; Ludwig & Ajmone-Marsan, 1975; Salanova *et al.*, 1991; Blume *et al.*, 1991; Williamson *et al.*, 1992). In most cases the elementary visual hallucinations are contralateral to the epileptogenic side.

These elementary visual hallucinations have been elicited by cortical stimulation of occipital lobe areas 17, 18 and 19 (Foerster & Penfield, 1930; Foerster, 1936; Penfield & Rasmussen, 1950; Penfield & Jasper, 1954).

Ictal blindness has been reported in as many as 40 per cent of patients with occipital lobe epilepsy (Holmes, 1927; Penfield & Jasper, 1954; Russell & Whitty, 1955; Olivier *et al.*, 1982; Salanova *et al.*, 1991; Williamson *et al.*, 1992), and in a few patients prolonged ictal blindness referred to as status epilepticus amauroticus has also been reported (Ayala, 1929; Barry *et al.*, 1985).

We reviewed 20 children under 16 years of age with occipital lobe epilepsy treated surgically at the Montreal Neurological Institute between 1930 and 1990, and found that 70 per cent had visual auras. In most children these auras consisted of elementary visual hallucinations; many of these patients also had ictal blindness during some of the seizures.

Other occipital manifestations include contralateral ocular movements, which are most often tonic; however, clonic eye deviation and nystagmoid eye movements have also been described (Gastaut, 1954, 1960; Takeda *et al.*, 1970; Talairach & Bancaud, 1974). These eye movements have also been elicited by metrazol activation in patients with occipital lobe epilepsy (Penfield & Jasper, 1954; Ajmone-Marsan & Ralston, 1957).

Munari *et al.* (1984) studied 16 patients who had ocular deviation during 10 s of the seizure onset with stereo EEG. In the majority of these patients the eye movement was tonic and in all it was contralateral to the ictal discharge. Many of these patients also exhibited bilateral blinking. The authors found that the seizures usually originated from the medial occipital cortex.

Contralateral head and eye deviation in patients with occipital lobe epilepsy has been reported by Penfield & Jasper (1954), and by Ludwig & Ajmone-Marsan (1975). More recently, Williamson *et al.* (1992) reported eye deviation with or without head deviation in 16 of their 25 patients, and bilateral blinking in 14 patients.

Rosenbaum *et al.* (1986) reviewed the literature relating to contraversion and occipital lobe epilepsy, and noted that in all reported cases head deviation was contralateral to the seizure focus. They also noted that the prevalence of adversion in patients with occipital lobe epilepsy was 20 per cent to 40 per cent.

At the MNI we found that 55 per cent of 20 children with refractory occipital lobe epilepsy exhibited contralateral eye and head deviation. Ten per cent had blinking and 5 per cent had nystagmoid eye movements.

A sensation of ocular movement at the beginning of the seizures has been reported by Holtman & Goldensohn (1977) and by Williamson *et al.* (1992).

Non-occipital clinical manifestations

Complex visual hallucinations usually preceded by elementary visual hallucinations have been reported by many authors (Huott *et al.*, 1974; Ludwig & Ajmone-Marsan, 1975; Munari *et al.*, 1984; Blume *et al.*, 1991; Williamson *et al.*, 1992). Russell & Whitty (1955) described complex visual hallucinations in 20 per cent of 60 patients with visual seizures, and Ludwig & Ajmone-Marsan (1975) noted psychic auras in 14 per cent of their patients with occipital lobe epileptic foci; half of these were visual.

Ten per cent of our 20 children with occipital lobe epilepsy exhibited elementary visual hallucinations followed by complex visual hallucinations. Gloor *et al.* (1982) have shown that experiential phenomena, including complex visual hallucinations, only occurred when the ictal discharge involved the limbic structures, suggesting that complex visual hallucinations in patients with occipital lobe epilepsy are due to seizure spread to temporal structures.

Oral alimentary automatisms typical of those of patients with temporal lobe epilepsy have been reported in 29 per cent to 88 per cent, and focal motor activity in 38 per cent to 47 per cent of patients with occipital lobe epilepsy (Ludwig & Ajmone-Marsan, 1975; Salanova et al., 1991; Williamson et al. (1992).

Ajmone-Marsan & Ralston (1957), using metrazol activation, showed that automatisms were due to spread of the ictal discharge to the temporal lobe. They also showed that suprasylvian spread resulted in somatic sensory, supplementary motor, and somatic motor manifestations. Subsequently, these spread patterns have been confirmed experimentally (Collins & Caston, 1979), and in patients studied with depth electrodes.

The patterns of spread are through the inferior longitudinal fasciculus to the ipsilateral temporal lobe, the superior longitudinal fasciculus to the superior frontal parietal region, and via the fronto-occipital fasciculus. These patterns of spread account for the non-occipital clinical manifestations and for the fact that many patients with occipital lobe epilepsy have more than one seizure type, which contributes to the difficulty in diagnosis.

Thirty-five per cent of our 20 children with occipital lobe epilepsy exhibited oral alimentary automatisms, and 45 per cent had focal motor activity.

Neurological examination

Preoperative visual field deficits have been reported in 20 per cent to 56 per cent of patients with occipital lobe epilepsy (Ludwig & Ajmone-Marsan, 1975; Salanova et al., 1991; Blume et al., 1991; Williamson et al., 1992). We found that 65 per cent of our 20 children had preoperative field defects, and in all cases they were contralateral to the epileptogenic side.

Radiological findings

Radiological abnormalities are found in 37 per cent to 72 per cent of patients with symptomatic occipital lobe epilepsy (Ludwig & Ajmone-Marsan, 1975; Blume et al., 1991; Williamson et al., 1992). More than half of our 20 patients had radiological abnormalities; most often these consisted of atrophic lesions involving posterior head region.

Aetiology of occipital lobe epilepsy

Rasmussen (1975) reported that of 23 patients with refractory occipital lobe epilepsy, one-third had a history of trauma or anoxia, 9 per cent had gliomas, 13 per cent had post-inflammatory brain scarring, and in 26 per cent the cause was unknown.

Ludwig & Ajmone-Marsan (1975) also described the presumed aetiology in 55 patients: one-quarter had various encephalopathies including birth injury, anoxia, and severe head trauma. Thirteen per cent had had encephalitis or meningitis, 14 per cent had vascular lesions and 7 per cent had expanding lesions. More recently, Williamson et al. (1992) found low grade neoplasms in 10 of 16 patients with occipital lobe epilepsy who then had resections of these lesions.

Fedor Krause (1912) in his book *Surgery of the brain and spinal cord based on personal experiences* discussed several patients with 'neoplasmata of the occipital brain'. One of the patients with a left occipital lobe tumour diagnosed as 'fibrosarcoma of the brain' had a right-sided hemianopsia, and 'optic illusions toward the right'. The patient complained of seeing coloured patterns which lasted 2–4 min. Following removal of the tumour the 'visual illusions' disappeared, and Krause referred to 'the brilliant results obtained in this case'.

In 1930 I.M. Allen reviewed the clinical features of 40 patients with occipital lobe tumours studied at The National Hospital, Queen Square, London. He found that 52.5 per cent of patients had 'epileptiform attacks or loss of consciousness'. In 30 per cent of patients, this was the presenting symptom, but in only one-third were the attacks preceded by a visual aura. He reported visual hallucinations in 25 per cent of the patients studied, and stated that in 15 per cent these were the typical 'unformed' images due to an occipital lesion. Surprisingly though, he stated that 'in only 10

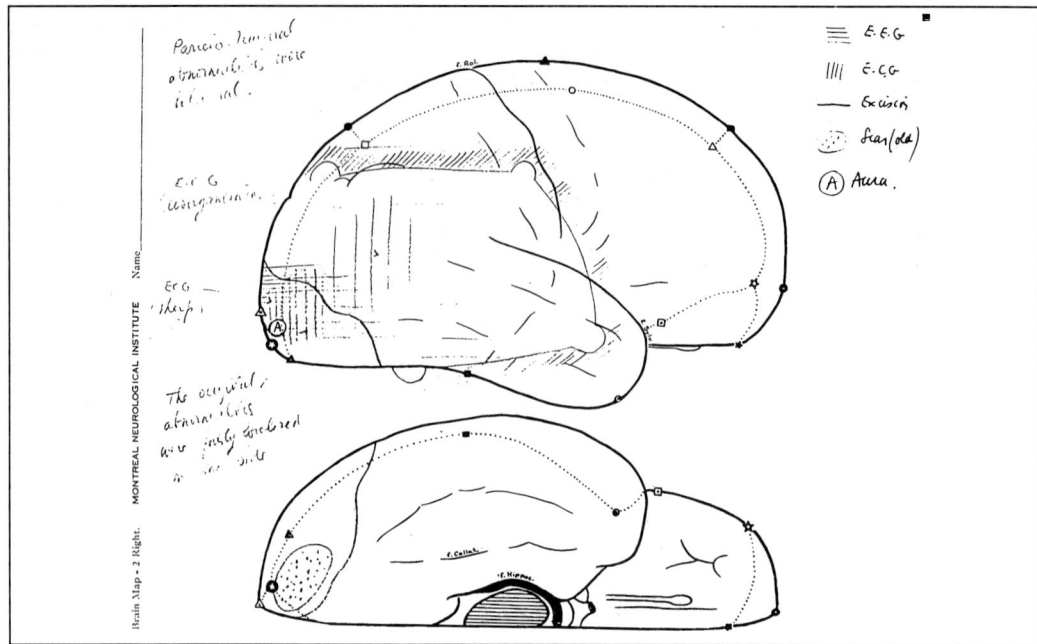

Fig 1. 11-year-old female (NM) with occipital epilepsy. Onset at 7 years of age. Visual aura described as 'colours' in left visual field, followed by familiar objects moving towards her and fear. Map showing extent of resection and site of aura elicited by cortical stimulation.

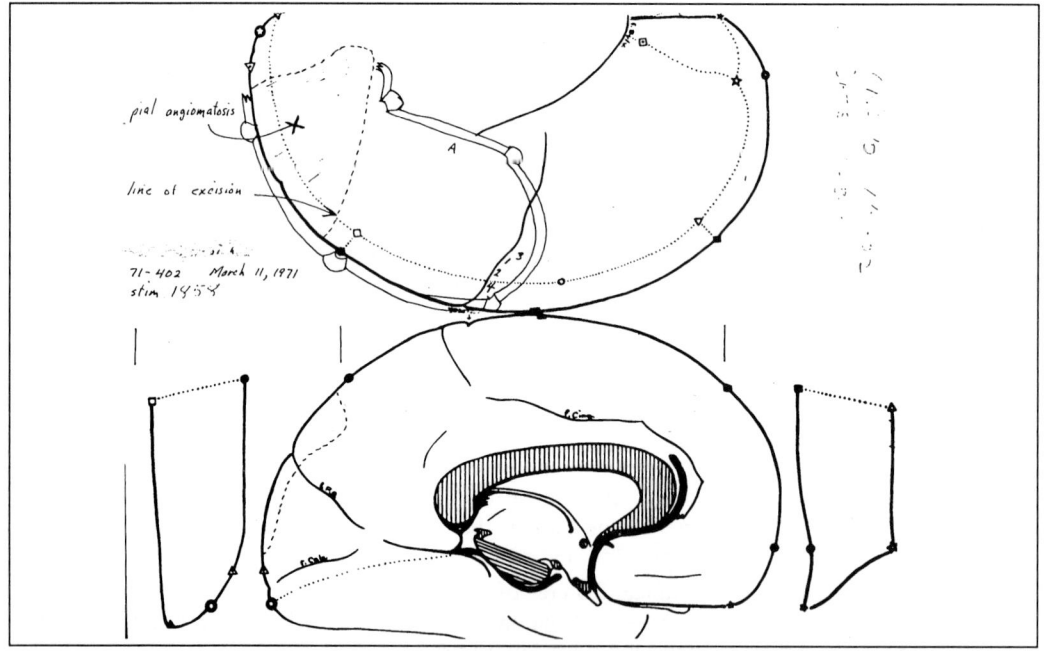

Fig. 2. 14-year-old female (CB) with occipital epilepsy due to pial angiomatosis without nevus flammeus or calcifications. Onset at 8 years of age. Aura described as 'flashes of light in the right eye'. Surgical map showing extent of resection.

per cent of cases did the visual hallucinations represent the aura of an epileptiform attack'. Allen (1930) described these unformed hallucinations as flashes of light, flashes of flame, a round ball of bright light, usually contralateral to the tumour. Two patients also had a 'formed visual hallucination' associated with auditory hallucinations. One patient described his teacher's voice speaking to him associated with a visual hallucination in the form of the teacher himself.

It is interesting that Allen (1930) reported that 'it was unusual' for the patients with these occipital lobe tumours to be aware of a visual field defect, and only 16 per cent of them could recall an experience which suggested visual impairment on one side, and 'in only one case did the patient state definitely that he could not see on the affected side'. However, he reported that detailed visual field studies were available in 80 per cent of patients studied and in every case but two there was some degree of homonymous hemianopsia.

Obviously this is the case with slow growing lesions, and highlights the importance of having detailed visual field testing of these patients. He also found that the epileptic attacks were less frequent when the tumour was confined to the occipital lobe, and more frequent when the parietal or temporal lobes were also involved.

Twenty percent of our children had a history of head trauma, and 25 per cent had a history of birth injury. Other aetiologies included porencephalic lesions, focal microgyria with cyst formation, pial angiomatosis, calcified abscesses and focal cortical dysplasia.

Differential diagnosis: benign occipital epilepsy

It is important to keep in mind that patients with benign occipital lobe epilepsy also have similar symptoms and age of onset of their seizures. Gastaut (1982, 1985), and Gastaut & Zifkin (1987) have reported this syndrome. The age of onset ranges from 15 months to 17 years, migraine can affect as many as 16 per cent, and 37 per cent had a family history of epilepsy. Elementary visual hallucinations have been described in 55 per cent and transient loss of vision in 65 per cent of patients. Complex partial seizures and focal motor activity indicating ictal spread to temporal and frontal lobe structures have also been described.

Most of these children have a normal neurological examination. Gastaut (1982) reported that 90 per cent of his patients were neurologically intact. Neuroimaging studies were also normal. The EEGs showed normal background and high voltage spikes over posterior head regions. It is important to differentiate these patients from those with mitochondrial encephalomyopathy with lactic acidosis and stroke-like episodes (MELAS) syndrome (Montagna *et al.*, 1988). These patients present with occipital seizures, which at first are infrequent and easy to control, and they also have migrainous attacks. However, as the disease progresses, stroke-like episodes with frequent bouts of epilepsia partialis continua, quite difficult to control, usually occur.

Surface EEG evaluation

Williamson & Spencer (1986), and Williamson *et al.* (1992) have reported that temporal epileptiform discharges were most often found in patients with refractory occipital lobe epilepsy, and stated that surface evaluation could be misleading (Williamson *et al.*, 1988). Bitemporal independent epileptiform discharges, and bilaterally synchronous epileptiform discharges over posterior head regions have been reported by several authors (Huott *et al.*, 1974; Ludwig & Ajmone-Marsan, 1975; Williamson *et al.*, 1992). This could be due to secondary bilateral synchrony, and/or secondary epileptogenesis (Tukel & Jasper, 1952; Morrell, 1959, 1985).

Ictal onsets can also be misleading; Williamson *et al.* (1988) found that in many of their patients intracranial recordings were required.

We found that interictal epileptiform discharges and ictal onsets were most often recorded over the posterior temporal and occipital regions. However, 21 per cent of our children had interictal epileptiform discharges confined to the occipital region.

Intracranial recording

Several authors have used intracranial recordings with depth electrodes to evaluate patients with refractory occipital lobe epilepsy (Bancaud, 1969; Bancaud et al., 1965; Takeda et al., 1969, 1970; Babb et al., 1981; Munari et al., 1984; Olivier et al., 1982; Williamson et al., 1981, 1987, 1988, 1992; Palmini et al., 1991).

Williamson & Spencer (1986) use stereotactically placed occipitotemporal electrodes, directed anteriorly toward the amygdala, which allow sampling from the long axis of the hippocampus, as well as from the occipital region.

At the Montreal Neurological Institute depth electrodes are usually implanted in the coronal plane, through the second temporal convolution and the lateral occipital region (Gloor, 1975, 1984). The two deepest contacts sample from the mesial structures and the superficial contacts from the lateral temporal and lateral occipital areas. Intracranial recording is often necessary in the evaluation of patients with posterior, temporo-occipital epilepsy (Palmini et al., 1991).

Electrocorticography and cortical resections

Penfield & Jasper (1954), Penfield & Rasmussen (1950), and Rasmussen (1979, 1984, 1987) have used intraoperative cortical electrical stimulation to elicit the patient's habitual aura, and electrocorticography (ECOG) in patients undergoing cortical resections to delineate the epileptogenic area.

We found large epileptogenic zones in many of the patients undergoing surgery for occipital lobe epilepsy at the MNI (Olivier et al., 1991). Pre-excision ECOG spiking was restricted to the occipital lobe in only 41 per cent of 17 children; the remaining patients had more extensive spiking extending into the posterior temporal and posterior parietal regions.

Fifty-five per cent of the children had either partial occipital resections or occipital lobectomies. The remainder had more extensive resections which were guided by the findings on cortical stimulation studies and electrocorticography (Gloor, 1975). Post-resection ECOG was performed in 12/20 children; 50 per cent showed no residual spiking and 25 per cent showed reduced spiking.

Neurological deficits before and after surgery for occipital lobe epilepsy

As mentioned earlier, 13/20 (65 per cent) of 20 children with refractory occipital lobe epilepsy had preoperative field defects. Following surgery an additional three patients developed a field defect. One patient had transient aphasia, and two had aseptic meningitis. One child died post-operatively, early in the series.

Surgical outcome

Thirty-two per cent to 50 per cent of patients with occipital lobe epilepsy treated surgically became seizure free (Wyler et al., 1990; Olivier et al., 1991; Blume et al., 1991). Williamson et al. (1992) reported excellent results with elimination of seizures in 14 of their 24 patients; all 14 patients had structural lesions.

Follow-up of 1–46 years (mean 18 years) was available for 18 of our 20 children operated on at the MNI. Thirty-three per cent were seizure-free since discharge and an additional 22 per cent became seizure-free after early attacks. Another 17 per cent had late recurrence of occasional seizures, or no more than two seizures per year. Thus, 72 per cent benefited from surgery. In our patients the factors correlating with a good outcome were the absence of epileptiform discharges on the post-resection ECOG and EEGs, and the presence of a structural lesion on imaging studies.

References

Allen, I.M. (1930): A clinical study of tumors involving the occipital lobe. *Brain* **80**, 194–243.

Ajmone-Marsan, C. & Ralston, B. (1957): *The epileptic seizure: its functional morphology and diagnostic significance*, pp. 211–215. Springfield, IL: Charles C. Thomas.

Andermann, F. (1987): Identification of candidates for surgical treatment of epilepsy. In: *Surgical management of the epilepsies*, ed. J. Engel. Jr., pp. 51–70. New York: Raven Press.

Ayala, G. (1929): Status epilepticus amauroticus. *Boll. Accad. Med. Roma* **55**, 288–290.

Babb, T.L., Halgren, E., Wilson, C., Engel, J. & Crandall, P. (1981): Neuronal firing patterns during the spread of an occipital lobe seizure to the temporal lobes in man. *EEG Clin. Neurophysiol.* **51**, 104–107.

Bancaud, J., Talairach, J., Bonis, A., Schaub, A., Szikla, G., Morel, P. & Bordas-Feré, M. (1965): Les épilepsies occipitales. In: *La Stereo- électroencéphalographie dans l'épilépsie*, pp. 93–103. Paris: Masson.

Bancaud, J. (1969): Les crises épileptiques d'origine occipitale (étude-stéreo-éléctroencephalographique). *Rev. Oto-Neuro-Ophthalmol.* **41**, 299–315.

Barry, E., Sussman, N.M., Bosley, T.M. & Harner, R.N. (1985): Ictal blindness and status epilepticus amauroticus. *Epilepsia* **26**, 577–584.

Blume, W.T., Whiting, S.E. & Girvin, J.P. (1991): Epilepsy surgery in the posterior cortex. *Ann. Neurol.* **29**, 638–645.

Collins, R.C. & Caston, T.V. (1979): Functional anatomy of occipital lobe seizures: an experimental study in rats. *Neurology* **29**, 705–716.

Foerster, O. & Penfield, W. (1930): The structural basis of traumatic epilepsy and results of radical operation. In: *Epilepsy and the convulsive state*, Vol. 7, Part II, pp. 569–591. Association for Research in Nervous and Mental Diseases.

Foerster, O. (1936): Sensible corticale Felder. In: *Handbuch der Neurologie*, Vol. VI, eds. O. Bumke & O. Foerster. Berlin: Springer-Verlag.

Gastaut, H. & Roger, A. (1954): Une forme inhabituelle de l'épilepsie: le nystagmus épileptique. *Rev. Neurol.* **90**, 130–132.

Gastaut, H. (1960): Un aspect méconnu des décharges neuroniques occipitales: la crise oculo-clonique ou 'nystagmus epileptique'. In: *Les grandes activités du lobe occipital*, ed. T. Alajouanine, pp. 169–185. Paris: Masson.

Gastaut, H. (1982): A new type of epilepsy: benign partial epilepsy of childhood with occipital spike waves. *Clin. Electroencephalogr.* **13**, 13–22.

Gastaut, H. (1985): Benign epilepsy of childhood with occipital paroxysms. In: *Epileptic syndromes in infancy, childhood and adolescence*, eds. J. Roger, C. Dravet, M. Bureau, F.E. Dreifuss & P. Wolf, pp. 159–170. London: John Libbey.

Gastaut, H. & Zifkin, B.G. (1987): Benign epilepsy of childhood with occipital spike and wave complexes. In: *Migraine and epilepsy*, eds. F. Andermann & E. Lugaresi, pp. 47–81. London, Boston: Butterworths.

Gloor, P. (1975): Contributions of electroencephalography and electrocorticography to the neurosurgical treatment of the epilepsies. In: *Advances in neurology*, Vol. 8, *Neurosurgical management of the epilepsies*, eds. D.P. Pupura, J.K. Penry & R.D. Walter, pp. 59–105. New York: Raven Press.

Gloor, P., Olivier, A., Quesney, L.F., Andermann, F. & Horowitz, S. (1982): The role of the limbic system in experiential phenomena of temporal lobe epilepsy. *Ann. Neurol.* **12**, 129–144.

Gloor, P. (1984) Electroencephalography and the role of intracerebral depth recordings in the selection of patients for surgical treatment of epilepsy. In: *Advances in epileptology*. XVth Epilepsy International Symposium, eds. R.J. Porter, R.H. Mattson, A.A. Ward & M. Dam, pp. 433–437. New York: Raven Press.

Holtzman, R.N.N. & Goldensohn, E.S. (1977): Sensations of ocular movement in seizures originating in occipital lobe. *Neurology* **27**, 555–556.

Holmes, G. (1927): Savill Memorial Oration on Local Epilepsy. *Lancet* **i**, 957–962.

Huott, A.D., Madison, D.S. & Niedermeyer, E. (1974): Occipital lobe epilepsy: a clinical and electroencephalographic study. *Eur. Neurol.* **11**, 325–339.

Krause, F. (1912): Neoplasmata of the occipital brain. In: *Surgery of the brain and spinal cord*, Vol. II, pp. 639–657. New York: Rebman Company.

Ludwig, B.I. & Ajmone-Marsan, C. (1975): Clinical ictal patterns in epileptic patients with occipital electroencephalographic foci. *Neurology* **25**, 463–471.

Montagna, P., Gallassi, R., Medori, R., Govoni, E., Zeviani, M., Di Mauro, S., Lugaresi, E. & Andermann, F. (1988): MELAS syndrome. Characteristic migrainous and epileptic features and maternal transmission. *Neurology* **38**, 751–754.

Morrell, F. (1985): Secondary epileptogenesis in man. *Arch. Neurol.* **42**, 318–335.

Morrell, F. (1959/1960): Secondary epileptogenetic lesions. *Epilepsia* **1**, 538–560.

Munari, C., Bonis, A., Kochen, S., Pestre, M., Brunet, P., Bancaud, J., Chodkiewicz, J.P. & Talairach, J. (1984): Eye movements and occipital seizures in man. *Acta. Neurochir.* **33** (suppl), 47–52.

Olivier, A., Gloor, P., Andermann, F. & Ives, J. (1982): Occipitotemporal epilepsy studied with stereotaxically implanted depth electrodes and successfully treated by temporal resection. *Ann. Neurol.* **11**, 428–432.

Olivier, A., Salanova, V., Andermann, F., Rasmussen, T. & Quesney, LF. (1991): Electrocorticography (ECOG) cortical stimulation and surgical outcome in 29 patients with occipital lobe epilepsy. *Neurology* **41**(suppl. 1), 202.

Palmini, A., Dubeau, F., Andermann, F., Olivier, A., Gloor, P., Quesney, L.F. & Salanova, V. (1991): Stereo-EEG study of occipital and temporo-occipital epilepsies: strategies of evaluation and surgical approaches. *Epilepsia* **32** (suppl 1), 120.

Penfield, W. & Erickson, T.C. (1941): *Epilepsy and cerebral localization*, pp. 101–102. Springfield, IL: Charles C. Thomas.

Penfield, W. & Rasmussen, T. (1950): Vision. In: *The cerebral cortex in man: a clinical study of localization of function*, pp. 135–144. New York: Macmillan.

Penfield, W. & Kristiansen, K. (1951): Seizure patterns. In: *Epileptic seizure patterns*. Springfield, IL: Charles C. Thomas, 16–84.

Penfield, W. & Jasper, H. (1954): *Epilepsy and the functional anatomy of the human brain*. Boston: Little, Brown and Company.

Rasmussen, T. (1975): Surgery of epilepsy arising in regions other than the temporal and frontal lobes. In: *Advances in neurology*. Vol. 8, *Neurosurgical management of the epilepsies*, eds. D.P. Pupura, J.K. Penry & R.D. Walter, pp. 207–226. New York: Raven Press.

Rasmussen, T. (1979): Cortical resection for medically refractory focal epilepsy: results, lessons and questions. In: *Neurosurgery*, eds. T. Rasmussen & R. Marino, pp. 253–269. New York: Raven Press.

Rasmussen, T. (1984): Results of cortical resection in focal epilepsy. In: *Advances in epileptology*. XVth Epilepsy International Symposium, eds. R.J. Porter, R.H. Masson, A.A. Ward & M. Dam, pp. 449–455. New York: Raven Press.

Rasmussen, T. (1987): Focal epilepsies of nontemporal and nonfrontal origin. In: *Presurgical evaluation of epileptics*, eds. H.G. Wieser & C.E. Elger, pp. 301–305. Berlin, Heidelberg: Springer-Verlag.

Rosenbaum, D.H., Siegel, M. & Rowan, A.J. (1986): Contraversive seizures in occipital epilepsy: case report and review of the literature. *Neurology* **36**, 281–284.

Russell, W. & Whitty, C. (1955): Studies in traumatic epilepsy. 3. Visual fits. *J. Neurol. Neurosurg. Psychiatry* **18**, 79–96.

Salanova, V., Andermann, F., Olivier, A., Rasmussen, T. & Quesney, L.F. (1991): Occipital lobe epilepsy: electroclinical manifestations in 29 patients treated surgically. *Neurology* **41** (suppl. 1), 365.

Talairach, J. & Bancaud, J. (1974): Stereotaxic exploration and therapy in epilepsy. In: *Handbook of neurology*, eds. P.J. Vinken & G.W. Bruyn, Vol. XV, pp. 758–782. Amsterdam: North Holland.

Takeda, A., Bancaud, J. & Talairach, J. et al. (1969): A propos des accès épileptiques d'origine occipitale. *Rev. Neurol.* **121**, 306–315.

Takeda, A., Bancaud, J., Talairach, J., Bonis, A. & Bordas-Ferrer, M. (1970): Concerning epileptic attacks of occipital origin. *Electroencephalogr. Clin. Neurophysiol.* **28**, 664–649.

Tukel, K. & Jasper, H. (1952): The electroencephalogram in parasagittal lesions. *Electroencephalogr. Clin. Neurophysiol.* **4**, 481–494.

Williamson, P.D., Spencer, S.S., Spencer, D.D. & Mattson, R.H. (1981): Complex partial seizures with occipital lobe onset. *Epilepsia* **22**, 247–248.

Williamson, P.D. & Spencer, S.S. (1986): Clinical and EEG features of complex partial seizures of extratemporal origin. *Epilepsia* **27** (suppl. 2), S46–S63.

Williamson, P.D., Wieser, H.G. & Delgado-Escueta, A. (1987): Clinical characteristics of partial seizures. In: *Advances in neurology*, Vol. 8, *Surgical management of the epilepsies*, ed. J. Engel Jr., pp. 101–120. New York: Raven Press.

Williamson, P.D., Boon, P.A., Spencer, D.D., Spencer, S.S. & Mattson, R.H. (1988): Occipital and parietal epilepsy. *Epilepsia* **29**, 682.

Williamson, P.D., Thadani, V.M., Darcey, T.M., Spencer, D.D., Spencer, S.S. & Mattson R.H. (1992): Occipital lobe epilepsy: clinical characteristics, seizure spread patterns, and results of surgery. *Ann. Neurol.* **31**, 3–13.

Wyler, A.R. & Herman, B.P. (1990): Surgical treatment of occipital lobe epileptic foci. *Epilepsia* **31** (5), 38.

Chapter 26

Evolution of the semiology of the childhood occipital seizures

Joseph Roger

Centre Saint-Paul, 300 boulevard de Sainte Marguerite, 13009 Marseille, France

Summary

Data concerning the outcome of the semiology of childhood occipital seizures are rare and uncertain. There are reasons to think that differences exist according to age and aetiology.

However, in the literature no study with a long-term follow-up provides a semiological analysis of the seizures at different moments. The relationships between the maturation of the visual cortex and the occurence and the clinical features of the occipital seizures should be taken into consideration by performing simultaneous clinical and neurophysiological investigations of the development of the visual system.

For several reasons it is not easy to answer the question of what is the evolution of childhood occipital seizures and epilepsies. Firstly, the data from the literature generally do not concern a sufficient number of cases followed up for a long time with an accurate description of the clinical and electroencephalographical ictal and interictal symptomatology from the onset on.

Secondly, one could reasonably think that this symptomatology and its evolution would be different between idiopathic and symptomatic occipital epilepsies (OE) but the authors often do not separate these two types.

However, from the recent data some points seem to emerge.

The clinical semiology probably changes according to age, which is coherent with the maturational changes in the visual system, particularly in the occipital cortex and its connections. Several authors have described these changes (Kivity & Lerman, 1989, 1990; Panayiotopoulos, 1989). In the infant and the small child, visual symptoms are rarely reported. Usually there are eye and head deviations, vomiting, unilateral motor manifestations, and a sometimes prolonged impairment of consciousness. In the older child and the adolescent, initial visual symptoms are common, after which the secondary propagation of the discharge appears slower and progresses towards the temporal lobe rather than toward the motor area. However, in this meeting, Vigevano et al. (Chapter 15) reported on a patient who has had the same ictal semiology without any change between 2 and 9 years.

The seizure differences between the idiopathic and symptomatic types of OE could be described as follows:

- Illusions, metamorphopsies, illusional perseveration of a visual perception would occur more often in the lesional forms;
- An ictal sequence with initial visual symptoms followed by automatisms would be also more often observed in the lesional forms, probably related to the temporal lobe involvement, whereas the motor cortex involvement would be more common in the idiopathic forms;
- The combination of other seizure types, such as tonic seizures and atypical absences, would exist only in the lesional forms.

But, in this discussion, one must keep in mind that some symptomatic epilepsies of childhood with occipital seizures at the onset depend on progressive diseases and progressive lesions: OE with bilateral calcifications (Gobbi *et al.*, 1988) with or without associated coeliac disease, mitochondrial myopathy, encephalopathy, lactic acidosis and stroke like episodes (MELAS) (Pavlakis *et al.*, 1984), Lafora's disease (Roger *et al.*, 1983).

Another problem is to explain why OE are more frequent than epilepsies with centrotemporal spikes among the idiopathic epilepsies of the small child.

A partial epilepsy can have its expression only in the cortical areas which have reached a degree of maturity and we know that the visual cortex has the earliest development as regard to the other regions. Nevertheless some anatomo-clinical correlations observed in adult patients do not confirm that the occipital cortex becomes epileptogenic easily. They tend to demonstrate the contrary.

For a similar lesion its epileptogenic potential is lower than in the other regions. This finding is evident in the epilepsies occurring after an open cranial injury: the risk for seizures is of 70 per cent in the rolandic injuries versus only 15 per cent in the occipital ones (Paillas & Bureau, 1982). The same difference is observed in the case of slowly evolutive tumors (Paillas *et al.*, 1982).

When the moment of the constitution of the cortical lesion is known, as in the post-traumatic epilepsies, the delay of occurrence of the seizures is very long in the occipital localization. That is true not only for the adults (Roger *et al.*, 1987) but also for the infants when the trauma has provoked an expansive fracture (Roger, 1984).

Of course these data should be compared with those observed in other types of lesions specific to infancy, such as brain malformation and ischaemic lesions, where this rule seems not to be found.

In this colloquium several authors reported on the occipital cortical maturation and the possible clinical and neurophysiological investigations of the visual system development in infants and children. May be there we have a tool allowing us to assess its degree of maturity and its functional advancement and to correlate them with the ictal semiology in children affected by an OE. The simultaneous performing of both these investigations could give us the answer to the questions we have tried to pose here.

References

Gobbi, G., Sorrenti, G., Santucci, M., Giovanardi Rossi, P., Ambrosetto, P., Michelucci, R. & Tassinari, C.A. (1988): Epilepsy with bilateral occipital calcifications: a benign onset with progressive severity. *Neurology* **38**, 913–920.

Kivity, S. & Lerman, P. (1989): Benign partial epilepsy of childhood with occipital discharges. In: *Advances in epileptology*, Vol. XVII., eds. J. Manelis, E. Bental, J.N. Loeber & F.E. Dreifuss, pp. 371–373. New York: Raven Press.

Kivity, S. & Lerman, P. (1990): Stormy onset with prolonged loss of consciousness in benign occipital epilepsy of childhood. *Brain Dev.* **12**, 632.

Paillas, J.E. & Bureau, M. (1982): Aspects cliniques de l'épilepsie post-traumatique: étude d'une série de 333 observations. *Boll. Lega. It. Epil.* **39**, 11–17.

Paillas, J.E., Toga, M., Salamon, G., Hassoun, J. & Grisoli, F. (1982): *Les tumeurs cérébrales*. Paris: Masson,

Panayiotopoulos, C.P. (1989): Benign childhood epilepsy with occipital paroxysms. A 15 years prospective study. *Ann. Neurol.* **26**, 51–56.

Pavlakis, S.G., Phillips, P.C., Di Mauro, S., De Vivo, D.C. & Rowland, L.P. (1984): Mitochondrial myopathy, encephalopathy, lactic acidosis and stroke like episodes. A distinctive clinical syndrome. *Ann. Neurol.* **16**, 481–488.

Roger, J., Pellissier, J.F., Bureau, M., Dravet, C., Revol, M. & Tinuper, P. (1983): Le diagnostic précoce de la maladie de Lafora. Importance des manifestations paroxystiques visuelles et intérêt de la biopsie cutanée. *Rev. Neurol.* **139**, 115–124.

Roger, J. (1984): Les sequelles neurologiques des traumatismes crâniens et l'épilepsie post traumatique chez l'enfant. *Rev. Franç. D.C.* **10**, 303–316.

Roger, J., Bureau, M. & Mireur, O. (1987): L'épilepsie post traumatique. *Rev. Franç. D.C..* **13**, 119–130.

Discussion

Mira

Concerning the first part of the Colloquium, the questions we have gathered from the audience address the issue of how much basic sciences have contributed to the understanding of seizures and to what extent they can clarify obscure issues about the mechanism of seizures.

The questions are:

- We heard that the inhibitory GABA system is not immediately effective: what inhibitory systems are active at an earlier stage?
- Can the excessive convulsiveness in the first year of life be explained by the maturational course of the inhibitory GABA system?
- Is there a consistent relationship between the age of rodents and the age of human beings, and, thereby, how should we interpret experimental data and to what human ages should we compare them?

Spreafico

Answers are not easy; I will start from the last question: it is extremely difficult to transpose all available experimental data directly to human pathology; they merely give us indications which should then be evaluated with comparative neuropathological studies. No clear relationship exists between the gestational age or postnatal development of many of the animals used in these kinds of experiments, and the respective human stages. The only comparable animal is the monkey, for which very few data are available.

What inhibitory systems might be active in place of the GABA system? I talked mainly about the GABA system because it was the main topic: other systems are not as directly inhibitory as the GABA system, but some data point to the fact that the intrinsic cellular activity of the cerebral cortex is not endowed with the same excitability as the cortex itself. In a sense it is more excitable, in another it is less excitable: for instance, spike and PDS (paroxysm depolarization shift) production is more likely in the tissue immediately after birth than in the adult animal, but in the newborn animal the system gets exhausted much more readily, and this can explain the fragmentation of discharges that we observe.

The other point is that the GABA system is undoubtedly a basic inhibitory system, but the cells try to protect themselves from excessive excitability in other ways as well. We should not forget that cells discharge not only because of neurotransmitters, but also because of their membrane characteristics. These are different in the embryonal tissue and in the tissue immediately after birth, as compared to the adult. On this issue, Wasterlain can talk about compartmentalization of intra– and extracellular ions, which certainly changes during ontogenesis and play a crucial role in the balance of membrane excitability.

Other systems are not strictly related to neurotransmitters, such as, for instance, all the so-called neuromodulators, which are also active in this field; and receptors themselves, both NMDA and non-NMDA (about which Wasterlain talked), certainly play a different role in the postnatal period.

Chiarenza

In man, in the newborn and infant, we can study directly the so-called evoked potential recovery function, by which, in varying stimulus frequency, it is possible to evaluate the inhibitory power of several sensory systems, though we cannot clearly identify the inhibitory system in play.

Spreafico

We know from experience that a fatigue system exists, corresponding to what is somewhat improperly called discharge 'refractory time', which is certainly much longer in the period immediately after birth.

Avanzini

I could add that, since discharge properties of the cell in fact depend on several currents, the calcium currents are well developed at birth, in the first week already, and tend to produce the cell discharge, but hyperpolarizing potassium currents are also well developed, and probably are even more active than in the mature animal. One of the most often observed effects (maybe Imbert might comment on this) is a very high spike frequency accommodation in the first weeks of life, that tends to restrict the discharge. This means that there are some basic mechanisms, apart from well identified neurotransmitters, as Spreafico said, that can modify excitability. Therefore, a reduction of effectiveness of GABA does not necessarily result in an excess of excitability.

Spreafico

I would like to add a further comment, regarding the relationship between animal and man: we should remember that in the animal the development after birth takes a very long time. That is true for man also, but it mainly concerns the complexity of axon branching. In fact, few data are available, but, for instance, we know that in an infant of 1 to 2 months of age the interneuron system is already present and functional in the cortex, and so is GABA, although the connections that will appear and develop in the following months are not fully present.

Beaumanoir

I found it very interesting when Imbert talked about re-information allowing restoration, and I would like to ask him to develop this point.

Imbert

Very briefly, when an animal has undergone a major sensory deprivation during the first weeks of postnatal life, the properties of the primary visual cortex look absolutely non-specific, but a few hours of visual experience are enough to establish, or re-establish the situation in a dramatic way, and restore the properties of the neurons as they would have been if the animal had had a normal development for its entire life. This means that the deprivation does not freeze, does not fix the system at a given developmental stage: the nervous system goes on in its development even if it does not fully express itself in the electrophysiological properties of its neurons. I think that this point is really important. This restoration depends on information which is not exclusively visual, as I said, but also motor or proprioceptive, therefore not originating from the retina.

I think that an equally important point is that in the primary visual system, at a very early stage of visual information processing, some non-retinal information plays a crucial role. In my opinion, this is not quite an intuitive notion. It is commonly held that multimodal, multisensory interactions between vision, audition, proprioception, etc., occur in associative areas, at the level of relatively higher processing. In fact, this is not so: there are multimodal interactions occurring at the very early stages of sensory information. This observation can have substantial implications for the function of the visual system.

Lagae

I want to stress this point, because it is very fascinating. I always believed that orientation selectivity develops by connections, by inhibitory connections; so, if you say that a few hours are enough to restore orientation selectivity, does it mean that these pathways are formed and that they become functional in a few hours?

Imbert

Exactly, I think so. You know that there is still much debate on the cellular mechanisms responsible for orientation selectivity. The almost classical theory by Hubel and Wiesel, according to which the cortical cells encode orientation by integrating information from the lateral geniculate body cells, characterized by a peculiar anatomical organization with respect to the visual field representation, has been opposed by other theories, stating that the property of orientation selectivity is settled at the cortical level, through the activity of interneurons and in particular of local inhibitory systems. As a matter of fact, I believe that the truth lies in the middle... There are both convergence phenomena and local intracortical inhibitory phenomena. But, in my opinion, our experience shows that, although all mechanisms may be present, they cannot express themselves at the level of neuronal functioning, because something is missing. A possible hypothesis is that a very short visual experience, just a few hours, is sufficient to trigger neuroendocrinological processes, in particular at the thyroidal level, producing a thyroxine pulse that allows the mobilization and fast polymerization of certain contractile proteins, necessary for establishing synaptic contacts. That is one possibility to think about.

Zagury

How can we explain the neurotrophic activity of sleep in this perspective? The same experiments have been made in the animal after deprivation of paradoxical sleep, and the resulting dysfunction was more severe. Can we explain this? The same experiments as Hubel and Wiesel's were done carried out with sight deprivation, that is, closing one eye by stitching the eyelids, and with sleep deprivation the results were much worse.

Imbert

This is obviously a complicated issue.

Beaumanoir

I would like a comment on about our knowledge on the PGO (ponto-geniculo-occipital) system.

Imbert

All these systems, the PGO system and the systems which allow activity-dependent changes of the properties of cortical neurons, are under the control of neurotransmitter systems, we can call them neuromodulators, in particular those localized in the brainstem, which act in the regulation of the various sleep stages.

The control mechanisms are quite complex, because all these systems – serotoninergic, cholinergic, catecholaminergic – in fact interact with each other; then (I am thinking of Kasamatsuda's and Berre's works, as well as other studies) all these systems interact during development and, moreover, they control the ontogenesis of sleep–wake cycles, but at the same time the 'plasticity' properties of cortical systems, in particular the development of specific, activity-dependent properties.

Avanzini

Is it still correct to speak of occipital seizures and epilepsy with occipital seizures? From the anatomical point of view, the occipital lobe does not have well-defined boundaries: representations are heterogeneous within it, and several visual areas lie outside. I would like to suggest, at least heuristically, that we speak of seizures with visual symptoms, or of epilepsy and seizures with visual symptoms, without linking them to a specific anatomical site which is not even anatomically defined. I think we have good reasons for doing this and the very heterogeneity of symptomatology, as discussed before, is suggestive.

Tassinari

I guess the frontal lobe, the parietal lobe, the temporal lobe, the occipital lobe would then disappear. That might be.

Andermann

I think that there is some truth in this; some visual phenomena are strictly linked to the occipital region, while others are not. That is all we can say. What is important is how the seizure starts, according to a first principle that has been valid for 150 years and still is valid: how it starts in time and how this starts in space. The first sign of seizure onset is always important. After several years, things may change and give way to different types of seizures, but we must be careful and go back to see how seizures began, whether they started from an occipital focus or altogether differently, from the beginning.

And the same holds for space. Does it all begin with a visual symptomatology which is necessarily occipital, or with phenomena which cannot be localized? That is the reason, I think, why we cannot overestimate the importance of lesions; the meaning of lesions has deeply changed the approach to all these problems. Franck presented the contribution of functional imaging tests. This does not diminish the importance of EEG, but I think that more than EEG, more than imaging, functional imaging is going to represent the next major step in the localization of these problems.

Roger

I was struck by the fact that these EEG abnormalities, of peculiar epileptic types recorded by occipital electrodes, are seen proportionately more often in cases of dysfunction of the visual system in a very broad sense, including myopia, squinting, etc., and without epilepsy, while such a situation is rarely encountered in the absence of other neurological deficits in children.

It would seem, therefore, that an early dysfunction, particularly of ocular motility, can modify the occipital cortex to the extent that it functions differently.

Beaumanoir

Among the subjects with occipital spikes that were presented, only 60 per cent had epileptic seizures and – in my own sample – 16 per cent had an early congenital visual defect, most often concerning ocular motility.

Imbert

Having listened to the various talks, I wonder whether, for instance, systematic studies on ocular movements, morphology have ever been carried out in children: accuracy of saccadic movements, nystagmus gain, possibility of pursuit, etc. Do we have adequate information? My prediction is that we would probably get interesting findings. That is a first point regarding ocular motility and visuo-motor behaviour, but the same question arises regarding visual hallucinations.

The variety of visual hallucinations is extraordinary. These hallucinations seem – I am actually exaggerating a little bit – the specular equivalent of neuropsychological deficits, that is, specific deficits of some aspects of visual function due to well-characterized lesions of cortical visual areas in a broad sense.

Would it be possible, through visual hallucinations, to study the areas that Avanzini showed yesterday as acting in the visual function?

Again, listening to you, another question comes up concerning the age-dependent nature of occipital epilepsy in childhood: are there significant differences between boys and girls, and are there systematic differences between males and females in onset time or in maximal expression of epilepsy? That would correspond to several suggestions made in particular about the development of binocular connections in the primary visual cortex, which would depend on neuroendocrine mechanisms related to testosterone and others.

Dalla Bernardina

In some clinical studies we read that, from the electroencephalographic and clinical point of view, the occipital lobes would mature earlier and a series of events would occur earlier in the occipital lobe. Then, when the child grows, the maturation would involve anterior regions and abnormalities would move forward.

What do basic scientists think of this? My opinion is that Imbert is right when he suggests to compare males and females, who can present differences in the timing of some maturational processes. Seizures may appear mostly at a given maturational stage. The occipital lobe, due to its earlier maturation, gets earlier to the critical stage, and then it achieves a maturation level at which it no longer has that susceptibility, if the form is functional (is not true for lesional forms, since in that case they remain occipital forever). It might be that the rolandic area comes to this stage only later, probably with a marked discrepancy between males and females; it presents a tendency to unilateral seizures and to lateral mal status.

At this point I would like to ask neurophysiologists whether they can provide some neurophysiological support for this clinical observation.

Avanzini

I think that in the first period of postnatal life there is in fact a maturational difference between the occipital lobe and, for instance, the somatosensory cortex, but I do not believe that this difference can fully answer the question.

Perhaps Tassinari has some evidence, or some idea, at least as far as the somatosensory cortex is concerned, about whether there is a transitory, age-dependent property accounting for the fact that in this period an epileptogenic pattern, though variable with time, manifests itself more easily.

Spreafico

Surely, at least in the embryonal stages and therefore, probably, in post-natal maturational stages, systems maturation is not homogenous at all. The evolutional stages of what I called 'cortex transitory structures' are different, too: the occipital, parietal and anterior cortices and what will later become the convexity cortex develop in completely different ways, in terms both of cell migration stages and, for instance, of inhibitory systems expression. This means that some nervous system areas develop earlier and, consequently, inhibitory systems also develop earlier, which could explain, at least in part, why some events occur for a given time and then move to other cortices.

In addition, I think – I do not know whether comparative data are available for animals – that the systems afferent to various cortices do not achieve the same maturational stage at the same time, so that, for instance, the thalamocortical pathways of different origin (that is, from the lateral geniculate body or from the ventro-postero-medial nucleus) are out of phase when they reach the cortex. This would play a considerable role.

Sokol

We must not forget the retina; we are talking about cortical maturation when in fact the retina is very immature: the cones are not at all densed, there is no fovea, so that while the cortex may be limited it is getting very limited information from the retina, from the retinal cells.

Imbert

What Sokol says is very important. We should not forget that while the primary visual cortex receives, at least in primates, almost all signals from the lateral geniculate body, the lateral geniculate body itself receives only 20 per cent of retinal signals. Therefore, 80 per cent of signals arriving at the lateral geniculate body are extraretinal. Consequently, even if the retina is not fully mature, that does not prevent the geniculo-cortical system from functioning. On the other hand (this is admittedly a rash generalization) there is a centre to periphery gradient in maturation. In particular, corticogeniculate projections from the primary visual cortex to the lateral geniculate body mature earlier than geniculocortical projections. The descending corticofugal system achieves maturity earlier than the corticopetal system.

Lagae

I want to comment on the question of maturation and possible epileptic phenomena. You certainly do not need full maturation of a brain area to have epileptic seizures originating in it. In neonates, for example, one can see a motor jerk without a fully developed motor cortex. In this respect, it is worthwhile looking at the developmental PET-scan studies of Chugani.

Concerning the other question: perhaps we do not see any seizures because we do not look close enough. If we were to test these infants carefully with a battery of specialized neuropsychological tests, we might discover more problems in children with occipital spikes and waves. We now call these infants asymptomatic because we only have a limited range of techniques to look at them.

Tassinari

I may not have an answer to Avanzini's question about some age-dependent property able to explain that in childhood an epileptogenic pattern presents itself more easily; but I can at least try to understand what he means. I guess you hinted at the fact that we are realizing, with regard to partial idiopathic epilepsies, that the focus is not well defined, i.e. restricted to one area, right rolandic or vertex, etc. From our study on gigantic evoked potentials, which in my opinion are equivalent to spontaneous spikes, it is quite clear that a subject at a given age (usually children who have rolandic epilepsy) may begin to show hyperexcitability areas, which we provoke and test with peripheral stimuli. If we follow up the evolution of this phenomenon, we see that, with time, the same subject does not show only one focus, but several foci, arising in the whole somatosensory area of hyperexcitability. This hyperexcitability slowly fades away, proving that it is not one focus, it is not an organic event, but an age-dependent tendency of certain areas.

On the other hand, it is difficult to establish whether it is a matter of maturation or non-maturation or peculiar organization. For sure these same regions show an extreme variability, that is, areas change within a short time; in fact, we have evidence that in a matter of days the cortical excitability changes. In addition, sleep studies prove that these phenomena change from wake to sleep, so the mechanism is essentially functional rather than anatomical or hormonal.

In conclusion, there must be some controlling factor of hyperexcitability capable of changing in few hours, or with sleep and wake, etc.

Ravnik

About different seizure patterns, I would like to mention that brief repetitive attacks in the visual or multisensory modalities may occur during and after infectious episodes in otherwise healthy children.

Visual phenomena are described as micropsia, macropsia and teleopsia in the two visual hemifields. Other sensory and perceptual modalities may be disturbed, though they usually do not occur at the same time as the visual trouble. In our small series of 10 cases, a child complained of hyperacusis and said that he felt the weight of the toy car he held in his hands had changed into very heavy. Another asked his mother to speak more slowly: 'Do not speak so quickly, I understand it all but you speak too quickly'.

The usual duration of the visual phenomena is about 10–15 s, with possible repetition. There are no disorders of consciousness. The child may be afraid when experiencing the disorder for the first time. There is no headache during or after the episode, though some of the children have been reported to suffer from occasional, probably migrainous, headache.

It seems that infection itself, whether viral (more often) or bacterial, does play a role; fever does not seem to be essential, as the episodes have been described during prodromal afebrile states. The first episodes may occur 2 to 5 days after the beginning of the illness when fever has abated. They may recur during convalescence or reappear with repeated infections of similar kind.

Neurological examination is normal; fundus oculi, lumbar puncture, CT scan and evoked potentials (interictal) are normal (all the investigations have not been performed in all cases). Interictal EEG is normal with no paroxysmal abnormalities.

The only ictal recording was performed in a girl aged 7. She had micropsia during which no paroxysmal abnormality was noted in the EEG. However, on eye opening there was no reaction of the background activity when she had micropsia. The reactivity was normal when she did not complain of the disturbance.

The question about the nature of the disorder remains open. In my opinion it is most likely due to an exogenous toxic influence by infection on a constitutionally migraine-prone 'territory'.

Mira

The audience has practical questions, too: what do we know and what can be said about fast rhythms in critical EEG in basilar migraine?

Then, a few questions concern the talk by Beaumanoir, asking to clarify the critical EEG in migraine and in occipital epilepsy, but mostly about the morphology and duration, in terms of days, of postictal abnormalities in seizures and migraine.

On migraine, again, there is another question: do we have data on blood flow and metabolism during epileptic seizures, in migraine attacks, and in their association?

About mitochondrial diseases: what is the physiopathogenetic basis of the predominance of occipital involvement in mitochondrial pathology?

A related question: what is the incidence in general population of occipital cortical dysplasia?

What is the HLA typing in occipital epilepsy with respect to other epilepsies?

Is there any explanation for the very marked sensitivity to ILS in patients with renal disease, and the incidence of occipital seizures in the same kind of diseases? And is the onset of occipital seizures in the child with renal failure related to the possible intake of drugs like erythropoietin for treatment of severe anaemia?

Then, a question on spasms: we saw spasms with a well-defined focal localization: when are spasms generalized seizures and when, on the other hand, are they a sign of partial seizures, or are both situations intertwined?

The last question is on epilepsies and coeliac disease: how is it that in other diseases with immune complex deposition and in vasculitis there are no calcifications? Are there no studies on calcifications in these situations, or studies we do not know about?

Andermann

I will try to answer the question on the predominance of occipital seizures in mitochondrial diseases, as it is easy: I do not know the reason for this predilection for the occipital region. Maybe Avanzini can answer this question.

This is a most important issue, probably one of the basic issues of this Colloquium, since it applies not only to mitochondrial pathology, but also to migraine and to certain occipital epilepsies. It is very difficult to know what is particular or special about them.

I also would like to comment on migraine: I think that the mechanisms and the reasons why people suffering from classical migraine also suffer from epileptic seizures are not very clear.

Though the matter is much debated, it is likely that the mechanism of aura in migraine is identical or analogous to the spreading depression of Leao. Terzano proposed the notion of intercalated seizures; my experience with intercalated seizures is different from his: these subjects start to present a migraine aura that can be visual or auditory; at a given moment they have a seizure, but it is a motor and not a visual seizure; it is not a sensory seizure. The spreading depression does not cross the great cerebral fissures, according to Leao and others. If, for one reason or another, the spreading depression were to cross the central fissure, producing a motor seizure, then this would also be the most likely explanation for the motor seizures seen in so-called 'intercalated' seizures – at least for lack of a better hypothesis, or until proven otherwise.

Avanzini

I think it is necessary to explain what the spreading depression of Leao is, and why a definition entailing depression could be related to seizure onset.

The spreading depression is a phenomenon observed in animals during experiments when the cortex is manipulated in certain ways; it is caused by a large amount of potassium leaking from cells, with a marked rise of extracellular potassium. This potassium wave progresses and spreads, depolarizing the cells: that is why the spreading depression is preceded by an hyperexcitability wave which could trigger seizures.

Beaumanoir

If the motor intercalary seizure occurs because the spreading depression crosses the fissure, then, shouldn't the time course of the seizure be slower?

Andermann

Not necessarily. The process is somewhat different.

When it reaches the motor area, it changes character, so that it causes an epileptic seizure instead of continuing the classical slow march of the spreading depression. This is admittedly no more than a hypothesis. We do not have any evidence, but this is the only satisfactory hypothesis which takes into account what we know about the march of classical migraine.

It is not necessarily the same mechanism. People suffering from confusional migraine can also have epileptic seizures at the height of the aura, but I do not think we can speak altogether of the same mechanism.

Terzano

This issue might be crucial. We have recorded migraine attacks with electroencephalographic aspects similar to those described by Beaumanoir: a slowing which can be limited only to the polar tip of the occipital lobe or can spread more or less extensively in the occipital lobe, but can also involve the whole hemisphere.

We know that in classical migraine the spreading depression does not usually cross the rolandic fissure, but when this does happen, it does not imply that we must necessarily have motor manifestations. All migraine attacks that get over the rolandic fissure provoke the so-called confusional migraine, basically because the frontal lobe, or the temporal lobe, is involved. We have recorded cases of confusional migraine and can further confirm these data: the slowing is generalized, there are also diffuse slow waves anteriorly, and therefore some central brainstem mechanism is involved, spreading this kind of abnormality.

We must say that these abnormalities, though dramatic, tend to clear up quickly, within 24 h, and most of the time they end with the subject falling deeply asleep. The sleep recorded at the end of the confusional state, after the disappearance of these hemispheric abnormalities, is perfectly normal.

Then, because of these aspects, the phenomenon of psychic and sensory, and actually electroencephalographic, manifestations in classical migraine is absolutely independent.

The spreading depression is a purely artificial effect, produced in the laboratory in the cortex of animals through several stimulation tests, but nothing prevents this phenomenon from having a somewhat clinical identification precisely in classical migraine.

At this point we cannot say that, if migraine triggers a seizure, it should be a purely visuomotor seizure. The seizure is a phenomenon in itself, deserving to be justified in its own terms, because, once the focus is activated, all mechanisms typical of an epileptic seizure follow. So, if other occipital seizures have motor manifestations, these can have them also.

We recorded two cases of basilar migraine; first of all, we must say that this is a real syndrome, which affects young people with an extremely severe symptomatology and has a very quick resolution. We never find fast rhythms, but slow posterior rhythms, projected anteriorly, and a marked instability of the EEG, with tendency to dozing. EEG instability can last for months after the complete disappearance of the episode.

Zagury

I would like to ask Andermann a question regarding the chapter of mitochondrial encephalopathies; the mitochondrial pathology very often predominates at the muscular and often also at the ocular level. Does an early ocular involvement explain, in relation to maturation processes, the fixation of epileptic problems in the occipital lobe? It might be an hypothesis.

Andermann

That is interesting, but quite unlikely: since these patients are usually deaf, they are often affected with neuronal deafness which sometimes is the only manifestation for several years; many people, particularly those with myoclonic syndromes, have optic atrophy, but most of them do not seem to have primary visual problems.

I think that Terzano presented the alternative point of view, that is Gloor's point of view, who insists that this has never been seen in man, and Rolando does not exist in man: so, here you have two alternative points of view, that it exists, and that it doesn't.

Other authors besides Terzano and Beaumanoir spent a long time recording migrainous patients. A series of very interesting observations substantially confirm what Beaumanoir described for the first time, subsequently confirmed by people in Bologna: discharges that are practically very similar to epileptic discharges show up occasionally during the migraine aura in several of these patients. For the first time it has been possible to evaluate their number and how often they occur: they occur in about 3 per cent of a population with migraine severe enough to require hospitalization for evaluation.

Roger

There was already enough debate about this, and there are other questions regarding migraine and the duration of postcritical abnormalities.

Beaumanoir

Yesterday I showed the case of a child who one day presented an epileptic seizure and a migraine, intercalated or not, and another day an occipital seizure with postcritical headache of long duration: the EEG during the migraine and during the postictal headache is not the same... That is the first thing to be underlined. The second thing is that the duration of postcritical abnormalities is also different. In fact, those with migraine show slow, monomorphic abnormalities, well localized in the occipital region, which actually last much longer than the postictal abnormalities of an epileptic seizure. The morphology of slow waves is different, too, being more polymorphic in postictal headaches. Therefore – in children, especially when they have migrainous phenomena without clear headaches and seizures with headache – it is possible to make a differential diagnosis a posteriori between an occipital seizure and a migraine.

Roger

This discussion comes from an historic problem, maybe an old quarrel between Marseille and Montreal.

Since the first observations were published by Camfield about a diagnosis of severe migraine with epileptic-type EEG abnormalities, Gastaut maintained that these patients did not have migraines, but epileptic seizures. This led several colleagues who have been studying benign occipital epilepsies to deny a relationship between them and migraine. Now these relationships are certain. They are true, but we must acknowledge that we still can say: 'this patient has an occipital epilepsy, this patient has migraine, this patient has both'.

In every instance we are able to say 'this was a migraine attack and this was an epileptic seizure', because Beaumanoir demonstrated that neither the clinical picture, nor the critical, intercritical and postcritical EEG are the same in the two cases.

Avanzini

I have a question for Gobbi: has anyone ever tried to test the presence of coeliac disease or HLA typing in Sturge–Weber?

Gobbi

I did, in three cases only. As a curiosity, I can mention that in our cases of occipital epilepsy DR5 is found in only two subjects of group 3, that is those with epilepsy and occipital calcifications without coeliac disease. I do not know what this means, but it is suggestive, because these two patients show both HLA typical of coeliac disease and DR5; perhaps, again, because of multifactorial genesis.

Roger

Somebody asked about the incidence of cortical dysplasias in the general population. Well, I think that nobody knows the answer. It is true that some neuro-imaging data demonstrate that it is far more frequent than previously thought: which I have known for a long time, from what neuropathologists explained to me. But I think that nobody knows what the proportion is in a general population. The second question regards the predominantly focal malformations, whether they are more often occipital and whether occipital malformations are associated to epilepsy more often than others. I should answer no: in fact, considering the group of malformations with great focal predominance, the peri-rolandic malformations are most frequently epileptogenic (and they almost always are), much more frequently than occipital malformations. This does not rule out that other large hemispheric malformations prove to be epileptogenic, without explaining exactly why. Andermann has shown this in a large number of cases. Maybe Avanzini has some precise ideas in neurophysiological terms: what is the exact relationship between the structure of a malformation and its epileptogenic potential? If we knew that, we would already know many things. It is true that some patients with large malformations are candidates to surgical treatment because it seems that only a portion of the malformation gives rise to seizures. And it is true that in these cases it is usually the occipital portion.

Andermann

Our series of over 50 patients with neuronal migration defects is selected in that the patients were referred because of intractable epilepsy. Of 30 patients with focal unilateral lesions, 26 had epilepsy so severe as to require surgical treatment. In only four was the epilepsy not invalidating enough to justify such an approach.

Marsel Mesulam at a recent meeting of the American Academy of Neurology described some pathological observations in subjects who had had learning deficits; in these individuals minor migration defects were found, which probably would not show on the MRI as it is available today. Our own experience suggests that the cortical disorganization is much more extensive than the visible lesion and that what we see on MRI is but the tip of the iceberg.

Many neuronal migration defects produce unusual ongoing sharp and slow wave discharges on EEG. Judging from the corticography they are capable in themselves of generating epileptogenic potentials unlike tumours or other structural abnormalities which are inert from this point of view.

A last brief comment on the topic of Gobbi: I was very surprised to hear that coeliac disease is so common in Italy. I think there is no justice that in the land which has the finest pasta in the world, you have the highest incidence of coeliac disease.

Guerrini

I would like to add something on cortical dysplasias: we collected a series of about 25 cases and in fact only one patient had occipital lobe involvement. When the originary abnormality is essentially a migration or post-migration defect, it surely predominates in periopercular and rolandic regions; when a cortical dysplasia is the origin, it can be everywhere (as a matter of fact we found one case with occipital dysplasia).

Besides, I would like to point out something I recently learned at a neuroradiology meeting in Padua, where a series of paediatric MRI was shown and the group from Padua presented their studies with high definition MRI in muscular dystrophy. Starting from the observation that in Fukuyama-type dystrophy the level of cortical disorganization predominated in the posterior regions, they carefully studied the occipital regions of patients with Duchenne disease and found an abnormality of gyri architectonics in about 70 per cent of cases. These data are probably still unpublished.

Dravet

I would like to go back to the semiology of seizures. My question is about the prolonged seizures described by Vigevano: the clinical semiology with eye deviation, vomiting and finally in most cases a unilateral clonic phase, critical discharges essentially in one hemisphere, always followed by a unilateral suffering. We have seen these kinds of manifestations in subjects in which no true occipital abnormalities had never been demonstrated outside seizures; during the postcritical phase the abnormalities are not necessarily more posterior than anterior. The seizure develops not only in the occipital structures: it involves a whole hemisphere, predominating usually in the temporal region. But the evolution of the seizures is the same, particularly inasmuch as they develop at the end of the night: these children are found in their bed, in the morning, with eye deviation and vomiting. The unilateral phase is generally prolonged and we must end it by injecting diazepam.

Then the question is: is it also possible to see this type of seizure with foci outside of the occipital region?

Vigevano

I think it is possible, the cases are very similar. What we know for sure is that our patients had only that type of seizures. In their evolution they never presented seizures with visual symptoms: this is the first remark, which explains why also in the cases presented by Panayiotopoulos, for example, the early form is in fact similar to my cases, to these cases; while the late form, with visual symptoms, is perhaps a completely different thing, as Dalla Bernardina pointed out.

As for the intercritical focus, out of 12 cases, three had a normal recording, that is, they did not have any abnormality, nine had roughly posterior abnormalities. Nobody had clearly temporal ones. But none of our cases had photosensitivity, for example, and so we did not see the typical evolution of classical occipital epilepsies; on the contrary, we could see the progressive appearance of rolandic foci or the appearance of spikes provoked by stimulation, a phenomenon that we are presently studying. Some of our cases are now presenting them.

Beaumanoir

I would like to ask Panayiotopoulos some comment on the seizures he described, to close the discussion.

Panayiotopoulos

I am very pleased that in this very successful symposium it has become apparent that the syndrome of 'childhood epilepsy with occipital paroxysms' is not restricted to children with visual illusions, as was originally recognized by the Commission of the International League Against Epilepsy. Other authors have confirmed the early onset variant with mainly nocturnal seizures, deviation of the eyes and vomiting. Prolonged seizures presenting as partial status epilepticus has also been confirmed, as I reported previously.

It has been difficult to have my results accepted on this early-onset variant: reviewers were reluctant to accept that vomiting might be a clinical manifestation of seizures; some considered it difficult to accept that a partial epileptic status may have a good prognosis, and others thought that this was a form of basilar migraine or that the evidence produced was insufficient for a new syndrome.

Nonetheless, an important question is whether or not to start medication. My view is that one should wait and then start, probably with small doses of carbamazepine, after the second seizure. Withdrawal may start one year after onset of seizures.

Dravet asked whether the syndrome may manifest without EEG evidence of occipital paroxysms. The answer is 'yes'. I have seen patients who did not have occipital paroxysms in their first EEG, but developed them later, or who had them in their first but not subsequent ones. I have also seen one child with characteristic clinical manifestations but all his EEGs were normal (see Panayiotopoulos in this volume). A syndrome requires a cluster of symptoms, signs and laboratory data which are not identical and of the same severity in all patients.

EEG occipital paroxysms are striking but not pathognomonic of the syndrome. Emphasis is given to their characteristics defined as high amplitude, long runs of repetitive occipital spikes/sharp and slow wave complexes which are often bilateral and attenuate on eyes open. Their shape and amplitude are similar to the centrotemporal spikes. Fixation-off sensitivity is frequently demonstrated. Ten per cent of the patients may also have in the same, or demonstrate in subsequent EEGs centrotemporal and/or frontal and/or somatosensory evoked spikes. Unfortunately, even today, any posterior abnormalities which attenuate on eyes open are considered by some authors as occipital paroxysms. They are not.

We live in a wonderful period for epilepsies and patients with seizures. It is one that requires a disease/syndrome diagnosis instead of a symptom/seizure identification or the unsatisfactory monolectic label 'epilepsy'. The French and Italian schools of epileptologists have made great contributions to this classification and we should be grateful to them. It is up to us to take advantage of this classification and try to improve it. It is not without its imperfections; this should, however, not be used as an argument against, but as a challenge in favour of the syndromic classification of epilepsies.

Synopsis

Anne Beaumanoir

The choice of the topic 'Occipital seizures and epilepsies in children' was brought about by the observation that an epileptogenic process common to all ages manifests itself differently according to the stages of evolution in cerebral functions.

Progress in research on epileptogenicity on one hand, and on the processes of visual system maturation on the other, suggested that the model of occipital epilepsy might be adequate to clarify some aspects of epileptic seizures and epilepsy in children.

The lectures and discussion clearly indicated that further meetings between specialists, both basic scientists and clinicians, are still required for a better understanding of the evolution of critical occipital symptomatology and occipital epilepsies in children.

It was pointed out that the normal maturation of the brain during the postnatal period largely depends on early sensory-motor experience, particularly in regard to the visual functions. Therefore, any alteration of the visual input in an animal during a critical period of postnatal development can cause profound modifications in the response properties of neurons in the striate cortex, suggesting a specific relationship between motor processes and vision during development. Such modifications are seen not only in animals, but in man as well.

On the other hand, the development of the ocular motor system is closely related to that of the visual system. In the young infant the visual system is immature, and the central retina undergoes developmental changes up to about the 20th week. Even if the retina is not fully mature, the geniculo-cortical system is not thereby prevented from functioning. The descending corticofugal system achieves maturity earlier than the corticopetal system.

According to Imbert, in the primary visual system some non retinal information plays a crucial role at a very early stage of visual information processing. This is not quite an intuitive notion. Some multimodal interactions occur at very early stages of sensory information, and this observation may have substantial implications for the functions of the visual system.

On the other hand, as Wasterlain pointed out (and as his co-workers Sankar *et al.* write elsewhere in this volume), experimental studies have shown great age-dependent variations in the nature and severity of brain damage associated with seizure activity. The immature brain is far more resistant than the adult one to damage induced by lactic acid buildup, or kainate-induced status epilepticus.

At the same time, the limited ability of the younger brain to transport glucose across the blood-brain barrier, the absence in some neurons of the calcium buffering capacity due to the calcium buffering protein calbindin D28k, the overexpression of NMDA and AMPA receptors and the adverse effect of inhibiting brain growth make it far more vulnerable than the adult brain to some types of insults.

It seems that in infants a particular oculomotor symptomatology can be the sign of a critical pathology in relation to the maturation of the oculomotor system.

It has long been known that the congenital deficit of oculomotion (in connection with the maturational delay of the oculomotor system) is correlated with the presence of spikes in the occipital areas recorded on the EEG of children at about 3 years of age. These spikes, as Lagae and Casaer pointed out, may reveal a deficit of perception and integration of visual inputs; these issues are currently hardly known, probably because they are still scarcely studied.

In view of the exceedingly deep modifications occurring in the maturing visual system during the first months of life, it is certainly very useful to study critical situations with regard to the maturational processes in very young children.

The studies by Lortie, Plouin, Pinard and Dulac represent the first attempt to define the occipital epilepsy in this age range. Some clinical characteristics have been identified, including ictal oculomotor signs, very early onset of seizures, early spasms, no tendency to spontaneous remission, and severe mental and behavioural disorders. Such features may be useful to recognize occipital epilepsy at this early age.

Early control of occipital seizures is therefore a prerequisite for the improvement of long term prognosis, particularly as to the cognitive and behavioural outcome. The observation that cognitive sequelae are proportionally related to number of seizures, and therefore to the severity of epilepsy in infancy, suggests that seizures subsided only when much of the brain had lost plasticity and therefore the ability to recover sensorial integration. When, on the contrary, there are no seizures, the same maturational deficits of the visual system and particularly of the oculomotor system do not prevent the recovery of integrative abilities of the child.

As Spreafico and Regondi explained, the GABAergic system should not be regarded, at least in the neocortex, as functionally homogeneous in the course of the development. The inhibitory effects of GABA, usually recognized in the adult cortex, are not evident in the early stages of development when the GABA system is subserving other processes, such as morphogenetic roles. This statement raises the problem of treatment, i.e. which antiepileptic drugs are useful and effective in the first stages of maturational evolution.

The characteristics of seizures and epilepsies in children have been outlined, but the interpretation of age-dependent idiopathic epilepsy with occipital paroxysms is still controversial; Panayiotopoulos, with the agreement of most authors, suggests a distinction between early onset and late onset syndrome.

The issue of the relationship between epilepsy and migraine, and particularly basilar migraine in the child, was next taken into account. Here many questions arise about the pathogenesis of seizures and migraine in children and about maturational processes at play in this age range, different from those concerning the maturation of the visual systems.

The discussion about this association offered the opportunity to speculate on the relevance of maturational factors and particularly of observations related to sex differences, but did not yield satisfactory answers. Therefore, many questions on the pathogenesis of seizures and migraine in children in connection with maturational processes still remain unanswered.

The age-dependent liability of occipital cortex to seizures was mentioned with regard to coeliac disease and mitochondrial disorders. Coeliac disease with occipital calcifications, and mitochondrial disorders such as MELAS and MERRF, share a bend towards the involvement of occipital structures. Clarification of the basis for this involvement must await progress in our understanding of the neurobiology of the occipital lobe.

In conclusion, since occipital seizures differ depending on age, an age-dependent epilepsy with occipital paroxysms exists, a preferential age for the association between epilepsy and basilar migraine also exists, and moreover newborns and infants may suffer from an occipital epilepsy with peculiar evolution: therefore the role played by maturational processes in these various aspects of epilepsy and occipital seizures in children is certainly important.

This Colloquium focused and clearly outlined these crucial problems, and attempted to suggest interpretations and gather evidence from the basic sciences; a great deal of work still lies ahead.

Author Index

Akira, T.	15	Lambertini, A.	189
Andermann, F.	111, 213	Lanzi, G.	87
Avanzini, G.	31	Lortie, A.	121
Baiona, M.	183	Lo Russo, G.	203
Balottin, U.	87	Malapani, C.	203
Battaglia, A.	165	Michelucci, R.	141
Beaumanoir, A.	1, 71, 101, 237	Minotti, L.	197
Bouquet, F.	189	Mira, L.	65
Bureau, M.	165	Munari, C.	203
Capizzi, G.	59, 183	Olivier, A.	213
Cappellaro, O.	173	Panayiotopoulos, C.P.	151
Caraballo, R.	173	Parrino, L.	93
Casaer, P.	43	Pengo, A.M.	183
Colamaria, V.	173	Pietrini, V.	93
Dalla Bernardina, B.	173	Pinard, J.M.	121
Darra, F.	173	Plouin, P.	121
Donati, E.	197	Poggioli, D.G.	197
Dravet, C.	165	Rasmussen, T.	213
Dulac, O.	121	Regondi, M.C.	9
Fontana, E.	173	Ricci, S.	133
Francione, S.	203	Roger, J.	221
Galli, L.	93	Rossi, P.G.	197
Gobbi, G.	189, 197	Rubboli, G.	145
Greco, L.	189	Salanova, V.	213
Genton, P.	165	Salvi, F.	145
Guerrini, R.	165	Sankar, R.	15
Hoffmann, D.	203	Santucci, M.	197
Imbert, M.	3	Sokol, S.	49
Kahane, P.	203	Spreafico, R.	9
Lagae, L.	43	Tarsi, E.	197

Tassi, L.	203	Vigevano, F.	133
Tassinari, C.A.	141, 189	Vigliano, P.	59, 1833
Terzano, M.G.	93	Wallis, R.A.	15
Thompson, K.	15	Wasterlain, C.	15
Tornetta, L.	59	Yang, C.X.	15
Van Lierde, A.	65	Zaniboni, M.G.	189
Ventura, A.	189	Zullini, E.	173

Subject Index

abducent nerve, sectioning	5–6
absence epilepsy	
and migraine	94
visual stimuli	142 (table)
action myoclonus, myoclonus epilepsy with ragged red fibres	118
acuity, visual	
development	60
measurement	44–45
threshold spatial vision, neurophysiology	52–53
adolescents, semiology of occipital epilepsy	221
afferent fibres to neocortex, development	10, 229
age	
brain damage from epilepsy	237
susceptibility	15–29
epidemiology of epilepsy	183–184
epileptogenicity	230
occipital epilepsy	
onset of seizures	130
semiology	221
Alice in Wonderland syndrome	90
Alpers' disease, case like	113
alpha waves, maturation, impairment in blindness	67
alternating hemiplegia of childhood	89–90, 106
amaurosis, occipital seizures	73
amblyopia, pattern VEP studies	62
Ammon's horn sclerosis	24
attention, development of	46
attention centres	44
auditory hallucinations, severe partial occipital epilepsy	205
aura, migraine	89
EEG	105
epileptic discharges	233
autoimmune endothelitis	194
automatisms, seizures in structures connected to visual cortex	74
autonomic symptoms	
basilar migraine	106
and benign occipital epilepsy with prolonged seizures	133–140
partial occipital epilepsy	71
axonal growth cone marker protein	26
basilar migraine	90, 97, 233
EEG	104–105
vs late onset variant benign CEOP	160
basket cells, cerebellum, development	25
benign childhood epilepsy with frontal spikes, incidence	156
benign childhood epilepsy with midline spikes, incidence	156
benign childhood epilepsy with occipital paroxysms	151–164
authors disputing existence	174
benign occipital epilepsy, *vs* refractory occipital epilepsy	217
benign paroxysmal vertigo of childhood	91
benign partial epilepsy of childhood	
with occipital spikes	133
with occipital spike-waves	197
with rolandic spikes	197
binocular interaction	3
behavioural studies on development	6–7
disruption of development by strabismus	4
postnatal development	5–6
blindness, *see* amaurosis; ictal blindness	
blinking, bilateral	214
blood vessels, possible role in MELAS	117–118
'blurred vision', occipital seizures	72
body image, disturbances	90–91
brain damage	
cases of occipital lobe epilepsy	217
causing occipital lobe epilepsy	215
correlation with seizure type	184
from neonatal occipital epilepsy	130–131
susceptibility, effect of age	15–29
brain growth, effect of neonatal seizures	24–26
brain stem involvement, occipital seizures	80
Brodmann, K., cytoarchitectural map of brain	31–33
bullet wounds, study of human visual cortex	36–37
calcification, cerebral	
bilateral, severe partial epilepsy with (Gobbi 1988)	198
with epilepsy and coeliac disease	189–196
occipital epileptic encephalopathy	201
calcium	
role in excitotoxic brain damage	17
role in neuron function	226
calmodulin kinase II	15, 17–18
carbamazepine, management of CEOP	236

vs phenobarbitone	201	behavioural studies on development	6–7
cataract surgery, late, study of perceptual deficits	4	step function in development	46
central vision		discrimination, visual	43–44
effect on idiopathic occipital epilepsy	184	distributed systems, cerebral function	33
elimination for testing	162	diurnal occipital seizures	72
centro-temporal epilepsy, *see also* idiopathic benign childhood epilepsy with centro-temporal spikes and migraine	94	DNA studies, mitochondrial disorders	117
		early onset variant of BCEOP	153–154, 156–160, 163, 167
		electroclinical studies, severe partial occipital epilepsy	203–211
cerebellum, basket cells, development	25	electrocorticography	218
cerebral atrophy, occipital lobe epilepsy	215	electrodes, in prosthetic implants	37
character features, migraine patients	89	electroencephalography	
chemotherapy (antimitotic), role in epilepsy and cerebral calcification	194	antiepileptic drugs, effect of withdrawal in CEOP	168–170
		benign occipital epilepsy with prolonged seizures and occipital symptoms	138, 139
childhood epilepsy with occipital paroxysms *see also* benign childhood epilepsy with occipital paroxysms; idiopathic childhood epilepsy with occipital paroxysms	236,	CEOP	236
		cryptogenic vs symptomatic	177 (table), 178 (table)
		marker for	165
antiepileptic drugs	197–199	interictal	94
constituent syndromes	94–96	migraine and epilepsy	101–110
prognosis	165–171	occipital seizures	75–80
clinical data, brain damage susceptibility	27	infants, A. Lortie *et al* series (1983–1991)	122–123
clobazepam, benign partial epilepsies of childhood	197	photoconvulsive or photoparoxysmal response	146
clonic attacks, CEOP	96	scalp	
coeliac disease		imprecision for occipital seizures	128, 217
cases, non-response to gluten-free diet	200	severe partial occipital epilepsy	208–209
with epilepsy and cerebral calcification	189–196	visual disorders	228
in Sturge Weber syndrome	234	visual pathway damage	65–70
colour, intermittent photic stimulation	149	electroretinograms	59, 60
colour information pathways (Macaque monkey)	35	elementary visual hallucinations, occipital seizures	72
complex cells, visual cortex	33	encephalopathies, causing occipital lobe epilepsy	215
complex hallucinations, occipital seizures	75, 96	'encoches', frontal, foetal EEG	66
'complex partial seizures'	210	endothelitis, immunocomplex-related	194
Condorelli, Luigi, on semiotics	87	epidemiology	183–188
cones, development of visual system	59	epilepsy	
confusional migraine	90, 233	connection with migraine	94
congenital ocular motor apraxia	62	lateral interactions	56
contrast sensitivity curve	45	epileptogenicity	
convulsions, seizures in structures connected to visual cortex	74	age	229, 230
		occipital cortex	222
cortex, resection	218	ergotamine, abuse	88
cortical blindness, neurophysiological studies	60	evoked potential recovery function	226
cortical dysplasias	234, 235	evoked potentials, *see* visually evoked potentials	
cortical infarcts, multiple, case of mitochondrial disorder	114	evolution of childhood occipital seizures	221–223
		excitatory amino acids, role in neonatal occipital epilepsy	130
cortical plate	10		
course of childhood occipital seizures	221–223	excitotoxic brain damage	16–17
cranial nerves, paralysis, ophthalmoplegic migraine	90	externality effect	46
cranio-cordinometer	37	extraocular muscle deafferentation, effect on binocular interaction	6–7
cryptogenic vs symptomatic partial occipital epilepsies	174–179, 221–222		
		eye closure	
Cuba, case of MELAS	112	EEG in photosensitive patient	151
cytoarchitectural map of brain (K. Brodmann)	31–33	passive, neonatal EEG	66
dantrolene, modifying excitotoxic brain damage	17	eye deviation, *see* ocular deviation	
darkness, effect on occipital paroxysms	151–152	eye opening, suppression of occipital discharges	176, 180
deafness, early symptom of myoclonus epilepsy with ragged red fibres	118	familial hemiplegic migraine	89
		family history	
dementia, myoclonus epilepsy with ragged red fibres	118	benign CEOP	174
demyelination, pattern VEPs	62	benign occipital epilepsy with prolonged seizures and autonomic symptoms	139
depth electrodes, *see* stereo-electroencephalography			
depth perception			

Subject Index

fast S rhythms, occipital seizures	75
fatigue, effect in MELAS	117
fatigue system	226
fixation	46
fixation off sensitivity (term), vs scotosensitive epilepsy	162–163
fixation off sensitivity spikes	102
case of late onset variant benign CEOP	162
flash electroretinogram stimulation	60
flash visual evoked potentials	59
flunarizine	97
foetus, EEG	66
folate deficiency, role in epilepsy and cerebral calcification	194
follow-up, CEOP	166, 177
fovea, development	59
frontal 'encoches', foetal EEG	66
frontal lobe type, seizures of occipital origin	210
Fukuyama dystrophy	235
fundamental component, pattern modulation	54
GABA$_A$ receptors, development	12
GABAergic system	225
immature brain	20
ontogenesis	9–13
GABA receptors, inhibitory, effect on visual acuity	45
GAD activity, discrepancy with GABA immunocyto- chemistry	11–12
GAP-43 (axonal growth cone marker protein)	26
geniculostriatal fibre damage	60
glucopoenia, in status epilepticus	20
glutamate, post-synaptic binding, vs high-affinity uptake, time lag	24
glutamate binding densities, vs Huttenlocher curve	27
glutamate receptors, role in excitotoxic brain damage	16
gluten-free diet	
non-response of coeliac disease cases	200
and prognosis for seizures	201–202
growth cones, metabolic effects	25–26
guanylate cyclase	20
hallucinations, see auditory hallucinations; visual hallucinations	
harmonic components, pattern modulation	54
headaches	
cryptogenic vs symptomatic CEOP	175 (table), 178 (table), 179 (table)
epileptic	74, 79
in migraine attacks	88–89
partial occipital epilepsy	71
postictal, CEOP	96–97
tension type, vs migraine	87–88
hearing loss, early symptom of myoclonus epilepsy with ragged red fibres	118
hemianopia, study of human visual cortex	36
hemiclonic attacks, CEOP	96
hemiconvulsions, seizures in structures connected to visual cortex	74
hemiplegic migraines	89
high-affinity uptake vs post-synaptic binding, glutamate, time lag	24
hippocampus, damage and status epilepticus	24
history-taking, migraine attacks	88-89
HLA typing	
coeliac disease and cerebral calcification	192 (table)
Sturge Weber syndrome	234
Holmes, G, and W.T. Lister, study of soldiers, World War I	37
human visual cortex	35-39
Huttenlocher curve, synaptic density vs age	27
hypercomplex cells, visual cortex	33
hyperexcitability, phase in development	230
ictal blindness, occipital seizures	73, 214
ictal strabismus	74
idiopathic benign childhood epilepsy with centro-temporal spikes	101–102
with BCEOP	156
incidence	156
idiopathic childhood epilepsy with occipital paroxysms	
benign, subdivision	180
cephalgic attacks	74
fixation off sensitivity spikes	102
oculomotor seizures	74
therapy study	198–199
infantile spasms (West syndrome)	27, 130
infants	
occipital epilepsy, A. Lortie et al series (1983–1991)	121–131
semiology of occipital epilepsy	221
infarcts, multiple cortical, case of mitochondrial disorder	114
infections	230–231
inferotemporal visual area (Macaque monkey)	34
information streams, visual	44
inhibitory systems	225
intercalated seizures	
benign occipital epilepsy	93–99, 232
vs benign occipital epilepsy with prolonged seizures and autonomic symptoms	139
interictal electroencephalogram abnormalities	94
intermediate zone	10
intermittent photic stimulation	
EEG response	66
effect of method	145–147
interneurons, see local circuit neurons	
interstitial neurons	11
intestinal obstruction, in case of MELAS	112
intralaminar thalamic nuclei (Macaque monkey)	35
Italian Working Group, series of calcification with coeliac disease	190
kainic acid	
excitotoxic brain damage	17
status epilepticus in immature brain	21
kinetic perimetry	46
Krause, Fedor, on occipital lobe neoplasms	215
Kufs disease	119
lactic acidosis, in mitochondrial disorders	117
Lafora type progressive myoclonus epilepsy	118
lambda waves	66
latency values, positive deflection waves, VEPs	59–60, 62
late onset variant benign CEOP	160–162, 167
incidence	156

lateral geniculate nucleus (Macaque monkey)	35	neocortex, development	9
lateral interaction, development	53	neonates	
Leber's amaurosis	60	EEG	66–67
light stimulation, CEOP	94	occipital epilepsy, A. Lortie et al series	
local circuit neurons, development	10–11	(1983–1991)	121–131
long-range lateral visual mechanisms	54	seizures, effect on brain growth	24–26
loss of consciousness		neoplasms, occipital lobe	215–216
nocturnal prolonged seizures	75	neurological deficits, after surgery for occipital	
in seizures, anatomical correlates	184	lobe epilepsy	218
loss of contact, *see also* absence epilepsy		neurological examination, migraine attacks	88
severe partial occipital epilepsy	205	neurons, membrane characteristics	225–226
macular sparing, brain injuries	37	neurophysiological examination, visual function	49–57
magnetic resonance imaging		nitric oxide, in seizures	18–20
in infants under 2 years	128	NMDA receptors	
MELAS	117	overexpression in immature brain	20, 21–24
with positron emission tomography	39	role in excitotoxic brain damage	16, 21–24
malformations	185–187	nocturnal prolonged seizures	72–73, 83
management		loss of consciousness	75
CEOP	236	nyctohemeral orientation, seizure occurrence	184
occipital epilepsies	197–202	nystagmoid eye movements	214
marginal zone	10	occipital epilepsy with photosensitive occipital	
matrix cells	9	seizures, therapy study	199
medial superior temporal visual area (Macaque		occipital epileptic encephalopathy, therapy study	200, 201
monkey)	34	occipital intermittent rhythmic delta activity	105
medial temporal area (Macaque monkey)	34	occipital lobe	
membrane characteristics, neurons	225–226	ontogenesis	3–8
methotrexate, role in epilepsy and cerebral		problem with definition	228
calcification	194	structures and functions	31–41
migraine	87–91	occipital lobectomy	218
confusional	90, 233	occipital seizures	162
EEG in attacks	104–109	definition problems	39–40
and epilepsy, EEG studies	101–110	difficulties in diagnosis	128
interference from occipital foci	97–98	patterns of spread	215
malignant, mitochondrial encephalomyelopathy		semiology	71–86, 121
with lactic acidosis and stroke-like episodes	116–117	occipito-visual areas (Macaque monkey)	34
mitochondrial abnormalities	118	ocular deviation	
symptoms in CEOP	166	benign occipital epilepsy with prolonged seizures	
migraine-epilepsy syndrome	93–99	and autonomic symptoms	139
migration defects	235	clonic	214
migratory waves, neuroblasts, cortical development	10	localizing value	210
mitochondrial disorders	111–120, 233	severe partial occipital epilepsy	205
predominance of occipital seizures	232	ocular movements	228–229
mitochondrial encephalomyelopathy with lactic		ocular pursuit, hallucinations, occipital seizures	73
acidosis, *vs* refractory occipital epilepsy	217	oculoclonic seizures, anatomical correlates	184
mitochondrial encephalomyelopathy with lactic		oculomotor seizures	73–74, 75
acidosis and stroke-like episodes	111	oculomotor system	
malignant migraine	116–117	defect	237
modulation, windmill-dartboard pattern	53–54	development	237
motor activity, development of occipital cortex	4	and development of occipital cortex	4
motor seizures, in CEOP	152–154	and development of orientation selectivity	5
muscular dystrophy, magnetic resonance imaging	235	ophthalmoplegic migraine	90
myelin, *see* demyelination		optokinetic nystagmus reflex	46
myelin-specific lipids, effect of seizures in		optotypes	44
immature brain	25	orientation selectivity	3, 45–46
myoclonic epilepsy, visual stimuli	142 (table)	development	227
myoclonus epilepsy with ragged red fibres	111, 116–117	postnatal development	4–5
RNA mutation	118	paradoxical sleep deprivation	227
National Hospital, Queen Square, cases of occipital		paraesthesiae, lateralized, severe partial occipital	
lobe neoplasm	215–216	epilepsy	205
natural history of childhood occipital seizures	221–223	parieto-occipital fissure	31

paroxysmal vertigo of childhood, benign	91
partial occipital epilepsies	173–181
pattern visually evoked potentials	49–57, 59, 62
peak latency, visually evoked potentials	51
perforant path, stimulation model of status epilepticus	24
periodic syndromes of infancy	90–91
personality, migraine patients	89
phakomatoses	185–187
phase of fundamental components of VEP, vs age	56
phenobarbitone, vs carbamazepine, in CEOP	201
phosphenes	
occipital seizures	72, 75
stimulation studies	37
phosphocreatine-organic phosphate ratio, migraine	118
photoconvulsive or photoparoxysmal response, EEG pattern	146
photosensitive epilepsy	141–144
myoclonus epilepsy with ragged red fibres	118
neurophysiological investigations	145–150
VEP abnormalities	62
visual stimuli	142 (table)
platinum electrodes, in prosthetic implants	37
pneumogram, in case of MELAS	112
polioencephalopathy, case of	113
ponto-geniculo-occipital system	227–228
positive deflection waves, VEPs, latency values	59–60, 62
positron emission tomography	
with magnetic resonance imaging	39
neonatal occipital cortex	130
postictal symptoms	
CEOP	96–97
occipital seizures	75
post-synaptic binding vs high-affinity uptake, glutamate, time lag	24
potassium	
neuron function	226
release in seizures	15
spreading depression	232
status epilepticus	20
preferential looking, testing vision	44–45
premature infants, provoked seizures	75
presurgical investigation, severe partial occipital epilepsy	204–205
primary visual area	33
primordial plexiform layer (term)	10
prognosis, occipital seizures	221–223, 238
progressive lesions	222
progressive myoclonus epilepsy, Lafora type	118
projecting neurons, development	10
prolonged photoparoxysmal response	146
prolonged seizures	235–236,
see also nocturnal prolonged seizures	
and autonomic symptoms, benign occipital epilepsy with	133–140
proprioceptive afferents, and development of orientation selectivity	5
prospective layer I	10
prosthetic implants	37
protein kinases	15, 17–18
pulvinar-lateralis posterior complex (Macaque monkey)	35
pyramidal cells, damage and status epilepticus	24
questionnaire, on intermittent photic stimulation procedures	147
radiotherapy, role in epilepsy and cerebral calcification	194
ragged red fibres	
in migraine	117
in mitochondrial disorders	117
rats, age vs human age	225, 226
reactive occipital epileptic activity (Bickerstaff)	184
receptive field sizes, vs phase changes in VEP	56
retina	
degeneration	60
development	237
effect on VEP waves	64
maturation	230
retinal migraine	90
retinitis pigmentosa	60
occipital focal spikes	68
retrolental fibroplasia, occipital focal spikes	68
RNA mutation, myoclonus epilepsy with ragged red fibres	118
rodents, age vs human age	225, 226
rods, development of visual system	59
scotomas	
CEOP	96
EEG in migraine	106
occipital seizures	73
scotosensitive epilepsy (term), vs fixation off sensitivity (term)	
seizures, brain damage from	15
self-limited photoparoxysmal response	146
semiology	87
sensory deprivation, restoration of CNS after	226
sex differences, occipital epilepsy	229
short-range lateral visual mechanisms	54
simple cells, visual cortex	33
simple hallucinations, migraine aura, EEG	104
single photon emission computed tomography, neonatal occipital cortex	130
sinusoidal modulation, windmill-dartboard pattern	53–54
VI nerve, sectioning	5–6
sleep	
occipital focal spikes	68
occipital seizures	75
as precipitating factor, benign occipital epilepsy with prolonged seizures and autonomic symptoms	138
sleep deprivation	227
slow wave sleep	
CEOP	94–96
occipital seizures	75
smile, visual, development	47
spatial frequencies, testing visual acuity	45
spatial ocular disparity calibration	6–7
sporadic hemiplegic migraine	89
spreading depression	97–98, 232–233
status epilepticus	
brain damage mechanism	17

effect on immature brain	20
status epilepticus amauroticus	214
status migrainosus	91
stellate neurons, rat	11
step function, development of orientation selectivity	46
stereo-electroencephalography	
occipital seizures with visual loss	76
refractory occipital lobe epilepsy	218
severe partial occipital epilepsy	204, 209
stereoscopic vision	3
stimulus orientation pathways (Macaque monkey)	35
strabismus	
ictal	74
occipital focal spikes	68
unilateral, and development of occipital cortex	4
stria of Gennari (Macaque monkey)	33
structural lesions, prognostic significance	27
Sturge Weber syndrome	
associations mimicking	190
HLA typing and coeliac disease	234
Sturge Weber syndrome	187
subplate	10, 11
substantia nigra, immature brain	20
suprasylvian spread, occipital seizures	215
suprathreshold spatial vision	50–52
surgery, occipital seizures in severe partial epilepsy	203–211
symptomatic occipital lobe epilepsies, therapy study	199–200
symptomatic vs cryptogenic partial occipital epilepsies	174–179, 221–222
synapses	
development in GABAergic system	11
effect of seizures in immature brain	25
synapsin I, in status epilepticus	17–18
synaptic density vs age, Huttenlocher curve	27
syndrome, of occipital epilepsy and migraine, evidence for	102–103
telencephalic vesicles	9
television-induced occipital seizures	141–144
temporal lobe type, seizures of occipital origin	210
tension headache, vs migraine	87–88
testing of vision, infants	43–48
thalamic nuclei, intralaminar (Macaque monkey)	35
thalamocortical pathways	
development phasing	229
Macaque monkey	35
thalassaemia, beta, trait, case with	115
therapeutic dissociation, migraine and occipital seizures	97
threshold spatial vision, acuity, neurophysiology	52–53
thyroxine pulse	227
Tolosa-Hunt syndrome	90
tonic body deviation	74
tonic-clonic epilepsy, visual stimuli	142 (table)
TORCH group disease, exclusion from coeliac disease study	190
transient structures, cerebral cortex	9, 229
trauma, open	222
trigeminal nerve, sectioning	5
unilateral prolonged seizures, epilepsy with	139
ventral intraparietal visual area (Macaque monkey)	34
ventral visual areas (Macaque monkey)	33–34
vertigo	
benign paroxysmal vertigo of childhood	91
cryptogenic vs symptomatic	
CEOP	175 (table), 178 (table), 179 (table)
vesicles, telencephalic	9
video-games	142
visual cortex	
Macaque monkey	33–35
map	33–34
visual disorders, electroencephalography	228
visual environment, development of occipital cortex	3–4
visual field, development	46
visual field deficits, preoperative studies, occipital lobe epilepsy	215
visual hallucinations	228–229
complex	214
epileptic, movement	40
occipital seizures	72
complex	75, 96
severe partial occipital epilepsy	205
simple	213–214
localizing value	210
migraine aura, EEG	104
visual loss	
EEG in migraine	106
focal spikes, occipital	68
visually evoked potentials	49–57
and damage to vision	59–64
EEG	66
testing visual acuity	45
visual pathways	
damage, electroencephalogram	65–70
Macaque monkey	35
visual prosthetic implants	37
visual triggering factors, epilepsy	141
visuomotor areas (Macaque monkey)	34
visuotopic representation, human cortex	40
vomiting	
basilar migraine, EEG	106
benign partial epilepsy of childhood with occipital spikes	135
cryptogenic vs symptomatic	
CEOP	175 (table), 178 (table), 179 (table)
epileptic	74, 79–80
war injuries, studies of human visual cortex	36–37
waveform, visually evoked potentials	51–52
West syndrome	27, 130, 5007
white light flash VEP studies	60–62
whole field flash ERG stimulation	60
windmill-dartboard stimulus	53–54